Beyond Talk Therapy

Beyond Talk Therapy

*Using Movement and
Expressive Techniques in Clinical Practice*

EDITED BY
Daniel J. Wiener

AMERICAN PSYCHOLOGICAL ASSOCIATION
WASHINGTON, DC

First printing May 1999
Second printing October 2001

Published by
American Psychological Association
750 First Street, NE
Washington, DC 20002

Copies may be ordered from
APA Order Department
P.O. Box 92984
Washington, DC 20090-2984

In the UK and Europe, copies may be ordered from
American Psychological Association
3 Henrietta Street
Covent Garden, London
WC2E 8LU England

Typeset in Goudy by EPS Group Inc., Easton, MD

Printer: Port City Press, Baltimore, MD
Cover Designer: DRI Consulting, Chevy Chase, MD
Project Manager: Debbie K. Hardin, Reston, VA

Library of Congress Cataloging-in-Publication Data
Beyond talk therapy : using movement and expressive techniques in
    clinical practice / edited by Daniel J. Wiener.
        p.   cm.
    Includes bibliographical references and indexes.
    ISBN 1-55798-585-5 (cloth: acid-free paper).—ISBN 1-55798-904-4
(pbk: acid-free paper).
    1. Arts—Therapeutic use.   2. Mind and body therapies.
3. Psychodrama.   I. Wiener, Daniel J.   II. American Psychological
Association
    [DNLM: 1. Art Therapy Case Report.   2. Movement Case Report.
3. Music Therapy Case Report.   4. Psychodrama Case Report.
5. Psychotherapy—methods Case Report.   WM 450 8573 1999]
RA489.A72B49   1999
616.86'16—dc21
DNLM/DLC
for Library of Congress   99-13104
                                                                    CIP

British Library Cataloguing-in-Publication Data
A CIP record is available from the British Library.

Printed in the United States of America

CONTENTS

ACKNOWLEDGMENTS

The seminal idea of creating this book rose from conversations with two close colleagues and friends: Adam Blatner and Howard Seeman. American Psychological Association acquisitions editor Margaret Schlegel provided encouragement and practical guidance in the early stages of the project. To these three, I offer great thanks.

An editor merely provides direction and reflective input to the work of the contributing authors. I acknowledge them all for their willingness to stay the course through the lengthy process of cocreating this book.

I also wish to express my appreciation for the contributions of chapter reviewers Jim Bitter, Jacqueline Carleton, Gerald Corey, Pamela Fairweather, Marc Goloff, Anne Hurley, David Johnson, Richard Kitzler, Helen Landgarten, Linda Oxford, Quinn Sale, David Waters, and Richard Whiting, as well as Gene Eliasoph and David Kipper, who reviewed the complete book. Their thoughtful comments aided me greatly in my editorial tasks.

Finally, I dedicate this book to the late Gloria Maddox, my beloved wife of 21 years and a great theater artist and teacher. Although she was stricken with amyotrophic lateral sclerosis (ALS; Lou Gehrig's disease), Gloria's valor and spiritual faith never wavered during the final three years of her life, which ended on May 11, 1998. I am grateful to our numerous friends and family, both temporal and spiritual, who supported us both during this dark time. Most of all, I am profoundly thankful for the inner support of my spiritual teacher, Hazur Maharaji Charan Singh Ji, which has enabled me to maintain mental and emotional balance.

CONTRIBUTORS

Adam Blatner, Austin, Texas

Cynthia A. Cook, New York Institute for Gestalt Therapy

Irma Dosamantes-Beaudry, University of California, Los Angeles

Bunny S. Duhl, Harvard Medical School

Renée Emunah, California Institute of Integral Studies, San Francisco

Michael Lee, Phoenix Rising Yoga Therapy, Housatonic, Massachusetts

Debra Linesch, Loyola Marymount University

Jean A. McLendon, Satir Institute of the Southeast, Inc., Chapel Hill, North Carolina

Janine Roberts, University of Massachusetts, Amherst

Benedikte B. Scheiby, New York University, Beth Abraham Health Service

Daniel J. Tomasulo, Princeton University and Brookdale College, Young Adult Institute

Daniel J. Wiener, Central Connecticut State University

Karyne B. Wilner, International Institute of Core Energetics, New York

Ruth Wolfert, New York Institute for Gestalt Therapy and Chrysalis Institute

INTRODUCTION

Ritual, drama, dance, and music have been used for healing purposes in the Western world at least as far back as antiquity. Such healing methods all involved the active participation of the person to be benefited. Starting in the late 19th century, however, Freud's contribution of "the talking cure" established psychotherapy as a verbal enterprise, a paradigm shift that had the effect of marginalizing action approaches (including the behavior therapies) in Western Europe and the United States until recently.

Nonetheless, there continued to be developments in the use of action methods. In early 20th-twentieth century Russia, for example, Vladimir Iljine's therapeutic theater (Petzold, 1973) and Nicholai Evreinov's theatrotherapy (Evreinov, 1927) used methods that were forerunners of contemporary drama therapy. Within the psychoanalytic camp, Sandor Ferenczi's active therapy, which was developed in the 1920s, combined verbal psychoanalysis with both in-session activities and role-plays linked to identified symptoms (Ferenczi, 1980). Wilhelm Reich, another early psychoanalytic "heretic," developed his "orgonomy" in the 1930s (Reich, 1949), which laid a foundation for many contemporary body psychotherapies that use action methods. Jacob L. Moreno developed psychodrama in the 1920s as an approach based on action methods that continues to the present (1980; also see chapter 6). In the 1950s action methods drawn from the expressive arts were incorporated into existing psychotherapy approaches (see the beginning sections of chapters 11, 12, and 13).

Twenty-five years ago an edited book titled *Active Psychotherapy* (Greenwald, 1973) was published that heralded the proliferation of "active psychotherapists" who went beyond promoting insight to focus on specific goals such as the elimination of symptoms. Until that time, the relatively few therapists who promoted active therapies were ignored by a therapeutic establishment that regarded insight as the sole legitimate goal of therapy. Today, the situation has changed greatly. The ascendance of managed care has made insight alone not reimbursable, and therapists are increasingly required to adhere to methods thought to produce observable, even measurable, results.

The proliferation of action methods has occurred partly as a result of a broadened definition of *psychotherapy*, which now encompasses symptom elimination, cognitive and social skills development, and interpersonal relationship improvement. Within some approaches, action methods were developed as a direct consequence of applying theory; in others, action methods were added as outgrowths of a founder's style, then later rationalized as integral to, or distinctive of, that approach. Some therapy approaches are theory-based systems that use and generate a depth and breadth of action methods, whereas others are names given to a principle or rationale linked to one or two techniques.

DEFINITION OF ACTION METHODS

As I define them in the context of psychotherapy, action methods are *those processes that have clients engage in purposeful physical activity at the direction of the therapist.* Action methods take a number of forms: (a) non-directive, expressive activity (as in the expressive arts therapies); (b) body awareness arising from movement (in the body psychotherapies); (c) use of representational objects (as in the Satir system); and (d) directed enactments (as in therapies using drama).

As used in this book, *verbal therapy* refers mainly to speech, but includes writing (e.g., of journals or letters, as in the narrative therapy of White and Epston [1990]) and reading (e.g., bibliotherapy [Pardecky, 1993]).

Experiential therapy, which may use verbal methods, focuses awareness on the here and now. All therapy redirects awareness; by directing awareness to the present (such as by using visual imagery), knowledge-as-concept can be tested by comparison with current experience. Action methods, then, are experiential, although not all experiential techniques are action methods.

Didactic therapy makes use of explicit teaching, such as psychoeducational approaches (e.g., working with families of schizophrenics [McFarlane, 1991]) and skills training, which can involve such action methods as realistic role-playing or simulation.

A distinction can be made between approaches that use action methods as metaphors for concepts that are then to be stated, defined, and processed verbally versus those approaches that use them to provide experiences that are deemed therapeutic apart from verbal mediation. This is the crux of the controversy between art-*in*-therapy versus art-*as*-therapy, discussed in chapter 5 by Renée Emunah, in chapter 11 by Debra Linesch, and in chapter 13 by Benedikte Scheiby.

WHY ISN'T TALK ENOUGH?

Words are not truth, nor the road to truth. They are flashes of lightning that illuminate the road to truth.

—Unknown

Primary experience, which exists apart from language, is described by language (a representation, or secondary experience). Language is that secondary experience created by verbalizing primary experiences. Verbal psychotherapy, then, is a procedure for the verbal processing of verbal descriptions of events. According to discourse theory (Fairclough, 1992), language constructs its own reality rather than corresponding to it.

Among those practitioners who use them for the purpose of representation, action methods generally are regarded as more vivid and memorable and having more impact than verbal methods. Action methods simultaneously engage cognition, affect, and behavior and better engage those clients who process information predominantly in visual and kinesthetic modes (Bandler & Grinder, 1975). When used as interventions, action methods provide novel ways to alter habitual patterns of thinking, feeling, and behaving.

According to some psychological theories, formative experiences that occurred at a preverbal stage of development can be accessed only by nonverbal methods. Also, there is evidence that traumatic experiences are stored or encoded differently than nontraumatic ones (Van der Kolk, 1996), suggesting that experiential therapies may have the potential to shift traumatic experience in cases in which verbal ones cannot.

As Korzybski (1958) noted, "the map is not the territory." Action methods get clients to venture into the territory of experience, enriching the experience of clients who have come to rely solely on the maps of verbalization. Experiencing these methods provides both a way of discovery in terms other than verbal ones and material that can be juxtaposed with verbally encoded representations. In sum, action methods put verbalizations to the test of experience.

Although psychotherapy will continue to be a verbally mediated process, the inclusion of action methods appears to promote significant clinical change in relatively short periods of time, making them particularly valuable in brief therapy and with populations not very responsive to talk-only therapy. The action methods discussed in this book go beyond isolated activities that might be used in the course of otherwise exclusively verbal therapy. Instead, these methods are integral to the process of therapy, constituting a way of discovering or altering a client's functioning that is unlikely to occur without their use.

EMPIRICAL SUPPORT FOR THE EFFECTIVENESS OF ACTION METHODS

Little or no rigorous research has been conducted to test or substantiate the clinical efficacy of action methods in general. This relative absence of clinical research, which is even more pronounced than for psychotherapy in general, appears to be the result of two overlapping factors:

1. *Researchers of therapy outcomes have not been inclined to study action modalities.* Rigorous psychotherapy outcomes research requires the investment of considerable resources. For the past 40 years, funding for such research has come predominantly from National Institute for Mental Health (NIMH) grants. For grant proposals to be accepted for NIMH funding they must include designs that standardize treatment protocols, a practice at odds with the way action methods traditionally have been used in psychotherapy. In contrast, verbal techniques can more readily be standardized, as can the classification and scoring of clients' verbal responses in comparison with action ones.

   Moreover, psychotherapy researchers predominantly have been psychologists whose clinical training, if any, has underrepresented action methods other than for behavioral rehearsal. Researchers are naturally inclined to investigate approaches with which they are more familiar (e.g., cognitive–behavioral therapy).

2. *Action method approaches have been developed and practiced by therapists untrained in or disinclined to conduct research.* This factor is the complement of the point made in the previous paragraph. The traditions and culture of psychotherapists using action methods, particularly those approaches within the expressive arts, have been, to a great extent, viewed as incompatible with measurement. And when research has been conducted, such methodological criticisms that research psychologists are used to making and receiving occasionally have been perceived within that culture as unfeeling, hostile, and evident of an intent to discredit their practices. As a result, many established, senior action method teachers and practitioners, accustomed to being marginalized within the larger

mental health care field, have conveyed an indifferent attitude toward research in their own fields.

Such a stance may have been viable in the era when reimbursement for psychotherapy was essentially unrelated to outcomes. This situation has clearly changed, as demonstrable results are increasingly becoming a precondition for third-party reimbursement. One pessimistic prediction is that favorable action method outcomes research will become essential to the economic survival of younger, less-established practitioners of such approaches. I do not share this view. For one thing, practitioners might note that such positive results of action method practice, reported on a case-by-case basis to managed care organizations, are truthfully and reliably justifying and receiving reimbursement at present. Also, it is accepted that many populations (particularly those individuals who are institutionalized) often do not respond effectively to exclusively verbal methods.

This is not to make a case for continuing the status quo regarding outcomes research on action methods. Research designs need not be methodologically narrow nor rigorously controlled to establish the potential of an approach's effectiveness. When research is done that finds even modest empirical evidence of reliable and large treatment effects for action methods, they will then assume a more prominent position in psychotherapy.

WHY THIS BOOK?

This book is designed both for students starting a psychotherapy career and for therapists wishing to revitalize their practice. Until now, clinicians interested in broadening their acquaintance with action methods typically have had to invest considerable time, first in selecting a single approach and then engaging in a study of its theory. This book will have greater appeal for practitioners and students whose interest is first stimulated by the methods of an approach, rather than by the elegance or plausibility of its theory.

Accordingly, this book's emphasis is on the action methods themselves as used in each of the approaches described. The methods featured in this book are representative both of the ever-growing variety and utility of action methods in use in individual, group, couples, and family therapy. Each action method is described in sufficient detail for the professional reader to place it in the context of theory and understand how it may be applied in clinical practice. This book also offers practical information regarding (a) the appropriate clinical conditions for the successful use of these action methods, (b) references to core writings in each approach, and (c) information on opportunities for training and certification, where available. It is hoped that readers may readily learn how to pursue further experience with those approaches that appeal to them.

There is an irony to using a verbal medium (such as this book) to acquaint therapists with action methods, which are distinctive precisely because they are experienced in ways other than verbal ones. It would be fair to say that studying this book will teach the reader a good deal about action methods in the context of particular approaches, but only direct experience with these methods will convey fully their value and impact in therapy.

An important issue is whether reading this (or indeed, any) book suffices as instruction for applying clinically the methods described. The general answer is "no." Even more than for exclusively verbal techniques, the effective and ethical practice of action methods requires observation and practice under supervision.

More specifically, the methods described range from those that a generically trained therapist could learn through brief exposure versus those that require fairly lengthy and specialized training. The appendix contains summarized, comparative information on the extent of training deemed necessary by the chapter's author to use each of the methods he or she describes.

ORGANIZATION OF THIS BOOK

The structure of this book and its chapters provide a good sense of its thematic direction. I want to illuminate this structure and provide a road map for the reader.

Chapter Format

The authors of all chapters except chapter 4 were asked to follow a format devised to cover key concepts of practical interest and facilitate comparisons across approaches. Each chapter begins with a brief overview of the approach, together with the rationale for using action methods as distinctive techniques within the approach. The chapters are not intended to expound theory in depth; this can be learned from referenced sources.

Following a survey of the differences between major proponents in the uses of the action methods within each approach, (usually) two brief case examples, the first simpler than the second, are presented. Some of these cases are composites; others are reports of actual clients. The names of all clients referred to in this book have been changed and facts altered to ensure confidentiality.

Case examples are formatted into two columns. The left, or *case narrative*, column contains the observations, instructions, and descriptions of what the client(s) and therapist did or said; the right, or *commentary*, column gives the therapist's rationale for how the session was structured, what the therapist looked for, and what was expected to occur. This structure allows the reader to follow the case narrative down the left column while refering to the right column to understand the therapist's thoughts and interpretation of events as they unfolded during the session. Following each case example, information regarding the population characteristics (e.g., age, level of functioning, or problem area) for which the action method is indicated or contraindicated and timing criteria for its use is given.

In brief sections the author then comments on how resistance (defined as divergent alignment of purpose between therapist and clients) is dealt with; next, the value of successive uses of action methods (including out-of-session "homework") is given; and, finally, the author comments on therapist characteristics desirable for the effective use of action methods within the approach. After this, the author summarizes empirical support, when such exists, for the efficacy of the action methods cited; where little or no research exists, the kinds of questions deemed important to help move the approach forward are offered. A description of the kinds of education, training, or experience needed to use effectively the action methods within the approach is followed by additional resources (e.g., key texts, journals, professional associations, and other resources) regarding further information on study, training, and certification.

Chapter Sequence

The approaches presented in this book range from those in which the action methods are adjunctive to verbal psychotherapy to those in which action methods are its vital core. They also vary from techniques that can be readily learned and interwoven into the work of most practicing therapists to those requiring extensive training and certification. I have chosen to organize the 13 chapters into 4 parts. The parts are ordered in a rough progression from action methods that may be integrated more readily into traditional talk therapy to those that emphasize talking less.

Part I, Psychotherapies That Use Action Methods, presents four predominantly verbal approaches: Gestalt therapy, Satir system psychotherapy, therapeutic rituals (which, because it is not a "school" with distinct training, is presented in more "how-to-do-it" detail than the others), and action metaphor (which intentionally departs from the standard chapter format to present the intimate connection between the thinking and style of the therapist and the action methods used).[1]

Part II, Therapies Using Theatrical Forms, includes four approaches that share their roots in drama: drama therapy, psychodramatic methods, group therapy for people with mental retardation (which details an appli-

---

[1] Not discussed in this book are action methods from three approaches that are well-represented in the clinical literature: behavioral rehearsal, cognitive therapy homework (used to test assumptions and challenge beliefs in vivo), and psychoeducational training.

cation of psychodrama to a special population), and Rehearsals for Growth. Readers will note both the obvious and subtle differences and similarities among these approaches.

A growing number of approaches integrate mind–body connections with elements of traditional verbal psychotherapy.[2] Part III, Body Psychotherapies, discusses two approaches, core energetics and Phoenix Rising Yoga Therapy, that in distinctive ways locate and work with mental and emotional patterns in the physical body.

Part IV, Expressive Arts Therapies, offers representative approaches drawn from the expressive and performing arts: art therapy, dance movement therapy, and music therapy. Lastly, an appendix summarizes comparative information about the action methods featured in the chapters.

CONCLUSION

Techniques do not bring about change; therapists and clients do. The successful use of action methods requires mature clinical judgment and the effective use of the therapist's self. When enacted by clients, action methods frequently stimulate clinicians' own physical, emotional, and cognitive process; it is useful to attend to those internal changes to enhance one's therapeutic effectiveness. Practitioners who make action methods an important part of their therapy work will find themselves personally enriched and enlivened by their use.

REFERENCES

Bandler, R., & Grinder, J. (1975). *The structure of magic: A book about language and therapy.* Palo Alto, CA: Science and Behavior Books.

Evreinov, N. (1927). *The theater in life.* New York: Harrap.

Fairclough, N. (1992). *Discourse and social change.* Cambridge, England: Polity Press.

Ferenczi, S. (1980). *Further contributions to the theory and technique of psychoanalysis.* New York: Brunner/Mazel.

Greenwald, H. (1973). *Active psychology.* Northvale, NJ: Jason Aronson.

Korzybski, A. (1958). *Science and sanity: An introduction to non-Aristotelian systems and general semantics.* Lakeville, CT: International Non-Aristotelian Library.

Kurtz, R. (1990). *Body-centered psychotherapy: The Hakomi method: The integrated use of mindfulness, nonviolence, and body.* Mendocino, CA: Life Rhythm.

---

[2]Other somatic approaches to psychotherapy that use action methods include bioenergetics (Lowen, 1984), Rubenfeld synergy method (Rubenfeld, 1992), Hakomi (Kurtz, 1990), and Pesso Boyden system psychomotor therapy (Pesso, 1991).

Lowen, A. (1984). *Bioenergetics*. Harmondsworth, England: Penguin.

McFarlane, W. R. (1991). Family psychoeducational treatment. In A. S. Gurman & D. P. Kniskern (Eds.), *Handbook of family therapy* (Vol. 2; pp. 363–395). New York: Brunner/Mazel.

Moreno, J. L. (1980). *The theater of spontaneity*. New York: Beacon.

Pardecky, J. T. (1993). *Using bibliotherapy in clinical practice: A guide to self-help books*. Westport, CT: Greenwood Press.

Pesso, A. (1991). *Moving psychotherapy: Theory and application of Pesso system/ psychomotor therapy*. Cambridge, MA: Brookline.

Petzold, H. (1973). *Gestalt therapy and psychodrama*. Nicol, Germany: Kassel.

Reich, W. (1949). *Character analysis* (3rd ed.). New York: Orgone Institute Press.

Rubenfeld, I. (1992). *Mind–body integration* [Videotape]. Berkeley, CA: Thinking Allowed Productions.

Van der Kolk, B. A. (1996). *Traumatic stress: The effects of overwhelming experience on mind, body and society*. New York: Guilford Press.

White, M., & Epston, D. (1990). *Narrative means to therapeutic ends*. New York: Norton.

I

PSYCHOTHERAPIES THAT USE ACTION METHODS

1

GESTALT THERAPY IN ACTION

RUTH WOLFERT AND CYNTHIA A. COOK

Gestalt therapy is a holistic approach in which action is regarded as the natural completion of awareness. Using any of a variety of techniques, Gestalt therapists focus on heightening awareness, actively experimenting to restore the spontaneous cooperation of sensing, feeling, and movement. The radical perspective of this therapy is that health is known and felt in the quality of the experience. Rather than seeking to adjust a person to an external standard of mental health, Gestalt therapy fosters the emergence of authentic being through contacting. This process of "touch touching something" is the self's ongoing creative adjustment in the moment (Perls, Hefferline, & Goodman, 1951/1994, p. 151).

Gestalt therapy sees all aspects of existence as interconnected, with meaning deriving from the whole situation; therefore, contacting always occurs in a field. Interactions take place at the contact boundary between the organism and the environment—a meeting of "me" and "not me" at a boundary that is formed in becoming aware of something other than oneself. The process of creative adjustment that then occurs at the boundary *is* the self: the finder and maker of meaning, or more precisely, the finding and making of meaning, the living of experience through the forming of *gestalts*. This German word has no truly adequate English translation; it refers to a structured, meaningful unity that stands out against a background in the organism/environment field.

As Gestalt therapists, we look for clear and lively gestalt formation, which indicates healthy contact. Whatever the content or meaning, there is a unity to the flow of experience in which awareness is focused and bright, sensing has clarity, and movement reflects and completes the emotion of the moment. It is only when there is an interruption in contacting that the fragmentation of the unity is evident: Energy does not flow; body and emotions seem at cross-purposes; and awareness is unclear, uncertain, and indirect. Then the work is to heighten awareness of the "how" of the interrupting, regardless of the content of the figures, for that is where the self is engaged. Interruptions indicate unfinished business in the background—the residue of failing to get a vital need met. Intolerable suffering has resulted in giving up and blotting out awareness of the need, which was a creative adjustment in a limited and difficult field. But a vital need always persists, and in the absence of new, more favorable circumstances, the suppression must also persist unawares, becoming a fixity in the background. The situation remains perpetually unfinished: draining energy from the foreground; requiring ongoing muscular constriction to maintain; and resulting in tension and numbness, postural distortions, restricted breathing, and inhibited movement. The self's ability to sense the field and form vivid new figures is impaired, so new, satisfying creative adjustments cannot be achieved. Over time, more and more unfinished business accumulates, creating more clutter in the background, requiring more energy to maintain suppression, with less available for contact.

Such a burden of unfinished business creates a chronic emergency in which certain self-functions that usually act to support contact now operate as interruptions. Each function organizes the boundary in a particular way. In confluence, there is no awareness of a boundary between organism and environment. In introjection, something of the environment is experienced as being in the organism. In projection, the reverse is true; something of the organism is experienced as being in the environment. In retroflection, the organism treats part of itself as though it were the environment. In egotism, the boundary is experienced as rigid and fixed, isolating the organism from the environment. In health, these functions enable individuals to respond flexibly to changing circumstances; however, when they have become unfelt habits because of background fixations, they interrupt contact. Healthy confluence, for example, occurs in those unions that enlarge people, that include the actuality of self and other. In contrast, neurotic confluence blots out the actuality; self and other are diminished.

In Gestalt therapy, we invite clients to become aware of what is now habitual, experiencing the automatic ways of thinking, feeling, moving, and expressing that function as interruptions. This basic experiment creates increasingly vivid and complete contact in the moment. As we continuously focus on the gaps in the client's experiencing, more and more of the unfinished business in the background becomes foreground and available for integration in the present. In these moments of contact, energy is freed from fixations; meaning, responsibility, and choice emerge. Even memory and expectation become fluid and alive, causing past and future to lose their fixed meanings. The client can now create new possibilities in the present and be more fully alive. Because interruptions indicate a break in the flow of the unity of sensing, feeling, and movement, an active approach is vital in restoring wholeness. And so we use experimenting. Starting with the basic experiment of focusing on sensations, emotions, muscular tensions, impulses, thoughts, fantasies, and recollections, therapist and client together generate more specific ones. The fundamental experiment is based, as indeed are all Gestalt experiments, on the paradoxical theory of change—that change is fostered by enabling contact with *what is*. Rather than having a goal in mind, we have an exploratory attitude, an openness to whatever emerges from the client's increasing awareness. In framing an experiment we are seeking a way to mobilize the self through contact, thus making it possible for the client to have a new experience and form a different creative adjustment. An experiment could involve anything from exaggerating something habitual to expressing something never dared before. Action completes awareness, whether the work is small and detailed or larger and more expressive.

The Gestalt experimental approach can be used with anyone, for the therapist tailors the method to each individual, working with the interruptions to contacting that emerge in the client–therapist interaction in the moment. Since alienation from the body is endemic in our culture, Gestalt therapists often offer experiments with body, breathing, sensing, and feeling. Clients who are kinesthetically oriented or find it easy to enter imagined realities are often relieved to discover an approach that values these dimensions. This makes them particularly good candidates for more active experiments with a body focus and role-playing, as are those clients who tend to split or dissociate. Clients without these affinities often require more graduated experiments to build a base of body awareness that then supports more expressive work. This is not a hierarchy, for some of those doing more expressive work at first will then need to do more detailed work later.

The style of experiment will also reflect the background, interests, and experience of the practitioner. Laura Perls often said that there are as many Gestalt therapies as there are Gestalt therapists. She, Fritz Perls, and other early practitioners had very different personalities and styles, which influenced the various approaches in the Gestalt community. Because Gestalt therapy values creativity, practices are continually evolving, incorporating what is new in the culture as well as individual inventions. We can use any technique so long as it is used in an experiential, existential, and experimental way. This makes it difficult to generalize about styles of work; nevertheless, some differences in emphasis can be identified.

The range of current practice in the United States can be seen by looking at some of the largest institutes. The New York Institute for Gestalt Therapy, where both chapter authors are affiliated, was founded in 1952 as the first organization devoted to Gestalt therapy. Laura Perls taught there until a few months before her death in 1990, and her influence is seen particularly in therapists who engage with their clients in movement, alignment, and breathing experiments. The New York Institute is unique in that it is a membership organization whose members continually recreate it in an ongoing experiment in group process, which provides one of the contexts for continuing training. Out of this collaboration, the Institute is developing Gestalt group therapy theory. Working from the classical field theory model, as presented in the text authored by Perls, Hefferline, and Goodman (1951/1994), members employ a full range of experimentation, including a focus on destructuring transference by introducing the reality of the therapist. Also in New York City is the Center for Gestalt Psychotherapy and Training, which carries the tradition of Fritz Perls, both in theory and practice, emphasizing empty-chair work; "how and now"; and expressive, body-oriented work. The Gestalt Institute of Cleveland has developed the "cycle of experience" model, which uses a systems approach and is known for offering a body-based track in its training program and for innovative work applying Gestalt therapy to organizational structures. Conversely, the Gestalt Therapy Institute of Los Angeles has a dialogic approach that emphasizes phenomenology, relying less on active, structured experimentation; instead, viewing the whole session as an experiment in relationship. The Gestalt Training Center—San Diego focuses on narrative and tight therapeutic sequences.

The growing edge of Gestalt therapy can be seen in the work of therapists who are exploring developmental issues, somatic modalities, and the integration of the transpersonal and who are broadening the therapeutic mandate by addressing community-based work and gender issues. For example, Ruth Wolfert has integrated the spiritual in her work, whereas Cynthia A. Cook currently is developing an energy model for Gestalt therapy. Ruth and Cynthia also share a background and interest in somatic work, which is reflected in the experiments that follow. Certain common assumptions underlie both Ruth and Cynthia's work: physical self-support is fundamental; emotions are experienced as bodily sensations that require physical energy to suppress; the body functions as a background of the self; and chronically conflicting desires cause a split that is encapsulated in this background.

Two case examples illustrate variations in the Gestalt experimental approach. In the first example, Ruth invites her client to locate and work with her opposing desires in her body as a way of accessing the deeper background split. In the second example, Cynthia asks her client to externalize and identify with her conflicting feelings to clear the background and support her sense of self.

EXPERIMENT 1: LOCATING FEELINGS IN THE BODY AND WORKING WITH WHAT EMERGES

Locating feelings in the body is a basic Gestalt therapy experiment. It addresses the fundamental mind–body split of our cerebral society. In the extreme, intellectualized individuals have limited access to their feelings because of their disconnection from their bodies. For the split to be healed, a person's body sense must be activated. This experiment is a gentle, nonintrusive way for someone to gain access to the depth of feeling that is held in the background. When a client has identified a feeling yet does not seem strongly connected to it, the therapist invites her to locate the feeling in her body and describe the sensation there. We then direct the client's awareness to the area and explore whatever arises—sensations, imagery, emotions, memories, impulses, etc. While honoring what seems bright and energized for the client, we also focus on the emerging process and the structure of fixations in the background. It is important to attend to the interruptions in physical self-support, such as breathing, posture, and relationship to the floor, because these reveal the fixations at a fundamental level. Staying with the body not only ensures the immediacy of the experience, it also enables a fuller integration of whatever material arises by involving more of the self.

This experiment, or one of its variations, can be used successfully with almost anyone and is often suggested early in therapy. However, if a person objects or has difficulty, it is important to let it go for the moment; most likely, returning to it at another time will have a better result. Responses such as the client's embarrassment at being witnessed as a body or anxiety about coming up with the "right" answer would indicate that more trust needs to be established in the therapy relationship, and these issues then inform the work. Experiments are always successful, whether completed the way we propose them or not. They always provide more information about the field and what is both possible and meaningful at the time.

In cases of severe disconnection from body and emotions, experimenting with locating feelings can be the focus of therapy for quite a while. For people who start out being more expressive, it can also be useful, but later in therapy, as a means for them to slow down and become more fully present with their experience. In the following example, Ruth's client is a good candidate for this experiment because she has great difficulty in accessing her body or feelings—a fundamental gap in her experiencing.

CASE EXAMPLE 1: JENNY

Jenny was raised in a developing country in conditions of extreme poverty, neglect, and physical abuse. Her mother died when she was young, and her drunken, violent father often disappeared for weeks or even months at a time. This left a sister not much older than Jenny to care for them both in a house with crumbling walls and floors, exposed pipes, and no separate bathroom. There were long periods when they were close to starvation. The two girls barely survived until they came to the United States to live with relatives, where they experienced the first stability they had known.

Despite her disgust for her father, Jenny became a scientist, the only profession he admired. Although she is very bright and apparently successful, Jenny lives in terror of being "found out" and struggles in agony for every small accomplishment. The only way she has managed to achieve anything has been by terrorizing herself. Throughout school and her previous career hurdles, Jenny has failed to function until the last possible moment and then only by forcing herself to accomplish the work. She was driven into therapy by her fear of losing her job.

In the few months Jenny has been in therapy with me (Ruth), an important theme of her work has been her helplessness and hopelessness about doing research, her most important responsibility at work. She has hidden out in her office for over a year—too incapacitated to organize her work on her own and too frightened of facing other people to enlist their help. Although her worry about losing her job has been mounting for some time, she frequently retreats from the pain and shame of her conflictual tangle by falling asleep at her desk. Compounding the situation, she has been spending an increasing amount of time rescuing injured animals from neglect and cruelty.

Case Narrative	Commentary
Jenny[1] starts the session by complaining about having done "no work" the previous week. She means that she has done little scientific research at her job, but rather has spent her time in cat rescue. She seems hopeless and helpless as she sits slumped in the chair, barely breathing, with her torso back, her chest hollowed and legs splayed, with the soles of her feet facing each other.	What stands out to Ruth is Jenny's lack of self-support. Her body seems to be communicating much that is outside her awareness, a split that seems to provide no direct access.

---

[1]Jenny's diagnosis would be borderline personality disorder in *DSM-IV*. Gestalt therapy does not use such diagnoses, as they cannot encompass the entire person and can be a barrier to being with the client in the moment—with all the possibilities for newness. It is included as a referent for those used to working with this terminology.

Sitting there with Jenny, my chest grows heavy and my breath diminishes. She seems encapsulated; I feel hopeless about reaching her.

I find myself sitting up straight in my chair and breathing more fully, giving myself the support to work with her.

I ask Jenny whether we should work on the split between wanting to do her job and cat rescue.

Jenny perks up at the prospect of a course of action and readily agrees.

I ask her to identify the two sides of the split. She answers without hesitation, "My desire to do cat rescue and my obligation to do research."

In response to further questioning, Jenny clarifies that it is her own sense of obligation and not something coming from her boss.

I invite Jenny to experience these two impulses in her body.

A first attempt leads to a flash of annoyance. "No, I can't!" she says peremptorily.

I appeal to her powers of observation and logic, and Jenny agrees that emotions are always bodily experiences.

She focuses again, and this time she feels her desire to rescue cats as a sense of crying in her eyes, a tightening around her mouth, and a feeling in her heart.

This is an example of somatic resonance, a form of healthy confluence in which the therapist resonates with the physical experience of the client.

Therapy would be difficult if Ruth remained confluential with Jenny in her hopelessness, so she differentiates by contacting herself more fully.

Ruth focuses on the background conflict so that it can become accessible to contact.

Her positive response affirms Ruth's choice of direction.

It is important that Ruth not interpret or define Jenny's conflict for her, but rather support Jenny in articulating her own experience.

Ruth determines that this sense of obligation is not an introject; Jenny has a conflict between two of her own wishes.

Ruth focuses on Jenny's body because feelings are bodily experiences, and suppressed feelings are suppressed physically.

Instead of taking Jenny's annoyance as resistance, Ruth experiences it as an increase in energy, confirmation that they are on a productive path.

Here Ruth is engaging the scientist, so that Jenny has more self to bring to bear. In calling on the other side of the polarity, Ruth lays the ground for further work.

Now Jenny is working with the experiment as her own and has begun bringing thoughts and feelings together.

I continue to probe, and Jenny senses her obligation to her job as a tightness in her chest. I inquire whether it is in the same place as the feeling in her heart.

Ruth wants to differentiate the fixations in the background.

Jenny flares up and pushes back at me, "I don't know! I was just guessing before."

In dismissing her own response, Jenny is retroflecting. However, the intense energy in her response indicates to Ruth that the background is emptying into the gestalt that is forming as Jenny's conflict is coming closer to the surface.

I again ask Jenny to experience these feelings in her body.

Ruth doesn't engage with the content, but rather stays with the process. Her invitation supports Jenny in undoing the retroflection and aligning with herself.

Jenny focuses more closely on the two sensations in her chest, finally distinguishing them—a heaviness, which seems related to her heart, and the tightness that feels as if it is in her lungs.

As soon as she comes into contact with the constriction in her lungs about her job, Jenny starts to cry. "When I was 14, I discovered science. What a feeling! At last I found something that could make sense of my world, could save me from the catastrophic turmoil of my life." She pours out her despair at not being capable of doing scientific research— at being thrown back into the chaos of her childhood, unable to understand the world and find her place in it.

Through step-by-step contacting, Jenny's suppressed feelings have emerged into full embodiment. Now there is a unity between what she is saying and how she is saying it. She comes alive as she faces her previously intolerable suffering. Something new and important can now emerge.

"I wanted to understand," she says. I support her with the quality of my attention. Jenny repeats the words, sensing more and more deeply her hunger for a world so clear and solid she could find a place to exist, her yearning for science to provide

This is the aftermath of contact, in which Jenny is assimilating her experience and making meaning of it. Jenny is very much with herself, so Ruth says nothing, but her presence is powerful and forms part of the ground for Jenny's assimilation.

it, and her grief at the loss of this hope.

"Literally to understand." Jenny takes a breath, "I wanted ground to stand on!" Her body straightens, and her fist adds an exclamation point to the vehemence in her voice.

I then ask her to be aware of her feet.

Ruth notices how Jenny is embodying her dilemma.

Jenny looks down, sees her feet resting on their sides, more in contact with each other than with the floor, and allows herself to sense them in this position.

I say softly, "And now it would be hard to stand," indicating the position of her feet.

Ruth invites Jenny to be present with her experience and become aware of how she is participating in creating that reality.

Jenny expels her breath and comes forward in her chair as she makes a new connection. "And now I have no place to stand," she says, facing her existential reality: her desperate, lifelong search for understanding, her creation of a postural inability to stand, and her current experience of loss of standing in her job. She finds new ground, coming to a balanced position in her chair with both feet momentarily resting lightly on the floor. The gestalt seems complete.

Shifting to the other aspect, I invite Jenny to focus on her bodily sense of her desire to rescue cats and ask her to give it a voice. This time the heaviness in her heart seems prominent, and she cries out from its weight. She weeps about the sad plight of the abandoned, diseased strays, especially "the poor creature" she rescued that is now staying in her office.

Ruth has sensed Jenny's openness to experiencing the other side of the polarity now that she has contacted one side so deeply.

When I ask her what is so sad about him, Jenny moans, "It's so awful that he doesn't understand—and I *can't make* him understand—that this is not his home, that he will be returned to the streets as soon as his infections heal." She sobs, "A person can understand, but a cat cannot. It's too much to bear!" She trails off and sighs.

Ruth is asking Jenny to explore more deeply the background to her feelings —the thoughts, beliefs, and projections about the cat that cause her to feel so sad for him.

Jenny's voice now sounds more distant as she talks of her identification with the pitiful state of the stray, saying that when she cries for him she is also crying for herself.

From her contact with her in the moment, Ruth realizes that Jenny does not have the self-support to reown the projection at this time. Attempting to do so would submerge her in her ungrounded state and leave the actual situation in the office, and the split unaddressed.

I ask Jenny to focus on what it is like for her to try to work with the cat in her office. She cannot work when she sees him, she realizes. "Each time, it is a blow to my heart!" she says, hitting her chest with her hand.

As a result of Ruth having asked her to contact the actuality of her situation, Jenny now understands why she has been unable to work.

I invite her to consider the realities of her mission of rescuing cats. Jenny gets in touch with how overwhelming her mission is, because no matter how many cats she saves, she cannot save them all.

Ruth considers it important to broaden the focus and look at the context so that Jenny does not sink into guilt she cannot support.

I underline the impossibility of this self-appointed mission, and Jenny begins to talk in a scientific mode.

Ruth chooses to focus on facts, which grounds Jenny in reality. Then Jenny can bring her observational powers to bear on the actual situation.

She takes a breath and raises her head to look at me, telling me crisply how many millions of cats there are in New York, more than the number of people.

Ruth's presence assists Jenny in staying with her experience, but little overt intervention is needed, for the contact is now nearly complete.

Then she remembers a plan she has created for a cat rescue organization

Jenny is now integrated.

that could save numerous strays. Jenny sits tall and smiles proudly. "This is what I'm good at. I can plan." Her chest expands, and her breath dissipates the heaviness in her heart—her scientific and compassionate aspects are now working together. Then she recalls how she likes standing and teaching beginning science students, another example of science and compassion cooperating in her life.

"In this moment, all the things that usually stop me from working—my sense of inadequacy, my guilt, my disorganization and helplessness—all that seems like so much horseshit from the past without any power."

For the moment, Jenny's split is healed. It undoubtedly will reappear because the deeper grounds of her childhood suffering have not been adequately addressed, but her achieving this integration, however briefly, is a milestone.

In the 6 weeks between the therapy session and the writing of this chapter, Ruth continued working with Jenny to heal the split by focusing again and again on her breathing and body in different ways. In each session, Jenny grew stronger and more integrated, but for the first few weeks, she still tended to become swamped between meetings by her desperate need to assuage the plight of the injured strays. This need is no longer so compelling that it drowns her. Jenny has now grown enough to start assimilating her deep grief and shame at having been left without the means of survival as a child and has diminished her projection onto the abandoned animals. Although she is still having difficulty doing her research efficiently, she has found a balance between working and rescuing cats.

EXPERIMENT 2: EMPTY-CHAIR WORK

Working with the empty chair,[2] a classic Gestalt technique developed by Fritz Perls, is a versatile structure for experimenting. The client is in-

---

[2]Jacob L. Moreno was the grandfather of the empty chair experiment in that he used role-playing to address clients' intrapersonal conflicts. Fritz Perls integrated this technique into Gestalt therapy as a way of exploring any polarity the client was experiencing as a sharpening of the awareness continuum. Unlike Moreno, Perls always had the client play all the parts and worked toward integration at each session.

vited to imagine someone or something in an empty chair to dialogue with it.[3] In its fully developed form, the client then moves between the chairs, embodying and speaking from each position, although many variations are possible. Anything can be placed in the chair—a person in the client's life, a personified feeling or attitude, an image from a fantasy or a dream, a part of the body, or an inanimate object. The person or object is then present experientially and is available for contact. The experiment allows the use of sensory awareness, fantasy, emotional expression, creativity, movement, and cognitive reframing. A rich, multidimensional experience is created in the moment that allows the individual to differentiate, identify, and own projections, introjections, and retroflections, illuminating the deeper background of the surface conflicts.

This type of experiment is appropriate when the client is caught up in strong feelings that seem out of proportion to the context, indicating that unfinished situations in the background are flooding the foreground. By working with the empty chair, the client can externalize and thereby differentiate the background into contextualized attitudes and feelings. Expanding the contact with each aspect in this way makes evident the underlying emotional perspective and existential stance. Now therapist and client can develop and explore the positions and the relationships between them. The Gestalt view is that all sides of an internal conflict reflect important aspects of the person and that to support them is to support the self. Rather than trying to pacify or solve it, Gestalt therapists encourage the conflict, thereby inherently affirming the person's wholeness and strength. We are always working with the structure of the process, not the content of the conflict, although it is an individual clinical judgment how much to support the client's splitting and at what pace to work toward integration. A valuable application of the experiment is with dissociative clients. It is particularly important to pay careful attention to the bodily experience of these clients, for this keeps them anchored in the room in the present. The experiment is then unifying, when it is otherwise potentially fragmenting. The client's body in effect becomes the chair, the container, and the bridge to the here and now, which creates fundamental support for tolerating memory, sensation, and emotion.

This experiment should not be seen as more advanced than the previous one. Rather than being two separate experiments, they mark the ends of a continuum. Either experiment can develop into the other. For example, locating feelings in the body could evolve into a dialogue between the feelings, or a dialogue with someone in the empty chair could be integrated as a feeling in the body. They are ways to grade an experiment up or down—*up* being more expressive and potentially involving more dimensions; *down* being more fine-tuned, detailed, and with a narrower

---

[3]See also chapter 6.

scope. Either could be appropriate at any stage of therapy, depending on the client and what is being presented. This illustrates the versatility of the Gestalt experimental approach.

Working with the empty chair uses emotional lability as a strength and is useful for those without a sharply defined sense of self. At the other end of the spectrum, a self-conscious person will have a harder time doing the experiment. In the following example, it was used many times with many variations.

CASE EXAMPLE 2: SHARON

Sharon was a pretty, girlish woman in her late 20s who hid her slender body under baggy clothes. She was referred to me (Cynthia) years ago by a student of mine who found her distraught and crying in a restaurant. Sharon's life was a chaotic series of unhappy relationships and what she viewed as demeaning waitressing jobs while she pursued her dream of being an actress. She had recently managed to end an abusive relationship with an acting teacher who had also become her guru and drinking buddy. When I inquired about her childhood, Sharon remembered little except her attempts to run away, which started when she was 5 years old and continued through her teenage years. It soon became evident that Sharon had an intense relationship with her critical and demanding father. Caught between hating and fearing him on the one hand and trying to please him and win his love on the other, she clung to a fantasy of herself as the problem in a supportive and accepting family.

What impressed me most about Sharon at the beginning of our work together was the extent of her fragmentation. Her winning smile could quickly dissolve into tears of rage and despair, and sometimes disappeared entirely for weeks on end. In the course of a session she could be energetic and self-confident, then crumble under a barrage of self-hatred, and then apparently get lost in a fragment of memory. I wondered from the start if sexual abuse had been part of her history, something Sharon herself alluded to without directly naming it. I had no interest, however, in chasing down those memories because Sharon was clearly not strong enough to assimilate even the shreds of recollection that were emerging on their own. Collapsed in her chair, not making eye contact, lost in a closed loop of circular thoughts, she seemed barely aware of being in the room with me. I felt that my first task was to help her into the room, into her body, and into the present with me, so that together we could find a way to contact and integrate all her fragments.

Despite how lost she seemed at times, Sharon also demonstrated strengths—vitality, resiliency, creativity, fighting spirit, and openness—that I felt Gestalt therapy could build on. For the first few years, much of our work consisted of one method: dialogues between various aspects Sharon could identify in herself, used over and over again. This process of sifting through her fragments felt like untangling threads and then reweaving a fabric. Each dialogue developed a different emphasis as each aspect of the tapestry that was Sharon emerged.

For example, initially Sharon had little sensation of her lower body and legs and felt a lot of shame and the need to hide her body. So we worked with dialogues in which she talked to her body and listened to it or listened to what her body had to say to someone in the empty chair. In all the dialogues, body-focused or not, I paid particular attention to increasing her physical support by including awareness of her breathing, the sensation of her feet and legs, and her experience of the chair on the floor. When Sharon was able to release her retroflected feelings and connect to her body, it became a powerful resource. She had been a track and field athlete as a teenager, and our work helped her reclaim that sense of power and competence.

Also, she had little sense of her own opinions, instead parroting the attitudes of her parents and the cultural framework in which she had grown up. As we worked, she was able to assert her own beliefs and preferences, particularly regarding her warm, affectionate, and supposedly "low-class" maternal grandparents.

The greatest benefit, however, was to Sharon's sense of self-esteem. Early on, she often berated herself for "being so stupid" and "such an idiot." One time when I asked her what it felt like to be yelled at and criticized in that way, she paused, seemed confused, and then in a small voice answered, "bad." I felt as though I was listening to a parent berate a child, one sign that I was hearing a parental introject and not Sharon's experience as a child. To support the child's perspective, I brought over another chair and asked her to place the critical voice in it so that she could have a dialogue between the two personas. This created the space for her to differentiate herself from the introjection and allow the background conflict to emerge. Taking the time in each chair to fully embody and experience herself as each part allowed a vivid experience to emerge.

Case Narrative	*Commentary*
In one chair, her arms wrapped around her chest, her face contorting into a sneer of disgust, Sharon told the Sharon in the other chair how she would never amount to anything and that she should just give up and stop trying. Suddenly she interrupted herself—OHMIGOD—frozen with	Identifying the critical voice, which she formerly thought of as her own, as an introject of her father freed Sharon to find her own voice.

her hands to her mouth as she realized she was hearing her father, indeed *being* her father. Now this chair became intolerable to stay in, and she fled back to the other one, crying for him to leave her alone.

Now more willing and able to identify with herself and her own experience, she then remembered how angry, scared, and humiliated she felt when he berated her. I encouraged her to stay with this experience—her breathing, her sensation of herself, the chair underneath her, her feet on the floor.

Directing Sharon's attention to these basics of her existence helped her reclaim the parts of her awareness she had blotted out to survive her father's assaults and supported the assimilation of a new experience in the present.

Her breathing grew calmer, her posture was upright, and she was thoughtful and animated as she reflected on what she had just experienced.

Another step came during a similar dialogue when Sharon was more able to tolerate the experience of identifying with her critical, abusive father. A door seemed to open as Sharon described wonderingly her father's sense of inadequacy, his fear of his own out-of-control anger, and his frustration at not being able to control her. Returning to the other chair, Sharon felt as if she were sitting opposite a person rather than a larger-than-life monster, and she began to have some empathy for her father's experience.

Contacting the introject was the beginning of a process of robbing it of its power and making it available for integration.

Empathizing with her father was not a goal, however; rather, the experience helped Sharon feel more like a full person. Now she could respond more as a whole instead of as a scared child, a mere fragment of herself.

At times Sharon experienced her father as looming over her, and I encouraged her to find what would help her feel safer or more protected. She folded over in the chair, clutching her belly, moaning and crying for him to leave her alone, telling me she just wanted to hide. "Where do you want to hide?" I asked. "Behind the chair." "So go ahead, let yourself hide," I responded.

Sharon is frozen in retroflection, disconnected from her energy and initiative, unable to act on her desire. Cynthia supports her longing for safety and her ability to create it for herself.

Pulling herself by her hands along the back of the chair, she dragged herself to stand behind it so that her body was then hidden from her abdomen down. Sharon was shaking, her legs were buckling, and she steadied herself by holding on to the chair. I urged her, "Feel yourself, find your feet, breathe."

Sharon is having difficulty supporting herself, so Cynthia encourages her to experience herself in relation to the environment in the moment and find what support is available.

As her breathing deepened and her legs strengthened, I asked, "And now, what do you want to say to him?" In a voice trembling with rage that seemed to come directly from her newly protected belly, Sharon told him to leave her alone—not a plea this time, but a demand. I encouraged her to find more words. "What do you want to say to him?" "Stop looking at me. Go away. Go Away. GO AWAY AND LEAVE ME ALONE!" And much to her surprise, he receded. I invited her to stay present to this new experience of peaceful and emptied space around her.

The amount of energy behind Sharon's first words to her father tells Cynthia that she is still holding back. Cynthia supports Sharon's assertion of the full force of her feelings and desire. In literally standing up to her introjected father, Sharon experiences herself for the first time as powerful in relation to him.

Sharon was empowered by this experience and was able to carry the effects of it with her into other situations. As she went into her acting class, for example, she left her father-introject outside and literally closed the door on him. She was becoming more able to identify and express her anger and otherwise protect herself, as well as to slowly let go of her doubt and self-questioning.

During this time we were also working with another dialogue that involved her relationship to what she identified as a young child in her. In working through her shame and disgust toward this powerless, bad little girl, she realized how this split served to contain the traumatic memories of her childhood. We worked with this dialogue internally, through imagery, body sensations, and emotions. This work further strengthened the adult in Sharon, a middle ground between the desperate, hysterical child and the domineering parent. Sometimes this adult was a mediator, sometimes an advocate for the child, at times agreeing with the angry, critical voice, but able to challenge its tactics and approach. The adult was ultimately able to tell the child that what she suffered was not her fault.

Case Narrative	Commentary

These two tracks came together in a confrontation with Sharon's father-introject as we were working with the persistent tie between them.

Cynthia is struck by how this introject keeps returning and recognizes it as a form of creative adjustment that is still serving a purpose. Therefore, there is something important that Sharon has invested in it.

In the middle of a dialogue with her father, I asked her if he had something of hers. She replied almost immediately, "a baby." This seemed very profound to both of us. As long as she felt that her father had "custody" of that part of her, her experience of herself always had to include him. I stood in front of her, holding a small stuffed monkey to represent the baby and asked her if she could take it back.

Cynthia chooses to stand in as custodian of the baby to allow Sharon to experience herself as separate, active, and adult. Watching Sharon take these steps was like seeing a disabled person struggling to walk.

Crying, her breath catching, her jaw set, her steps stiff and halting, she came toward me as if she were walking into a fire, pulled the monkey from me, clutched it to her, and fell back into her chair.

This was a pivotal session. Showing great determination and courage, Sharon was able to follow her own initiative for the first time without coaching. For someone whose relationship to her body was so damaged, experiencing herself physically as powerful and strong, particularly in relation to her father, was a tremendous change—a sign of growth and healing.

In the aftermath, I invited her to be in contact with the monkey–baby, and she described the infant's openness and trust in her as they sat there peacefully together.

Cynthia facilitates the completion and assimilation of the experience.

Sharon has been sober for 4 years. After moving through several relationships, each more self-respecting than the last, she has been alone for the first extended period of her life. She has recently taken her first steps in group therapy, indicating how much she has healed her shame, and has begun expressing her anger at me. She is auditioning well and has been cast in three shows over the next several months. Her periods of crisis and depression pass more quickly and do not reach the depths of those early days of despair. She is able to claim both her sweetness and her strength and to choose whom to trust with her vulnerability.

RESISTANCE

The focus in Gestalt therapy is not on resistance or compliance; we look instead at the interruptions to contacting. All interruptions are seen as archaic creative adjustments that were the person's best effort at that time and place. And we assume that now as well people are doing the best they can for themselves in the moment. Regardless of whether clients seem to be resisting or not, our task as Gestalt therapists is to remain steadfastly present and use our skills to keep opening opportunities for contact through creative experimentation.

Assertions of any kind are seen as instances of vitality, the life force in action that needs to be respected and allowed to bloom. In the case of someone as compliant as Sharon, Cynthia nurtures every shred of genuine assertion. For example, when Sharon says she wants to hide, Cynthia sees this as an active stance and affirms the strength in it. Jenny, on the other hand, is often oppositional, and the authentic vitality in this attitude must also be affirmed. Thus, when Jenny bristles and apparently "resists" the experiment, Ruth does not experience this as a conflict. Rather, she feels the rising of Jenny's energy, which is now available for deeper work. By responding to the quality of energy being expressed instead of the content of her words, Ruth gives Jenny support that enables her to redirect her energy. In another context, an alternative might be to support and encourage the expression of the client's objection to the experiment. Clients are not seen as resisting when they refuse to do an experiment but rather as being assertive in a way that is to be supported.

REPEATED USE OF AN EXPERIMENT

Rarely is an experiment a one-time solution to a client's predicament. Typically, the same experiment is repeated and varied over time, as it was in both of the cases described previously. For example, the same track was followed over the course of many sessions with Sharon. Through continuously dialoging between whatever fragments she presented each time, Sharon moved from feeling lost and overwhelmed by her emotions to being able to explore her conflict with her father and question her identification with him. This method ultimately enabled her to develop her assertiveness, differentiate and clarify her own attitudes, and have a growing experience of confidence and strength in her body. In general, repeated use of an experiment allows for fuller exploration of the client's background issues and restoration of the holistic unity of experiencing: the integration of perceiving, feeling, thinking, moving, and expressing.

EXPERIMENTS AS HOMEWORK

Along with the structure of any particular experiment, the therapist is also teaching the experimental attitude itself. As clients integrate this attitude, they are more able to approach any situation in an open, exploratory manner. In addition, we often will suggest that specific experiments be done as homework. This is both a way of supporting clients' continual expansion of self-awareness and of empowering them with resources to explore new possibilities in difficult situations. The type of experiment suggested for use outside a session generally provides a balance of support and challenge without being too anxiety provoking. For example, Ruth invited Jenny to focus on her breathing throughout her workday as an experiment in staying in touch with herself, particularly her impulses to avoid her work and escape into sleep. This experiment was both a challenge, requiring openness to her feelings, and supportive, increasing her physical self-support. It grew out of Ruth's observation that Jenny was able to productively focus on her breathing in session, strengthening her scientific mode, which she located in her lungs. Conversely, Ruth concluded that the experiment of locating feelings in her body would be destabilizing to Jenny as a homework assignment—producing too much emotion to be assimilated on her own. The experiment of focusing on feelings in the body, however, is often successfully given by both Ruth and Cynthia as homework in other cases in which the client's tolerance for feelings is greater.

EMPIRICAL EVIDENCE

Gestalt therapy is holistic and does not tend to classify by "variables" or even diagnose using the categories of the *Diagnostic and Statistical Manual of Mental Disorders* (American Psychiatric Association, 1994). Therefore, relatively little emphasis has been placed on research historically, although there is a growing body of empirical evidence (see the Frederick and Laura Perls' Collection and Gestalt Therapy Archives at Kent State University Library).

Two overviews of the Gestalt therapy research show a good deal of evidence for its efficacy (Bretz, Heckerens, & Schmitz, 1994; Harman, 1984), and Greenberg, Rice, and Elliot (1993) discuss the empirical evidence. Gestalt therapy has been shown to be effective with specific issues, such as phobias (Johnson & Smith, 1997) and body image (Clance,

Thompson, Simerly, & Weiss, 1994) and also with special populations, such as hospitalized individuals with schizophrenia (Serok, 1983), hardcore criminals (Serok & Levi, 1993), and psychotherapy trainees (O'Leary et al., 1998). In addition, there are studies in which Gestalt therapy compares favorably with other methods, such as psychoeducation (Paivio & Greenberg, 1995), and other experiential therapies (Greenberg, Elliott, & Lietaer, 1994).

QUALITIES OF THE GESTALT THERAPIST

All of the methods of Gestalt therapy are grounded in faith in the client–therapist field and the premise that contact results in growth. In this existential–phenomenological approach, we focus on what can be sensed and felt in experiments that highlight areas of unawareness and heighten holistic experiencing in the moment. This is a process that relies on the creativity of the therapist in meeting the client and opening opportunities for contact. Instead of having specific exercises or structures, and without any predetermined sequence, the Gestalt therapist applies herself in and to the actual situation as it unfolds with whatever professional skills and life experience she has accumulated and integrated.

Together, therapist and client invent and discover their relationship and themselves, creating ways to facilitate growth. Therapists are always participants in the process of contact with clients. We do not act as authorities or projection screens but rather interact as equals with clients. We have "beginners' minds" and allow ourselves to be moved and changed by our clients, growing as they do in the contact of the moment. We focus on our own gestalts as they emerge, on what stands out as most important to us, because we are part of the field and our responses to the client are pertinent. These emerging gestalts are different from interpretations in that they involve responding to the client from "the inside," from a unity of seeing, hearing, and feeling that is understood as our own experience. Gestalts occur in images and bodily sensations as well as words and, of course, include the background of life experiences, skills, and style the therapist brings to her work—the mix that is the creative wellspring for Gestalt work. As Laura Perls said, "In Gestalt therapy, there are as many styles as there are therapists and patients. The therapist . . . continually surprises not only his patients and groups, but also himself" (1992, p. 133).

Being present and responsive without extrinsic structuring is extraordinarily difficult and places special demands on the therapist. She must suspend preconceptions and be open to being surprised in each moment she and the client meet. With flexibility and creativity, she responds with experiments that enable the intrinsic structures to emerge and shift. As the dialogue with the client evolves, the Gestalt therapist must be able to relate in a real way—being open to feedback, directly responsive, and comfortable acknowledging and expressing limitations. The capacity to tolerate intense emotional expression is a crucial ability, which is enhanced by having developed an integrated body-based awareness.

TRAINING REQUIREMENTS

Skill in Gestalt therapy is the result of personal therapy experience as well as training in the theory and the structure of process. A trainee must have done enough of his own personal Gestalt therapy work to be sufficiently aware of his issues and not project them on to clients. The therapy also creates familiarity with, and faith in, the Gestalt process that cannot be gained any other way.

Training is offered at Gestalt therapy institutes, sometimes in the form of 3- or 4-year programs and sometimes in more open-ended formats. Time and a supportive community are required to learn experientially and integrate theory with practice. Trainees learn how to drain the background into forming figures, heighten awareness of the interruptions to contact, and construct experiments to assimilate them. They develop the ability to stay present and responsive through grounding in their own bodily awareness. By continually addressing their own background issues, they deepen their capacity for contact. Training usually occurs in theory groups, practica in which trainees get feedback on their work, and supervision groups for those beginning to practice. Many people come to Gestalt therapy training from other modalities, such as bodywork, the expressive therapies, and even psychoanalysis. Gestalt training supports individual strengths, and students are encouraged to recognize and develop their own styles of learning and working.

CONCLUSION

Working at the boundary in the therapist–client field, the Gestalt therapist attends to interruptions in contacting, structuring experiments that support new creative adjustments. Together, client and therapist find and invent meaning as they bring background fixities into awareness, enlarging self-functioning in the present moment. Continuously sensing and attending to the details of experience gives immediate, ongoing feedback on the effectiveness of the therapy. This is the autonomous criterion by which we guide our work. When there is a separation into parts—resulting in dull, weak figures, confused feeling, and inhibited movement—more work must be done. But when there is a unity and flow of spontaneous gestalt formation, when awareness is sharp, feeling vivid, and movement energetic and graceful, then contact is occurring and growth ensues.

REFERENCES

American Psychiatric Association. (1994). *Diagnostic and statistical manual of mental disorders* (4th ed.). Washington, DC: Author.

Bretz, H. J., Heckerens, H. P., & Schmitz, B. (1994). Eine Metaanalyse der Wirksamkeit von Gestalttherapie [A meta-analysis of the effectiveness of Gestalt therapy]. *Zeitschrift fuer Klinische Psychologie, Psychopathalgie und Psychotherapie, 42*(3), 241–260.

Clance, P. R., Thompson, M. B., Simerly, D. E., & Weiss, A. (1994). The effects of the Gestalt approach on body image. *Gestalt Journal, 17*(1), 95–114.

Frederick and Laura Perls' Collection and Gestalt Therapy Archives. Kent, OH: Kent State University Library Special Collections and Archives.

Greenberg, L. S., Elliott, R. K., & Lietaer, G. (1994). Research on experiential psychotherapies. In A. E. Bergin & S. L. Garfield (Eds.), *Handbook of psychotherapy and behavior change.* New York: Wiley.

Greenberg, L. S., Rice, L. N., & Elliott, R. K. (1993). Facilitating emotional change: The moment to moment process. New York: Guilford Press.

Harman, R. (1984). Gestalt therapy research. *Gestalt Journal, 7*(2), 61–69.

Johnson, W. R., & Smith, E. W. L. (1997). Gestalt empty-chair dialogue versus systematic desensitization in the treatment of a phobia. *Gestalt Review, 1*(2), 150–162.

O'Leary, E., Purcell, U., McSweeney, E., O'Flynn, D., O'Sullivan, K., Keene, N., & Barry, N. (1998). The Cork person-centered Gestalt project: Two outcome studies. *Counseling Psychology Quarterly, 2*(1), 45–61.

Paivio, S. C., & Greenberg, L. S. (1995). Resolving "unfinished business": Efficacy of experiential therapy using empty-chair dialogue. *Journal of Consulting and Clinical Psychology, 63,* 419–425.

Perls, F. S., Hefferline, R., & Goodman, P. (1994). *Gestalt therapy: Excitement and growth in the human personality.* Highland, NY: The Gestalt Journal Press. (Original work published 1951)

Perls, L. (1992). *Living at the boundary.* Highland, NY: The Gestalt Journal Press.

Serok, S. (1983). An experiment of Gestalt group therapy with hospitalized schizophrenics. *Psychotherapy: Theory, Research and Practice, 20*(4), 417–424.

Serok, S., & Levi, N. (1993). Application of Gestalt therapy with long-term prison inmates in Israel. *Gestalt Journal, 16*(1), 105–127.

ADDITIONAL RESOURCES

Books

Feder, B., & Ronall, R. (1980). *Beyond the hot seat: Gestalt approaches to group.* New York: Brunner/Mazel. Readings in various forms of Gestalt groups.

Feder, B., & Ronall, R. (1996). *A living legacy of Fritz and Laura Perls: Contemporary case studies.* New York. Collection of case studies, including a long-term case by Ruth Wolfert.

Kepner, J. (1989). *Body process.* Cleveland, OH: Gestalt Institute of Cleveland Press. Description of theory and practice of body-based Gestalt therapy.

Oaklander, V. (1988). Windows to our children: A Gestalt therapy approach to children and adolescents. Highland, NY: *The Gestalt Journal* Press. (Original work published 1978) Classic book on Gestalt therapy with children.

Perls, F. S. (1969). *In and out the garbage pail.* Moab, UT: Real People Press. Fritz Perls's autobiography.

Perls, F. S. (1973). *The Gestalt approach and eye witness to therapy.* Lomond, CA: Science and Behavior Books. Fritz Perls's last work, edited after his death.

Perls, F. S. (1992). *Ego, hunger and aggression.* Highland, NY: *The Gestalt Journal* Press. (Original work published 1947) Clear, early statement of the Perls's innovations that would soon develop into Gestalt therapy.

Perls, F. S. (1992). *Gestalt therapy verbatim.* Highland, NY: *The Gestalt Journal* Press. (Original work published 1969) Transcripts of dreamwork in the "hot-seat" style.

Perls, F. S., Hefferline, R., & Goodman, P. (1994). *Gestalt therapy: Excitement and growth in the human personality.* Highland, NY: *The Gestalt Journal* Press. (Original work published 1951) The basic theory text, which has never been surpassed and is considered the bible of Gestalt therapy; also contains 18 experiments and people's reactions to doing them.

Perls, L. (1992). *Living at the boundary.* Highland, NY: *The Gestalt Journal* Press. Elegant collection of essays on topics in Gestalt therapy by its codeveloper, including a transcript of a piece of therapeutic work.

Polster, E., & Polster, M. (1973). *Gestalt therapy integrated: Contours of theory and practice.* New York: Brunner/Mazel. Fundamentals of the therapy from second-generation Gestaltists.

Zinker, J. (1977). *Creative process in Gestalt therapy.* New York: Brunner/Mazel. Discussion of how to structure experiments.

Journals

The Australian Gestalt Journal: An International Journal Based in Australia. 7A Chesterfield Road, Epping, New South Wales 2121, Australia. A semiannual journal with a wide range of philosophical, practical, and artistic contributions from American, European, and Australian authors.

The British Gestalt Journal. PO Box 2994, London N5 1UG, England. A large, semiannual journal that includes a mix of contributions on philosophy and practice from American as well as British and European authors.

Gestalt! URL: http://rdz.stjohns.edu/gestalt!/. An electronic journal available on the Internet with links to other sites.

The Gestalt Journal. Center for Gestalt Development, PO Box 990, Highland, NY 12528-0990. The original journal of Gestalt therapy, which has been published semiannually for 20 years.

The Gestalt Review. The Analytic Press, 101 West Street, Hillside, NJ 07642. A quarterly journal specializing in dialogue between authors and respondents.

Professional Associations and Organizations

Association for the Advancement of Gestalt Therapy
4 Highview Court
Denton, TX 76205
E-mail: bruboo@aol.com
Web site: www.g-g.org/aagt

International Gestalt Therapy Association
c/o *The Gestalt Journal*
PO Box 990
Highland, NY 12528-0990
(914) 691-7192
Web site: www.gestalt.org/igta.htm

Institutes[4]

Gestalt Center for Psychotherapy and Training
26 West 9th Street
New York, NY 10011
(212) 387-9429

Gestalt Institute of Cleveland
1588 Hazel Drive
Cleveland, OH 44106
(216) 421-0468

Gestalt Therapy Institute of Los Angeles
1460 7th Street, Suite 301
Santa Monica, CA 90401
(213) 458-9747

---

[4]There are more than 30 other Gestalt therapy institutes in the United States and many throughout the world. A list is available in *The Gestalt Directory*, which may be obtained from The Center for Gestalt Development, PO Box 990, Highland, NY 12528; (914) 691-7192.

Gestalt Training Center—San Diego
PO Box 2189
La Jolla, CA 92038
(619) 454-9139

The New York Institute for Gestalt Therapy
PO Box 238, Old Chelsea Station
New York, NY 10011
(212) 864-8277

2

THE SATIR SYSTEM IN ACTION

JEAN A. McLENDON

After reviewing a videotape of therapists under her supervision, Virginia Satir (1916–1988), founder of the Satir system of therapy, remarked that there was no way to know they were Satir therapists. Her reason: The therapists sat in their chairs the whole time; no one moved. During the next videotaping session, there was so much movement the therapists looked like monkeys! For Satir, Satir therapy had to have life. It had to contain the seeds of action necessary for addressing the real-life situations clients would encounter outside therapy.

HISTORY

Satir, who was known as the "Columbus of family therapy," trained academically as a clinical social worker. After receiving her degree in 1948, she learned psychodynamic and Freudian-based theories. Always eager to

---

I studied with Satir for nearly 20 years. I was a member of the Satir team that participated in the 1991 Family Therapy Research project directed by Joan Winter. In addition, I staffed with Virginia and other Avantans for a number of the summer Process Community Institutes. Unreferenced anecdotes, quotes, and so forth come from notes taken during this time and also from personal communications with Satir.

understand the workings of being human, Satir put her academic theories to work in a private clinical social work practice in which she often said she accepted the cases other therapists did not want. She was an experiential learner and relied heavily on her direct experiences with clients to deepen her understanding and assumptions about change. She began including families in her therapy sessions to better understand the resources available to and challenges facing clients. By the late 1950s, Satir was receiving widespread recognition as one of the foremost practitioners of a new approach to change called *family therapy* (Simon, 1989).

Time spent cofounding the Mental Research Institute (MRI) in Palo Alto, California, circa 1958, gave Satir the opportunity to work with colleagues and refine her theoretical premises. Those ideas were presented in the groundbreaking 1964 text *Conjoint Family Therapy* (Satir, 1964). Satir left MRI in 1964 and became director of training for Esalen, the human potential growth center in Big Sur, California (Robert Spitzer, personal communication, Jan. 25, 1999). While there, her humanistic beliefs and her experiential action methods crystallized (Goldenberg & Goldenberg, 1991). After leaving Esalen, Satir published the first edition of *Peoplemaking* (1972).

The Satir system, with its strong roots in communication and family systems was referred to by Satir as a human validation process model. For the thousands who observed her workshops and video demonstrations, Satir's evolving approach to change was humanistic, brief, experiential, strategic, structural, and, above all, genuine, caring, creative, and active. In short, it is process driven and outcome guided.

Wherever Satir presented it was likely that the room, no matter its size, would be filled. Before her death in 1988, she covered much of the world demonstrating and espousing her strong belief in the centrality of self-esteem for improving relationships, health, and performance. Inexperienced practitioners saw magic. Experienced professionals saw mastery. Her explanations to clients and students were spoken in simple terms and with authority. Notes taken by Satir during the 1980s for what was to become her next book, *The Third Birth*, reflect her memories and appreciation for journeying with about 30,000 people who sought her help for an array of professional and personal challenges. She noted, "I remembered the carefulness and patience with which I needed to proceed so that while they were facing the pain and uncertainty that often goes along with making change, there would be no injury to their self-esteem along the way" (Suarez, 1998, p. 11).

GOALS OF THE SATIR SYSTEM

The primary goal of Satir system therapy is high self-esteem. The outcome sought is congruence, a here-and-now internal mind–body–spirit harmony that is expressed outwardly. Congruent communication reflects high self-esteem. The client's unique mental, physical, emotional, and spiritual identity provides the primary resources the Satir therapist uses to help the client change. Acceptance and appreciation of one's unique self at these levels is the basis for self-esteem.

Congruence is often confused with consistency. However, it is much more complex. It requires consideration for oneself, the other person, and the context that provides the "container" and purpose for the relationship. The approach is not just about cognition. Congruence is not so much a way of speaking but a way of being. Socializing people to congruent speech is not sufficient to help clients grow. Nor is this approach just about affect. Languishing in a pool of emotion may reflect internal experience, but change requires action to face internal demons or those in someone else. The action approach to congruence is about achieving greater mind–body–spirit synergy so one's personal resources can be accessed for meeting life's challenges. Satir believed that the body was least likely to lie about a person's level of self-esteem and harmony. Having a client take a moment to reflect on internal signals the body might be sending was often a prelude to inviting the client to risk expressing the internal message.

HOW THE SATIR SYSTEM WORKS

Satir system therapists work from a system of beliefs and values that guide their involvement with clients and students. In general, Satir system practitioners believe that behavior is connected to one's internal experience of oneself. Behavior has purpose, and no matter how dysfunctional, it has value that can be developed. The problem is not the problem; it is the coping that is the problem. Coping is learned and influenced by one's level of self-esteem. All people are created with the birthright of self-esteem and have the resources needed for growth and change. There is a unique spirit and essence in all humans. Accessing this soul-filled inner place promotes growth and increased self-esteem.

Much of the work of the Satir system therapist is in facilitating awareness and acceptance and externalizing the conflicts associated with universal longings. When the client's internal experience is externalized, a new perspective is made possible, offering the client an experience to be studied and dealt with directly. Satir was ingeniously creative at transforming cognitive and emotional constructs into spontaneous opportunities for movement, and rather than verbal analysis, her action modes involved symbology using tools such as the self-esteem tool kit (Satir, Banmen, Gerber, & Gomori, 1991); communication stances (Satir, 1988); role-playing, especially as a part of family sculpting and parts parties (Satir et al., 1991); and "conversation" with family members through vehicles such as family-of-origin mapping and family reconstruction (Satir, Bitter, & Krestensen, 1988). Although acquiring background as context was important, action brings the client closer to behavioral change. Satir wanted to bring clients into the challenging "here and now" of their problem dynamics. There, she could give them the support they needed to access their personal resources. Her invitation for moving into the action, or enactment, usually included permission and a reminder for the client to breathe consciously, acknowledging his or her body and sense of wisdom. She might also give a supportive touch at the moment of the invitation.

KEY METHODS IN THE SYSTEM

Satir's mastery and magic were in creating engagement. She taught her students the art of human contact (Satir, 1976; Winter, 1993). She was superb at building a genuinely caring relationship that enabled a balanced focus on inner awareness and outer action. The Satir model is grounded in the importance of activating awareness, understanding behavior, authoring new choices, and practicing new behaviors.

Sculpting

As thousands of practitioners observed time and time again, Satir was very still and quiet when she was trying to get a picture of a client's experience. Once she had that picture, she moved into action, often getting people to take physical poses and postures that presented a human sculpt. Sculpting (Satir et al., 1991; see also chapter 4) offers a three-dimensional picture of the essence of each role-player's mode of operating as well as a depiction of the interpersonal dynamics of the system as a whole. The sculpts serve diagnostic and strategic purposes. The problem or dysfunctional coping can be sculpted as can trial runs at applying new ways of dealing with situations.

A client unfamiliar with sculpting usually picks up the idea quickly if shown a few ways in which people can be positioned, moved, or arranged to express feeling states. "Let me see," Satir might say, "YOU (indicating the husband), stand here trying to look unruffled, and YOU (indicating the wife), get down around his knees and pull on his pant leg. Is that what you are talking about?" She would work with the sculpt until each person felt their experience had been fully expressed and understood. She would then identify the positive and purposeful intent of the behaviors with wit and common sense, leaving the clients with an expanded version of the current situation and an opening for how to shift the dynamics. She knew affect and action were connected, and she knew where there was: "that place deep inside yourself where you keep the treasure that is called by your name" (Banmen & Gerber, 1985, p. 23).

Family Mapping

Family mapping, Satir style, is an active and creative process for eliciting and capturing facts and feelings about a client's life on a chart pad using colored markers. The choice of color and kind of markings depict the inner system of the person and show the quality of the relationships. Rather than being horizontal, as is the case with most genograms, the family map is vertical (Carlson & Kjos, 1998). The birth family is in the center of the page, with each member represented by a circle and a designation for male or female. The maternal family is shown on the right side of the paper above the symbol for the star's (the client's) mother; the paternal family is on the left above the symbol for the star's father. Adding adjectives to describe personalities, communication stances, goals for therapy, family rules, and other important data that helps externalize the full experience of awareness and acceptance facilitates articulation and authorship and helps clear the path for new behavioral applications (McLendon, 1997).

Satir's Self-Esteem Tool Kit

Satir system practitioners frequently use Satir's self-esteem tool kit (Satir et al., 1991) to work with self-esteem. These tools represent the elements of a self-esteem "maintenance kit" that merely requires awareness and use. The kit contains a detective hat, *yes/no* medallion, courage stick, wishing wand, golden key, and wisdom box. Although I never saw Satir have icons for the tools available for clients to see and hold during therapy sessions, she did have people imagine the objects and had group or family members role-play parts of someone's tool kit. Satir therapists now often create and personalize their tool kits for use in their professional and personal lives.

Although the heart was not an element of Satir's kit, I have made that addition. It is used to represent human emotion and compassion that deepen one's ability to make human contact. Without heart, there can be no congruence. I imagine it was an oversight and that Satir did not think her students needed to be reminded of the heart's value. The heart, representing emotion, is both an invitation and permission for a client to dip into his or her feeling states. McLendon demonstrates and discusses this action method using the heart icon in the *Family Therapy With the Experts* video series (Carlson & Kjos, 1998). Some individuals need better access to and use of their detective hat, the tool for analysis and logic. The golden key, symbolic of new possibilities, opens awareness to alternative options without the perceived invitation of emotionality that can be easily elicited with the wishing wand and the heart. The courage stick may encourage action even though there is the awareness of fear. In addition to promoting awareness, the therapist can use the tools to work with the mind and body to encourage movement.

The self-esteem tools can embody a sense of internal support for the client. Once contact has been made between a therapist and a client, the self-esteem tool kit can be used with any client who can comprehend simple concepts. To be effective, the client must be willing to participate in a learning context, have some desire for positive change, and have trust in the therapist's intentions and competence. With these requirements met, there are no problem areas that would not be fertile ground for developing a fuller use of the tools for building self-esteem. Clients with unusually low self-esteem will need patience as they practice ways of creating the safety needed to open themselves to something new, be it an idea, a feeling, or an action. In a time-limited educational class, the self-esteem tool kit can be introduced quite early. In a therapeutic setting, the tool kit can be introduced when the therapist feels enough rapport has been established with the client.

No doubt there are many Satir therapists who do not explicitly use the self-esteem tool kit; they do, however, know that multisensory learning promotes openings. They may not all use sculpting, do elaborate family-of-origin mapping, or use stand-ins for an inner child, but they know that the quality of the therapy outcome will be directly affected by the therapist's ability to relate to and to engage the client. Sensitive to two popular polar stereotypes, many Satir system therapists disclaim being labeled as "gimmicky" or "new age mystics."

CASE EXAMPLE 1: THE CHALLENGE OF DIVORCE

A couple entering a separation and divorce requested therapeutic assistance for their three daughters, aged 12, 10, and 7. They wanted to minimize the harm that could come to their children from the anger between them and the major changes the family was facing. Although this case focuses on the use of the self-esteem tool kit, it also presents uses of metaphor, sculpting, family mapping, and psychodramatic enactment.

Case Narrative

I began the first session with the parents while the girls waited outside in the waiting room. A request from me to hear how things were going quickly led to two intensely discrepant stories about who had done what to whom, over what period of time, at what cost, and with what likely legal recourse. I reminded the parents that they were not there for marital therapy, but for their girls. I asked if they believed they could focus on cooperating as parents even though their marriage was ending. They both quickly said, "yes."

I then invited the children in from the waiting room to join the therapy session. I gathered everyone around a flip chart pad and began by standing by the easel. I drew a circle to represent each of the family members. I then asked for the full name and age of each family member and wrote them on the pad. The parents' circles were drawn next to each other with a connecting line that symbolized their marriage. I drew the girls' circles vertically underneath the marital line.

Once everyone was on the chart, I drew a dramatic, dark red, zigzag line through the marital line and said, "I understand that we are here today to help you girls deal with what this means." There was silence. It seemed as if everyone stopped breathing.

I pointed to the red zigzag line, looked at the girls, and asked, "How are you doing with this?" The eldest daughter, E, jumped up, went to the other side of the room, and picked up a large golden key hanging visibly

Commentary

Because the parents moved so quickly into antagonistic positions with each other, I had to take charge early on and redirect the interaction. I believed little could come from further conversation with them absent their children. I could not be a safe therapist for the children if the parents used me for one side or the other.

Bringing in the children created a different context. The purpose was clearly not to deal with mending the marriage. The family, and particularly the children, became foreground. Moving immediately to the family map gave the family something to do and put the therapist in charge.

By explicitly drawing the "fight line" between the husband and wife circles, I sent the message that I would not avoid the core issue: the marital fight. Everyone was now reading from the same sheet: a family map with lots of pain.

from a coatrack. She walked back to the group, pointed the key into her chest, and said, "I feel like my heart has been opened up and ripped out." The other two girls nodded in agreement. The father got up, took a handkerchief out of his pocket, and walked into a smaller adjacent room to compose himself.

The father's need to leave the room to compose himself was a clue to move on. Had these parents not been embroiled in a fight, I would have dealt with what was happening with the father and how the others were dealing with his exit and his show of feelings. This couple could not have dealt successfully with each other in this manner, so I again redirected the session by structuring another working context.

When the father returned, I invited the girls to join me off to the other side of my large therapy room. I said, "I think you girls and I need to talk. Will you join me on the floor?" They followed me as I moved away from the easel. I walked over to the corner of the room, where I chose from a pile of stuffed dolls, animals, and other assorted therapy props a long pink rope and four small, soft, red, cushioned hearts.

I intended to use the pink rope to lay out a circle on the floor to indicate a boundaried space.[1] I wanted to create a place of protective distance from the marital tensions and a place where the focus could be healing. The hearts would speak the message that both their parents and I cared about how and what they were feeling.

They seemed relieved to have a place to go away from the tensions between their parents, and all seemed interested and curious as I gathered up the rope and hearts. I laid the rope in a circle on the floor and sat down on the floor, picking up and holding the rope in front of me. The girls smiled and followed suit. I handed each a heart and kept one for myself. The eldest, E, asked, "What are we doing?" I chose that time to make a

---

[1]See also chapter 4 regarding other uses of boundary sculpture.

stronger connection with them. Dropping the rope in my lap, I extended my open hands to the two younger girls, M and S, sitting on either side of me. They responded to my gesture and extended their hands to their older sister. I said, looking into each of their eyes, "I think your parents want you to have a safe place to talk about how you are doing and what you are feeling as you go through this big change in your life. What do you think about this idea?"

The rope, the circle with hands now held, and the red hearts in our laps were symbolic of what we would do in therapy in the weeks to come. It was done in the presence of the parents to ensure that all knew the plan and that the parents sanctioned our relationship and our agenda.

I wanted them to know that I saw their parents as capable people and as the people who would ultimately take action on their behalf. Parental permission to have this special space for the therapist and the children needed to be real. The picture of the rope, the hearts, and our holding hands let the parents and the children know what to expect and what was intended.

Each girl in turn talked about being scared and how sad it was going to be the following week when their parents did not live together. I explained that the pink rope meant that we had created a special group. What was said would stay within the boundary of our group, with two exceptions: They could talk with their parents, or if I feared harm would come to them, then I would talk with their parents.

At the second session, the girls entered the office with a lot of energy and went looking for the rope and hearts. With their help, I selected a rag doll for each that could represent their "little girls." I explained that we all have an inner child that needs our attention and love. They seemed to accept the idea and explanation. Without any words of instruction or

The second session was important. Would the girls feel comfortable to enter without their parents? That they could return to the pink rope, the hearts, the circle, and now the rag dolls gave them a sense of returning to something known and safe. I chose a rag doll for myself for modeling. The rag dolls are a useful way to provide a distanced perspective about request, we sat in the same kind of circle as the week before. Each of us had a doll to hold and a heart for each doll. I inquired about how they were feeling and what they were doing to help their "little girls" inside to deal with the difficulties of their situation.

By the third session, they were ready to explore beyond the pink rope and to add discussion about things in their school and friendship lives. I wondered if they would like to learn more about the self-esteem maintenance kit. They were interested. I shared my idea that it would be good to invite their parents for that session. They smiled, indicating approval.

The parents returned for the next session. I asked each of the girls one at a time to walk across the therapy room showing what she felt like when she was having a hard time and then what it was like for her when she was feeling good.

The eldest girl, E, stomped across the room, slammed herself into a chair, crossed her legs and arms, said, "I hate you" in the direction of her parents, and then turned her back to them. When asked to show what life is like for her when she is feeling good on the inside, E pranced across the room with a big grin on her face. The youngest girl, S, showed her negative state by sitting on the floor with her head in an exaggerated low position, her face hidden. She expressed her "feeling good" state by twirling with open arms and giggling. The middle girl, M, went to the easel, moved it away from the others' view, and drew miniature pictures that could not be seen by anyone

what one may be feeling and needing. The dolls provide a right-brain message that all of us, including the therapist, have an inner world that is important to who we are, how we feel, and how we behave.

I wanted another opportunity to observe the parents' skill at connecting with their daughters, and I wanted their support in reinforcing the use of the tools at home. My goal was to improve the girls' ability to accept their feelings and to recognize that they had choices about how they dealt with them. I felt we had spent time in the awareness, acceptance, and articulation phases and were now ready to work at the authorship level (McLendon, 1997).

I wanted to acknowledge that each of the girls deals with times when things are hard and times when things are good. The tools could be used as a method for enhancing esteem when dealing with the low times.

The sculpts and dramatizations disclosed the unique coping patterns each child was using when things were going badly. Few words were needed for clarification.

else. Her sculpt and portrayal of feel
ing good had M turning the easel to
the group and drawing a big, colorful
circle symbol.

I said I wanted to give the family
some tools to help them deal with
their feelings. I explained that the
tools were to help them take good
care of themselves and perhaps reduce the havoc their feelings might
have on their relationships and their
schoolwork. The family gathered
around the easel as I presented each
of the self-esteem tools, discussing
them and answering questions. As
part of introducing the self-esteem
tool kit tools, I asked the parents to
validate, through example, ways in
which the children owned and had
used the various tools. For example,
M had previously needed a medical
procedure, and the parents commented on her display of courage in
allowing the doctors and nurses to do
what they needed to do. Once all
the tools were presented and passed
around for each family member to
hold, I asked if anyone wanted to use
any part of the self-esteem tool kit to
help them deal with something that
might be bothering them.

E, the eldest, wasted no time. She
gathered up her rag doll, a heart, and
a courage stick from the self-esteem
tool kit. She looked over to me for
support and encouragement. I smiled
warmly and asked her what she
wanted help with. She began to talk
about how she worries about her parents. "They seem unhappy all the
time," she said. I asked if she believed that as the eldest she was responsible for helping her parents not
feel pain. She acknowledged that was
true. I gently touched E's rag doll
and explained that there was no way
her parents could avoid feeling pain

The family did well in the academics
of understanding the self-esteem tool
kit. However, they needed to practice using the tools.

I wanted the parents to hear this
message, no matter what E might
add. I realized that E was choosing a
difficult arena in which to practice:
her parents' pain. We would work at
whatever depth we could.

and that she was asking too much of her "little girl." I asked if she would be willing to let her parents deal with their own burdens so she could focus on helping the "little girl" inside her. She agreed. I added, "It is not the responsibility of the children to relieve their parents' pain."

I asked E to find symbols of her parents' burdens so that she could return them to her parents. She wasted no time in selecting a shawl and a blanket that lay on the sofa. I said I knew this was a hard thing to deal with and that maybe she would feel more of her personal power if she stood on one of the small footstools in the office. She liked the idea. I indicated that we were all very interested in hearing from her. Holding the heart, the courage stick, and her doll, she gave the shawl to her mother and the blanket to her father, saying, "You have to take care of these." The parents needed little coaching to respond positively and protectively to their daughter, assuring her that they could handle their own burdens and pain.

The session ended with my giving them a graphic handout of the self-esteem tools for the refrigerators at their parents' homes. I offered as homework that whenever anyone in the family was feeling low they would practice putting on their detective hat so they could figure out what tool might be needed.

This enactment allowed important dynamics to be brought to the surface and responded to. However, E did not appear to be fully congruent. She spoke the correct "healthy" words, but she was not fully present. She has a performer, bravado part that she uses to help her hide from her vulnerability and her fears. She had tucked her emotions away, unlike in the session the week before when she held her "little girl" and talked about loneliness, letting her tears come. Even so, she was able to say words that were important for her parents to hear. An important theme was now out in the open, and the younger girls were able to see their sister take a risk and not be judged.

I believed that groundwork had been laid but that much practice was needed.

CASE EXAMPLE 2: THE ATTORNEY AND THE HEART

A more complex application of the self-esteem tool kit in group therapy involved Bob, an attorney, as the star (i.e., the individual who is the focus of the therapeutic attention in a family or group). The complexity of this method is related to the number of people and systems reflected in the work. First, there are role-players who bring their unique emergent perspectives. Second, there are three different systems that are introduced: (a) the star's work system, (b) the star's family of origin, and (c) the star's current family, which in this example consists of the star's wife and children. (The therapeutic context included other group members working to improve balance in their personal and professional lives. Bob's wife was a member of the group and was brought into Bob's work.)

This kind of therapeutic intervention can be used in a broad variety of problem domains, but it is contraindicated for people who are already flooded with emotion. In choosing the timing for introducing such a dramatic intervention, the therapist must consider the star and the group members who will be role-players. A tremendous investment is required from both for success. An assessment must be made of the group's readiness to support the member selected as the star as it takes much empathy and emotional energy. Role-players must be open to giving that gift. Both the family of origin and the workplace are fertile ground for the tender human feelings of shame, humiliation, isolation, failure, and longing. The family of origin and the workplace also contain the seeds of support for healing.

Clients who are not ready to share themselves in a group context cannot benefit from this type of work. The exposure is too great and elicits their defenses. When their vulnerabilities are hidden behind their protective defenses, they cannot act positively from their right brain or their emotional and spiritual parts. They can go through the motions, accepting instruction and coaching, but it will be an exercise rather than an experience. If the embedded emotions in the system are to be brought to the surface, the star must stay present and must not disassociate. This was very difficult for Bob, the star in this example, who had an overused detective hat and an underused heart. Integration and sustainability of the changes that emerge within the psychodrama require that the star have support beyond the group experience. The star will have material to digest for months to come.

Considerable use is made of sculpting in this case. For the most part, it was used diagnostically to help recreate visually and experientially the wounding dynamics of the star's childhood, which continue to be repeated in his current work life. Before beginning my work with Bob I discussed quickly and superficially themes such as dominance and submission, extroversion and introversion, warm and cold, rigid and flexible, happy and sad, and angry and relaxed as a way to help stimulate ideas about characteristics that can be depicted in postures. Discussing polarities helps generate ideas and feelings for stars and role-players. Satir's incongruent coping stances: placating, blaming, superreasonable, and irrelevant, also can be taught quickly and can provide a starting place for sculpting (Satir, 1976).

Case Narrative	*Commentary*
Before beginning the sculpting, I asked Bob, the star, what he wanted to have happen for himself. He	

spoke of being overextended, feeling tired much of the time, and being irritable at home and work and said he felt he had been unable to create change in his situation. I surmised that this kind of living had not brought him very close to his loved ones. He glanced toward his wife, who was seated near where he and I were standing. His eyes showed the truth in this statement, but his voice was flat and stern when he acknowledged agreement.

I asked Bob to select from the group members a stand-in for himself so that he could view the sculpt from the outside. I suggested that this person be someone Bob felt could understand and support him. I also at this time began to refer to the stand-in as "little Bob." I explained this as the part of an individual that is still resonant with the true experiences of his or her childhood.

I asked Bob to select group members to play members of his family of origin and key members of his law firm. I requested that he put each role-player in a pose and place them in a picture, making them a part of either the family or work system. When he was puzzled about what posture to suggest, the role-players and observing group members readily offered ideas. Bob seemed comfortable accepting, as well as rejecting, the various ideas.

I instructed the two sculpts to move adjacent to each other so that "little Bob," the stand-in, could step into the sculpt, simultaneously existing in both systems. There were visible simi-

I felt I had enough data to begin his work. My impression was that he was well defended and he very much wanted to see and have a new way to live his life.

The quality of the relationship between the star and the stand-in helps create safety, making for more openness to connections for the star. There is useful data for the star from both inside and outside the sculpt. Taking in the picture from the outside offers the guide the opportunity to dialogue with the star about what he or she is noticing, what meanings he or she is making, what feelings he or she is having, and what he or she is doing internally with those feelings (Satir et al., 1991). Moving into the sculpt allows the star to experience the old dynamics directly but with support and new resources.

The sculpts should always reflect the star's ideas and feelings at the beginning.

Once there are interactions among the players, they can be given permission by the guide to change their positions to flow with the action.

I thought connecting the two system sculpts would help make the intra- and interpersonal dynamics clearer for Bob.

larities in the two systems. Both had dominant patriarchal father figures, and Bob was down on all fours, looking up, strained and twisted at his torso. The hands and arms of members of both sculpts were either stretched out requesting something of Bob or extended forward judging and blaming him.

I asked Bob if he would give "little Bob" permission to have and share his feelings. He said "yes," and I asked the role-players in the sculpt on the count of 3 to let out whatever sounds would reflect their inner experience. The human sounds that came conveyed great frustration and despair.

I coached Bob to move closer to "little Bob" and to share what was happening with him. Bob talked in parental fashion about "little Bob's" need for protection against encroachment and the ever-growing expectations on him from all directions. But Bob was not able to speak from his heart to his role-playing "little Bob."

I suggested that Bob move into the sculpt in the exact posture held by "little Bob." I requested that "little Bob" stay near Bob. From inside the sculpt, I invited Bob to speak about his experience, both in terms of his family and work. Although he believed the sculpt reflected accurately his experience, Bob could not talk with feeling or from his heart.

I requested the heart from the self-esteem tool kit. At this point, I was seated on the floor very close to Bob. I placed the heart firmly against Bob's chest and held it in place. At first,

Given that I was working with a well-schooled, superreasonable star, I needed to maximize the input of the role-players' experience without allowing them to become too verbal.

This often is the point at which the star can drop into a compassionate place for his inner child or the child he was, but Bob remained in his head.

Dealing with this kind of robust defensiveness and resistance was exacting all my deepest compassion and skill. Although the work to this point had value, it would not produce the level of mind–body–spirit transformation needed to open Bob to his deepest longings and resources. It was obvious that he was not in a place of self-esteem. The feeling state of being trapped and impotent that was portrayed in the sculpt was surfacing in his work with me. I knew Bob was not accessing his self-esteem tools.

I wish now I had also chosen the courage stick. Time was ticking away, not only in Bob's life, but also in this group session. The role-players were looking fatigued and discour-

Bob leaned back. I moved closer, looked him squarely in the eyes, and said, "Bob, be aware of your beating heart and the very tender part of the 'little Bob' who lives inside of you. He needs you to care about him." The role-players were relaxed but still in their positions. Bob looked up and around at his family and workplace and then looked down, shaking his head as if to say "I can't." I asked Bob's wife to come join us. She came. I had her sit in front of Bob. He continued to shake his head despondently.

I continued to hold the heart to Bob's chest, but this time, his hand also helped hold the heart in place. I moved squarely in front of him and asked him to select role-players to represent his three sons. His pupils dilated, color came to his face, and his mouth dropped. His body spoke that a shift was happening. The first son to speak said, "Dad, don't let the partners chew you up. We love you, and we don't want you so unhappy." Bob melted and wept. He held his sons while they too cried. I asked Bob to share with his sons his struggles and his hopes.

Once he had spoken with each of his sons, I asked him to speak to his parents and his senior partner. This went well. Bob's role-playing sons were like a cheering section for Bob for each congruent statement he made about himself and his plans for the future.

Role-players were deroled and asked to share what the experience meant to them in their own lives. The star was at this time sitting next to his wife, holding hands, and looking tired, warm, and cuddly. He thanked the group for their "hanging in" with him, and the session was closed.

aged, much as Bob looked. Inviting dialogue with a nurturing grandparent or sometimes a parent helps loosen the rigid constraints to feeling.

In this case, I decided to bring forward to Bob the feelings of his three sons.

Once there is an affective shift, dialogue with role-players can have significant benefit. When the star can speak from a congruent place, deeper connections are possible. These connections can have real significance for the role-players.

Bob, like many adults, was not able on that day to fully commit to his growth and healing until he connected his problems with his children's pain and the disconnection of his heart to theirs.

Failing to have the role-players articulate their awarenesses as they relate to their own lives tends to leave the star in the position of patient. Satir work is about the universals of being human, not about pathology.

Satir developed the model of the change process shown in Figure 2-1. One begins the process of change when something happens to disrupt the status quo. Satir called this "something" a *foreign element*. The foreign element disturbs the calm of the status quo and initiates the stage called *chaos*. In the first example with the three girls, the marital crisis was the foreign element. For Bob, the attorney in the second example, his sons' pain acted as a foreign element, allowing him to begin the change process and enter his chaos—or meltdown. During the chaos, clients experience simultaneous highs and lows, their behavior becomes erratic, and their performance unpredictable. At times, they do better than in the old status quo, but there also are times when things become perhaps much worse.

There are two paths of escape from the throes of chaos. One may simply return to the old status quo. With that choice, the change process is aborted, and individuals move back to business as usual. The second path occurs when clients break through the chaos and move into the change process with a transforming idea. The impetus for this path may be a fight for survival or hope for a better future. The meanings that the

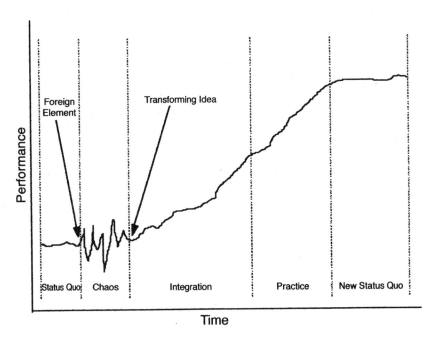

Figure 2-1. The Satir change process.

girls made of the pink rope, hearts, rag dolls, and self-esteem tools offer potential transformative ideas. The support and encouragement offered Bob by his sons was transformational. They enabled Bob to move to the integration and practice phase, where he practiced authoring new messages to his role-played family and law firm members.

The transforming idea leads into the phases of change called *integration* and *practice*. In this phase, clients may take ownership for the change and its associated new behaviors and begin the task of making those new behaviors a part of themselves. With ownership and practice, the new behaviors become a part of their lives, and the change process completes as clients arrive at a new status quo. This change model is cyclic. The new status quo replaces the former status quo, and individuals are again poised for the constancy of change.

Homework and Successive Uses

When a client is able to put an awareness into action successfully, he or she is accessing a transforming idea. Therapy helps the client discover these openings and facilitates the integration of the new with the old. Practice, which is successive application of the tools to real-life situations, is done for the most part outside therapy. Homework can be a useful way of conveying the therapist's commitment to helping to create real change in the client's life. The handouts of the self-esteem tool kit to the girls and their assignment said, "I care about you even when I am not with you." Assignments can be transitional objects that connect the client to the therapist between sessions.

Because the therapist is available to act as a safety net, in-session practice can be designed with more complexity and should be made challenging enough to stretch clients toward expanded possibilities and awarenesses about their core dynamics. Out-of-session homework should be designed for success. Incremental shifts in degree of challenge for both in-session work and out-of-session work should pace the client's readiness for chaos and motivation for practice and integration.

Resistance

With any action method, there is vulnerability. Once we move to action, we expose more of ourselves. It is easier to hide awkwardness, not knowing, and so on, when we are still. It is a problem of safety (Satir et al., 1991). Satir likened the issue of safety and resistance to the experience of crawling out from under a warm blanket into a cold room. Rather than incur resistance by removing the blanket, one might consider warming up the room.

Using the self-esteem tool kit as a teaching tool or as an aid in a psychodramatic action for therapy clients is contraindicated with clients who are overwhelmed with emotion or too fearful to expose themselves to risk taking. Reverent stillness with a client's feelings is deeply healing and a necessary step for change. When a client's past experiences leave him or her sensitive to criticism, failure, shame, or humiliation, he or she needs time to create safety before he or she is ready to risk stepping into a therapeutic action mode. However, a therapist might ask, "What would you need to take the next step?" With clients who show high resistance, even that question might be interpreted as blaming, pushing, criticizing, or trivializing. These clients need to be shown a lot of acceptance and allowed to take their time. If the therapist is leading from too far ahead, even gentle coaxing from a caring coach can evoke feelings of inadequacy. Satir talked metaphorically about leading from a half step behind, positioned close in so she could see where the client was headed, feel what the client might be feeling, and support the client's vulnerable back side.

A specific Satir method for dealing with resistance is reframing. As the look of a painting can change dramatically when placed in a different frame, so a client's view of a situation or issue can change when viewed from another angle. Such a change in view can open options and recall forgotten resources. Reframes that are embedded in the client's truth are empowering and can be good methods for overcoming resistance.

Externalizing an internal stressor is also helpful in creating emotional distance from one's demons. The externalization can use any object that can symbolize for the client the fearful issue, feeling, or relationship. The family map can serve this purpose. Various things can be indicated on the map that are too difficult to confront directly. For example, one client began for the first time to grieve for her grandfather's death when I crossed him out on the family map. For nearly a year, she would sit down, look at her family map, enter a trance, cry, and begin her work. Her map became my cotherapist. I came to know her family well through the mapping. Whenever she needed more support or more challenge, I could call on some member of her family. She had no difficulty bringing them to the session in her mind. I, however, no longer use an "X" on the map to indicate death; instead, I draw horizontal lines in the circle.

Even family mapping, perhaps one of the more cognitive methods of the Satir system, can trigger resistance. I have had more than one client who refused to have her family map visible to her during therapy sessions. Rather than giving her a safe distance from which to confront her many losses, one woman felt trapped, as if looking at the map placed her back in the painful past. It had not been safe to grieve her many losses as a young person when they occurred, and now, in middle age, she feared that were she to start the grief process she would never recover. She remained in therapy for about 2 years and never gave permission for the map to be present. In this case, I now believe the family mapping was begun before there was sufficient safety established for her.

Satir knew resistance was purposeful in its origin. When she felt it was present, she wanted to explore its meaning. She wanted her clients to have the freedom to make choices about their responses. Satir did not get into power struggles about what somebody should or should not do or about what step a person should or should not take. For Satir, resistance was just about the moment in time; it was not about forever. She stated, "Resistance is a survival resource for most members of an unhealthy system. It is an important basic belief of the Satir model that people do the best they can with what they know and what they perceive. Understanding this allows us to accept people's positions as a starting place and then help them move from there" (Satir et al., 1991, p. 101).

EMPIRICAL EVIDENCE OF EFFICACY

The most significant research to date evidencing the efficacy of the Satir human validation process action model was done by Joan Elizabeth Winter (1993) for her doctoral dissertation. Winter's research compared the results of the family therapy approaches of Murray Bowen, Jay Haley, and Virginia Satir. Each of these master therapists and teachers selected therapists to represent their particular approach. Each team of therapists was provided initially between 57 and 68 court-referred families of a delinquent youth. Definitive in this study are several key elements to successful therapy: the ability of the therapist to initially engage clients in therapy (or to make contact, as a Satir therapist would say), to work toward mutual completion of the therapy (or to prevent dropouts), and to have clients feel satisfied with both the person of the therapist and the treatment outcomes. The Satir system excelled in each of these areas. The Satir dropout rate was 5.1%; the Bowen rate was 36.5%; and the Haley rate was 60.9%. The Satir team experienced more success than the other two groups at engaging their referrals (93.7%); the Bowen group engaged 63.5%; and the Haley group, 67.6%. Similarly, the Satir group completed treatment with 88.8% of the originally referred sample; the Bowen group followed with 57.9%, and the Haley group trailed with 26.5%. On the Satisfaction With Outcome subscale, family members in the Bowen and Haley groups were significantly less satisfied with treatment than those in the Satir group. Satisfaction with therapist across family members was ranked in the following order: Satir, Haley, Bowen. The Satir model adolescent clients were significantly more satisfied with their therapists than were the adolescents in the Bowen and Haley groups (Winter, 1993).

BECOMING A SATIR SYSTEM PRACTITIONER

It is now obvious that one does not have to have had direct training with the master to have mastery of her system. Satir's legacy, now a decade old, continues to take shape in various ways. In 1977 Satir selected about 35 people she had trained extensively to help her create AVANTA, the primary clearinghouse for Satir materials, which is located in Burien, Washington. Many of these practitioners travel throughout the world, as she did, teaching the Satir system. Although there currently is no formal certification program, these practitioners and their students teach the system in academic, private, and public arenas. They have been instrumental in getting more of the system into print and in expanding its acceptability for use beyond traditional therapy into large, system-change projects.

It is not known at this time what percentage of practitioners identify themselves as Satir system therapists, and it is difficult to comment on how they differ in their use of action methods. There has been no large-scale research identifying the influence of the various schools of therapy on practitioners since the work of Quinn and Davidson in 1984. The national office of the American Association of Marriage and Family Therapy provided a list of all clinical, associate, and student members (N = 1008) residing in the state of Texas, the second largest chapter at that time, to the research team. A single mailing of surveys resulted in a 42% response rate. At that time, the orientations used most frequently were, in order, communication (Satir), strategic (Haley), experiential (Whitaker), and structural (Minuchin).

AVANTA, The Virginia Satir Network, along with its regional affiliate institutes and the International Human Learning Resources Network are the formal organizations that continue to develop and teach the Satir model. To date, they have no nationally recognized certification program for Satir system practitioners. AVANTA and The Satir Institute of the Southeast cosponsor programs and workshops designed to model and teach how the Satir system is used for developing individuals, couples, families, clinicians, leaders, and organizations. These programs are built on years of experience the director of training had with the Crested Butte, Colorado, training programs, the most in-depth training offered by Satir and her AVANTA colleagues until her death in 1988. Information about these and other programs is available from AVANTA, The Virginia Satir Network, and The Satir Institute of the Southeast, Inc. (see Additional Resources section).

AVANTA and the Library and Oral History Program of the University of California established a Satir Archives at the University's Santa Barbara campus. The archival collection includes audiotapes, videotapes, articles, and notes. A finder's guide can be purchased from AVANTA. AVANTA and The Satir Institute of the Southeast established two smaller resource centers, one in Columbia, South Carolina, and the other in Chapel Hill, North Carolina. AVANTA currently is involved in developing specific Satir curricula for diversity work with communities and corporations.

PERSONAL DEVELOPMENT OF THE THERAPIST

Satir believed that the humanness of the therapist was more important than any specific content expertise the therapist might acquire, and she knew that developing one's humanness was challenging work (Satir & Baldwin, 1983). Obviously, a major personal development component is required for becoming an effective Satir system practitioner. Satir wrote, "Therapy is an intimate experience. For people to grow and change they need to be able to allow themselves to become open, which makes them vulnerable. . . . Very little change goes on without the patient and therapist becoming vulnerable" (Baldwin & Satir, 1987, p. 21).

Without the stability and nurturance of grounded support in their personal and professional lives, therapists put themselves and their clients at risk when they work in the Satir system. Therapists must know the internal and external issues related to creating safety, both for themselves and for their clients. Otherwise, they emit messages through their voice, tone, and gestures that are contradictory to the messages they intend. Satir wrote, "The only times that I have experienced difficulty with people are when I was incongruent. I either tried to be something I wasn't, or to withhold something I knew, or to say something I didn't mean" (Baldwin & Satir, 1987, p. 22). Incongruence reduces safety and increases resistance. Clients often are very sensitive to the therapist's emotional and ego needs. Therapists need a high degree of emotional maturity, self-awareness, and self-acceptance to be emotionally honest and competently responsive to their clients. Given the dynamic nature of therapy and the ever-increasing litigious and management care challenges to therapists, Satir's words take on special significance: "We started out knowing that the person of the therapist could be harmful to the patient. We concentrated on ways to avoid that. Now, we need to concentrate on ways in which the use of self can be of positive value in treatment" (Baldwin & Satir, 1987, p. 25).

CONCLUSION

Satir was a practitioner and a teacher of practitioners, not an academician. This has been true, in large part, of her students. Her methods were widely promulgated during her lifetime because so many practitioners were able to experience her work demonstrated directly in her large workshop settings. They could literally see and feel the transformative power of the way she worked. However, if her system of therapy is to last much beyond the current generation of Satir practitioners, there needs to be published research. To begin with, a regional or national survey to find out how many people identify themselves primarily as Satir-influenced therapists would be helpful. From there, therapists' and clients' experiences with the model could be studied. Research on using Satir methods for effecting large-scale community and organizational change is also needed.

REFERENCES

Baldwin, M., & Satir, V. (1987). The use of self in therapy. *Journal of Psychotherapy*, 3(1), 17–25.

Banmen, J., & Gerber, J. (Eds.). (1985). *Virginia Satir: Meditations and inspirations*. Berkeley, CA: Celestial Arts.

Carlson, J., & Kjos, D. (1998). *Family therapy with the experts: Satir therapy with Jean McLendon* [Videotape]. Needham Heights, MA: Ally & Bacon.

Goldenberg, H., & Goldenberg, I. (1991). *Family therapy: An overview* (3rd ed.). Pacific Grove, CA: Brooks/Cole.

McLendon, J. (1997). The Tao of communication and the constancy of change. *Journal of Couples Therapy*, 6(3/4), 35–49.

Quinn, W. H., & Davidson, B. (1984). Prevalence of family therapy models: A research note. *Journal of Marital and Family Therapy*, 10(4), 393–398.

Satir, V. (1964). *Conjoint family therapy*. Palo Alto, CA: Science and Behavior Books.

Satir, V. (1972). *Peoplemaking*. Palo Alto, CA: Science and Behavior Books.

Satir, V. (1976). *Making contact*. Berkeley, CA: Celestial Arts.

Satir, V. (1988). *The new peoplemaking*. Mountain View, CA: Science and Behavior Books.

Satir, V. (n.d.). *The third birth* [Bound notes]. Burien, WA: AVANTA.

Satir, V., & Baldwin, M. (1983). *Satir step by step: A guide to creating change in families*. Palo Alto, CA: Science and Behavior Books.

Satir, V., Banmen, J., Gerber, J., & Gomori, M. (1991). *The Satir model: Family therapy and beyond*. Palo Alto, CA: Science and Behavior Books.

Satir, V., Bitter, J. R., & Krestensen, K. K. (1988). Family reconstruction: The family-within-a group experience. *Journal of Specialists in Group Work*, 13(4), 200–208.

Simon, R. (1989). The legacy of Virginia Satir [Special feature]. *The Family Therapy Networker*, 13(1), 26–56.

Suarez, M. M. (1998). *Virginia Satir*. Burien, WA: AVANTA, The Virginia Satir Network.

Winter, J. E. (1993). *Selected family therapy outcomes with Bowen, Haley, and Satir*. Unpublished doctoral dissertation, College of William and Mary, Williamsburg, VA.

ADDITIONAL RESOURCES

Books

Banmen, A., & Banmen, J. (1991). *Meditations of Virginia Satir*. Palo Alto, CA: Science and Behavior Books. Great resource to learn the underlying assumptions and beliefs of the Satir system.

Englander-Golden, P., & Satir, V. (1990). *Say it straight: From compulsions to choices*. Palo Alto, CA: Science and Behavior Books. Useful text for applying the Satir system to the field of addictions.

Loeschen, S. (1998). *Systematic training in the skills of Virginia Satir*. Pacific Grove, CA: Brooks/Cole. Simple and relevant exercises for students wanting to develop the basic skills of the Satir model.

Nerin, W. F. (1986). *Family reconstruction: Long day's journey into light*. New York: Norton. Narrative explanation and introduction to Satir's most complex action method, the family reconstruction.

Satir, V. (1978). *Your many faces*. Millbrae, CA: Celestial Arts. Introduction to the basic beliefs underlying the development of Satir's powerful psychodrama vehicle, the parts party.

Satir, V. (1988). *The new peoplemaking*. Mountain View, CA: Science and Behavior Books. Updates *Peoplemaking* and adds new chapters on spirituality, the later years, and the family in the larger system.

Satir, V., & Baldwin, M. (1983). *Satir step by step: A guide to creating change in families*. Palo Alto, CA: Science and Behavior Books. Provides reasons behind Satir's interventions and explicates Satir's worldview.

Satir, V., Stachowiak, J., & Taschman, H. (1975). *Helping families to change*. New York: Jason Aronson. Satir's early conceptions of congruence, including her beliefs about the use of self in therapy.

Schwab, J. (1990). *A resource handbook for Satir concepts*. Palo Alto, CA: Science and Behavior Books. Supplement to *The Satir Approach to Communication*.

Schwab, J., Baldwin, M., Gerber, J., Gomori, M., & Satir, V. (1989). *The Satir approach to communication: A workshop manual*. Palo Alto, CA: Science and Behavior Books. Useful guide for professionals wanting to teach the Satir system; provides exercises for learning basic concepts.

Weinberg, G. (1991). *Quality software management: Congruent action*. New York: Dorset House. An excellent explanation of congruent communication and illustration of the relevance of congruence to effectiveness for managers.

Journals

Brothers, B. J. (Ed.). *Journal of Couples Therapy*. New York: Haworth Press. Very readable journal that focuses on the process issues of therapeutic work with couples and frequently features the work of Virginia Satir.

Bula, J. (1991). Virginia Satir's triad theory for couples. *Journal of Couples Therapy, 2*(1/2), 43–57. Discussion of Satir's foundational ideas about systems, the dynamics of triads, and Satir's use of the concept of the "nurturing triad."

Carlson, J. (Ed.). *The Family Journal*. Thousand Oaks, CA: Sage. Official journal of the International Association for Marriage and Family Therapy. Readable journal with a mix of articles, interviews, reviews, and case consultations and a goal of the promotion of systemic thinking in academic and clinical practice settings.

Dodson, L. (1991). Virginia Satir's process of change. *Journal of Couples Therapy, 2*(1/2), 119–142. Presentation of how Satir viewed the process of change and placement of her ideas in the larger psychotherapeutic philosophies.

Simon, R. (Ed.). *Family Therapy Networker*. Washington, DC: Networker. Readable and enjoyable periodical that keeps pace with the realities of current clinical practice and focuses on societal issues affecting the therapy world.

Walsh, F. (Ed.). *Journal of Marital and Family Therapy*. Washington, DC: American Association for Marriage and Family Therapy. Solid source of information about marriage and family therapy, providing research studies and theoretical and applied articles.

Winter, J., & Parker, L. R. E. (1991). Enhancing the marital relationship: Virginia Satir's parts party. *Journal of Couples Therapy*, 2(1/2), 59–82. Discussion of the underlying principles and methodology for guiding parts parties for couples.

Professional Associations and Organizations

AVANTA, The Virginia Satir Network
Executive Director
2104 Southwest 152nd Street, Suite 2
Burien, WA 98166
(206) 241-7566
E-mail: avanta@foxinternet.net
Web site: www.avanta.net

AVANTA, The Virginia Satir Network, is an international educational organization whose mission is to support, connect, and empower people and organizations through the Satir growth model to respect differences, resolve conflicts, develop possibilities, and enable people to take responsibility for their lives, health, work, and relationships. Every few years, AVANTA holds conferences that are open to the public. It has a current membership of over 250 people from 18 different countries.

Institute for International Connections
5617 Oakmont Avenue
Bethesda, MD 20817-3529
(301) 530-1679
E-mail: mabsm@erols.com

Northwest Satir Institute
13787 Northeast 65th Street, Apartment 565
Redmond, WA 98052
(425) 869-2292
E-mail: jong@gte.net
    Offers membership and workshops.

Satir Institute of the Pacific Northwest
647 Moss Street
Victoria, BC, Canada, V8V 4N8
(250) 388-0447
E-mail: mtcallag@bcs02.gov.bc.ca

Satir Institute of the Southeast, Inc.
87 South Elliott Road, Suite 203
Chapel Hill, NC 27514
(919) 967-2520
E-mail: institute@satir.org
Web site: www.satir.org

Produces a subscription newsletter and, with AVANTA, sponsors Satir system training workshops throughout the year on a wide range of applications for the Satir approach.

Other

Archives: Library, Oral History Program
University of California
Santa Barbara, CA 93106
(805) 893-3062
Contact: David Russell .

Satir Resource Collections: University of South Carolina's College of Social Work
Columbia, SC 29208
Contact Person: Miriam Freeman, PhD
(803) 777-3290
E-mail: miriamfreeman@sc.edu

Chapel Hill Satir Resource Center
87 South Elliott Road, Suite 203
Chapel Hill, NC 27514
(919) 967-2520
E-mail: satirsystems@compuserve.com
Web site: www.satir.org

3

BEYOND WORDS: THE POWER OF RITUALS

JANINE ROBERTS

All rituals have symbols and symbolic actions. They are what give our rituals depth, meaning, and values. They express what words alone cannot. Simply seeing or remembering a symbol can evoke all of the memories and feelings attached to a childhood ritual. (Imber-Black & Roberts, 1998, p. 140)

As illustrated in the case study below, rituals in therapy move beyond words to tap the power of symbols (like Bobo the giraffe) and symbolic actions (passing the pain to Bobo) to help initiate change.

Melanie, age 7, had been experiencing severe stomach pains for 6 months. Numerous visits to the doctor, changes in diet, and a range of tests had found no physical problems. Her parents came with her and her older sister and younger brother to therapy. Melanie was missing a lot of school, and her parents were consequently missing a lot of work. She and her mother and father had gotten into a cycle of being connected through her stomach pains, which was not working well for any of them. In the second session, the therapist, Ben, asked Melanie to bring to their next meeting her least favorite stuffed animal. She brought in Bobo, her giraffe, because, "he's not that cuddly."

Ben coached Melanie and her parents on ways to pass the pain from Melanie's stomach onto the giraffe. He told Melanie, "Bobo can hold the pain easier than people can because stuffed animals don't have the

With deep appreciation to the many families and colleagues I have worked with over the years, especially Evan Imber-Black and Richard Whiting.

same kind of nerve endings as we do." They then set up times before and after school for close, connected contact between Melanie and her parents to practice letting go of the pain and sending it into Bobo. The stomach pains rapidly diminished. The parents continued the special times with Melanie, turning them into cuddling and story-reading times.

All clients have rituals, whether they are the daily ones of hello and goodbye, mealtimes, and bedtimes; family traditions such as birthdays, anniversaries, and vacations; holiday celebrations; or life-cycle rituals such as baby-naming ceremonies, weddings, and funerals. Because rituals are already known to clients, they are an easily accessible resource in therapy. Looking at rituals opens a window onto clients' beliefs, what is important to them, and ways in which they are connected or not in their community. The cultural and ethnic background of clients often is evoked and expressed in rituals, and working with them offers many opportunities for therapists to learn more about clients' unique histories.

RITUALS AS A RESOURCE IN THERAPY

Because rituals are so closely tied to life experiences and not to a rigid set of theoretical constructs, they can be used with any model of therapy. Rituals are available to a wide spectrum of ages of clients. Even a very young child picks up, for instance, the excitement of a birthday cake lit up with candles. Rituals can facilitate connection across generations because they can work on several different levels simultaneously. For example, an adoption day party can communicate to a young adopted child the welcoming of him or her by his or her parents and community while at the same time marking to older members of the family the transition of the family from one without children to one with a child and reflecting subsequent changes in other generations (e.g., the parents of the parents now become grandparents).

Rituals are both fun and elegant at the same time. They are evocative and can pique the interest of clients and therapists. Sandy and Lynne, a lesbian couple who had recently had their first child, Jamila, were frustrated looking at the baby books available in the stores to record memories, milestones, and make a family tree. As Lynne said, "All the books are built around a father and mother at the core of them. We'd have to cross out 'father.' It's right up in our faces that we're not a 'normal' family."

Their therapist suggested to them, "Why not make your own book?" "Why not?" Sandy said. They got a blank scrapbook and put in their own titles and headings. Friends enjoyed it so much that they encouraged Sandy and Lynne to write a description of it and put it in a gay and lesbian newsletter to encourage other families to make baby books reflective of their membership.

Working with rituals is about creating protected time and space to support clients in finding and expressing the meaning of key shifts and changes in their lives. Because rituals often call on known symbols and actions, they offer continuity that can create a sense of safety and facilitate movement into the unknown.

RITUALS IN THE FIELD OF THERAPY

Early work on rituals in therapy focused on therapeutic rituals designed by therapists. Rituals often were rigidly set up and came from a position of the therapist "knowing better" than the client what he or she should do. For instance, Selvini Palazzoli (1974) defined ritual in family therapy as "an action, or a series of actions, accompanied by a verbal formula and involving the entire family. Like every ritual, it must consist of a regular sequence of steps taken at the right time and in the right place" (p. 238). In this same book, Selvini Palazzoli and her colleagues in Milan gave a brief case example of work with a so-called aggressive boy. The ritual was prescribed to the family down to the exact words they were to say. (See Roberts [1988b] for a more complete description of this early work.)[1]

Van der Hart (1983) brought a more open approach to rituals and often made links to anthropology. He drew heavily on the work of Van Gennep (1960) and other anthropologists who looked at rites of passage. In his later work (van der Hart, 1988), he and his coauthors looked particularly at the role of ritual when there has been significant loss for individuals or families.

Wolin, a family therapist who has worked a great deal with alcoholism and resilience in families, and Bennett, an anthropologist, introduced a cognitive frame useful to therapists regarding a typology of ritual styles (Wolin & Bennett, 1984). I and my colleagues Evan Imber-Black and Richard Whiting expanded on this typology (Roberts, 1988b) and later reworked it from more of a resource perspective (Imber-Black & Roberts, 1998). Also, after several years of work with rituals and seeing the creative range of ideas and adaptations that families made to their daily and life-cycle rituals and other traditions, we focused much more on the rituals that family members already had available to them rather than designing new therapeutic rituals. We also moved into training therapists to look at

---

[1]Luigi Boscolo, one of the original Milan group members, and Paolo Bertrando describe some of their more recent work with these kinds of prescribed rituals in chapter 8 of their book, The Times of Time (Boscolo & Bertrando, 1993).

their own rituals as a way to help them understand the power of rituals (Roberts, 1988a).

Others have examined what happens physiologically to individuals when they are experiencing rituals. d'Aquili, Laughlin, and McManus (1979) drew on studies of ritualized animal behavior as well as the neurobiology of the brain to hypothesize that the active parts of rituals produce positive limbic discharges and that as different parts of the brain are stimulated, the two main hemispheres of the brain spill over into each other. This may be experienced as a "shiver down the back."

Kobak and Waters (1984) encouraged therapists to look at the process of therapy in and of itself as a ritual. They took the three stages proposed by Van Gennep (1960) as commonly found in rites of passage (separation, transition, and reintegration) and used them as a framework to examine the beginning, middle, and end-of-treatment phases of therapy. Bodin (1989) expanded on this work to look at minirituals as a resource in treatment to help therapists make transitions for themselves between therapy sessions.

Narrative therapists White and Epston (1990) also used the rite-of-passage analogy to look at crises in clients' lives as offering new possibilities to take on other roles and status. Combs and Freedman (1990), working from an Ericksonian perspective, presented a range of ways to creatively construct what they call *ceremonies*: from designing rituals with an ambiguous function to enacting the presenting situation in a ritual using metaphor.

FINDING RITUALS: FOUR ARENAS

Throughout the rest of this chapter, rituals in four different arenas will be referred to: (a) creating therapeutic rituals; (b) assessing families by examining the rituals they are already doing; (c) intervening by modifying these rituals when needed; and (d) looking at the ritual life of therapists. Fluidity in moving between these arenas provides synergy and creative input to work with rituals in therapy. For instance, having a good understanding of the way in which rituals have worked or not in their own lives can aid therapists in developing the kinds of questions they then ask of clients.

Asking about rituals in clients' lives is a good joining tool and a nonthreatening way to move into treatment. *Joining* is a common therapeutic term from Salvador Minuchin's structural model (first written about in the family therapy literature in 1974). Here, *joining tool* means a way for the therapist to connect with clients. In descriptions of rituals, key relationships and interactions are quickly highlighted. Rituals that already exist can be used as a foundation to modify and introduce change into clients' lives. There may also be situations (as in the case example at the beginning of the chapter) in which new rituals need to be brought into daily living. Finally, the therapist's ritual life, including ritual aspects of therapy (e.g., how people are greeted), is another resource. In the following section, 10 examples of ways to begin working with rituals in therapy are outlined. Examples are given from each of the four arenas identified above.

BEGINNING WORK WITH RITUALS

Work with rituals can be initiated in a number of small ways that will help the therapist learn how to bring rituals more into the therapy process as well as learn more about how they work for people and how they may have become interrupted, hollow, rigid, skewed, or obligatory. Another central means of exploring rituals is for the therapist to look at them in his or her own life.

It can be useful to think about rituals and participating or reflecting on them in three different ways. The first is actually doing the ritual. This brings into the therapeutic process all the stimulation of the ritual elements, such as symbols, foods and the smells associated with them, words, special clothing or locations, or symbolic actions, whatever they may be. These active parts of rituals can contribute to the significance of the event by providing many possibilities to make meaning of whatever changes are happening in clients' lives.

A second way of thinking about rituals and therapy is talking about them. This can provide clients with time and space to reflect on, name, and learn about intricate interactions. This can be a key part of working with rituals, both so that clients have a wide repertoire of rituals to draw on (not just those enacted in therapy) and because planning and processing rituals can be as important a part of the rituals as the event. Relationships can be reworked and events structured in such a way as to acknowledge dynamic shifts. In talking about rituals, clients can stay focused on what they can learn from them without the distraction of either doing the ritual or representing it in some way.

A third way of thinking about rituals and therapy brings together both action and protected space to think back over a ritual or imagine it in the future. Exercises, such as the ones described in the following section, can trigger memories and ideas about rituals in ways in which words alone cannot. This third format offers the benefit of time to examine aspects of rituals while simultaneously having the stimuli of other media to access different information as well as express a range of feelings.

Below are 10 examples of ways of bringing rituals into therapy:

1. Ask clients to describe their daily rituals, draw where people sit for meals, think about how they say hello and goodbye, and so on.
2. Bring in photos of life-cycle rituals, especially ones that reflect issues being worked on in therapy.
3. Bring in symbols of emotions, issues, and changes being worked on in therapy.
4. Pick up on key words or phrases used by clients that evoke symbolic actions (e.g., "We're at our wit's end" or "I'm all knotted up").
5. Ask about upcoming family holidays or traditions.
6. Use clay, paint, or other art materials to draw, paint, or represent visually various ritual times or make symbols to use in therapy.
7. Draw a floor plan of living space that a client grew up in or is currently living in to trigger memories about rituals.
8. Collect and share stories of other families' rituals.
9. Add questions about rituals to work with genograms.
10. Articulate ways the therapist can use rituals to aid in the process of doing therapy (e.g., meditating for a few minutes after a session to make a break between clients [Bodin, 1989]).

"I never thought of that as a ritual." One easy way for a therapist to introduce rituals into the conversation in therapy is for the therapist to ask clients about their daily rituals. For instance, the therapist can inquire about who sits where for meals and have the client draw it out, or if the therapist is working with a family, he or she can have them seat themselves that way. What roles are enacted by who shops for food, prepares it, serves it, cleans up? What is expressed about family beliefs with the rules that go along with mealtimes (e.g., eat everything on your plate or no elbows on the table)?[2]

People often do not realize the range of daily rituals that they have or their significance. Questions about them can help clients see their importance and introduce them as resources that can help articulate complex interactional patterns.

Pictures and Rituals

A good way for a therapist to learn about other kinds of rituals that do not happen as frequently, such as life-cycle rituals or family traditions, is to ask clients to bring in pictures of them. Depending on what is being

---

[2]For more extensive questions in this area, see Imber-Black and Roberts, 1998, pp. 163–165.

addressed in therapy, it may be desirable to see pictures of events that went well or ones that were problematic, or both to compare and contrast them. Most people have pictures of birthdays, vacations, weddings, and so forth, and if they don't, this can also be key information. Belinda, who had no pictures of her college graduation and was having trouble launching herself from her family and into a career, said, "You know, only my sister came to my graduation. That's one reason I don't have pictures. But it was like my parents, by not coming, didn't see me as a person moving more into adult-hood."

The therapist may also ask about life-cycle rituals that may be germane to the work being done. For example, with a remarried family with a lot of conflict between stepchildren and stepparents, the therapist asked them to bring in wedding pictures from this second marriage to stimulate discussion about what it meant to create this new family.

Bring on the Symbols

Another way to introduce some of the tools of ritual into therapy is to ask clients to bring to sessions symbolic objects that represent for them emotions, issues, or changes they are working on in therapy. For instance, Terence, who was very ambivalent about being in therapy, was asked to bring in two objects—one that represented his wish to be there and the other that represented his desire not to be in therapy. In the next session, Terrence first took out of a bag his son's Etch-a-Sketch with lines drawn all over it like a maze. "This represents wanting to be here," he said. "I want to find my way through these alleyways and dead ends. And this," he said, taking a lemon out of the bag, "represents not wanting to be here because lemon juice burns and stings in open sores, and there are a lot of things that are hard for me to open up."

With a group of young adults in day treatment, all of whom had been hospitalized, the tone of their meetings was quite down. The two group leaders asked each member to look around his or her living space and think about what objects were in it that symbolized hope. They were then asked to bring in the object they found most hopeful. Liz brought in a white technician's jacket with her name embroidered on it. "This gives me hope that I'll soon be able to go back to my job at the medical center." Seppo brought in a cordless telephone. "This is a symbol of being able to talk anytime, anywhere," he said. "And I know that's what's helping me to stay calm right now." These symbols and the other ones brought in were put out on a low table in the middle of the group, and the group leaders encouraged group members to use them as props. What symbol or symbols might group members want to hold as they talked to help them gather hope? What happened when one symbol met another? What did the symbols have to say to each other? How could they be arranged differently?

The tone of the group became much more animated and playful with the introduction of these objects.

Listening for and pulling out verbal references clients make to symbolic actions (e.g., "These feelings of despair wash over me" or "I need to set this aside for a while") can be another way to work with ritual elements. These phrases can be cues for symbolic actions that may be a building block for a ritual. Kay, a woman in her late 20s, said, "I feel hemmed in by 'shoulds' in my life. Things I 'should' do for my family, for my friends, and at work. Further training to get ahead in my career. I have little sense of what I want to do." The therapist asked her if she had any old clothing that she would not mind cutting up. "Yes," she said, somewhat surprised. "But why?"

"You know how hems go all around, so neat and orderly, all the edges sewn up—I was thinking you might want to cut off a hem or two, tie them into bows or make streamers, ribbons, or whatever out of them."

"I have it!" Kay said.

"What?" asked the therapist.

"An old beige suit. I got it for my first job, thinking I should dress up. I was a teacher's aide at a school. I was way overdressed. It cost me most of my first month's salary." As a symbolic way to play with the "shoulds" in her life, Kay cut the hem of the skirt and jacket, tied them into different knots, bows, and flower shapes and draped them over the mirror she used each morning to remind her that she could change the "shoulds" into other shapes and forms.

Upcoming Rituals

The therapist can also ask clients about upcoming holidays or traditions. This can be an excellent way to learn more about their relationships, their cultural and religious backgrounds, and the communities to which they are connected. Most people like to talk about these kinds of events and what they are looking forward to as well as what is hard about them. In one group that was just starting, the winter holidays (Thanksgiving, Hanukkah, Christmas, Kwanzaa, Three Kings' Day, New Year's, Chinese New Year's, etc.) were about to begin. After the group facilitator talked a bit about how holidays can affect people, she asked group members to share something about their own experiences with holidays. Group members learned things about each others' cultural backgrounds that they did not know before (e.g., the significance for Puerto Ricans of January 6th, Three Kings' Day) as well as their family relationships. They also began to connect with each other around how to deal with the stress of holidays and strategies to manage the pressures that they felt at that time. Links were created between people in the group at the same time that new content was introduced to support psychological growth and change.

Art Materials and Rituals

The use of clay, markers, crayons, and paints in session can help clients share their rituals. Clients can draw pictures or make figurines to depict family vacations, holidays, or bedtimes. New rituals that are being created can be imagined and drawn out as a way to help people visualize and think through what they would like to do. Things can be created that are essential parts of a ritual.

For example, in a third-grade classroom in which a child died suddenly after being hit by a car, each student was encouraged to make a card or picture to give to the dead child's parents showing something they would remember about their classmate, Fran. The parents were then invited into the classroom to receive from each child what he or she had made. It helped each child to have some way to mark this very difficult transition, and the parents received information that was very unique—the memories of 8- and 9-year-olds.

Triggering Ritual Memories: The Floor Plan

If a client is having trouble remembering rituals from either his or her current life or, for an adult, his or her childhood, an adaptation of the family floor plan often can stimulate memory. The client is asked to draw the plan of the house or apartment he or she lives or lived in as if from the air looking down (Coppersmith, 1980). This concrete representation of living space seems to provide a way for people to remember earlier events.

To focus the floor plan exercise primarily on rituals, the therapist should ask the client to draw the space in which he or she experienced the most rituals or the space where he or she most wants to remember rituals more vividly. As the client draws, the therapist should ask him or her to think about rituals in different parts of the house, like mealtimes in the eating area, bedtime rituals in the sleeping areas, and saying hello and goodbye near the entrance. While the client is drawing, the therapist can intersperse some of the following questions and ideas. He or she should speak slowly and in a soothing voice, with lots of pauses. Where were birthdays, holidays, special meals celebrated? Who gathered for these events? Imagine people coming into the apartment or house, or in a particular room. Look at their faces, their hair. What kinds of expressions do they have? How are they carrying their bodies? Who invited people, organized ritual events? What gender roles are expressed in that? What is the feel of the air in that space—the textures of the walls, the floors, the furniture? What smells are there? How might some of these things be shown on the drawing with color or a word or phrase?

What symbols are part of the rituals? What is their meaning? How can you show this? What actions, movement, music, or words are important? Who is *not* there for different rituals? What is the significance of that? If you wish to, draw this in some way. How would you wind down from rituals? Who would do the putting away, the cleaning up? What pictures or symbols are left from the rituals? Are they kept in any particular space in this house? Who is the organizer of them, the keeper of them?

To finish off the ritual floor plan exercise, the therapist can ask the client who drew the floor plan to take someone on a tour through his or her space and share ritual remembrances. If in a group setting, they could then reverse roles and go for a tour through the other person's floor plan. (Depending on the setting, the client might take another group member, other family members, or the therapist on the tour.) People going on the tour should feel free to ask open-ended questions of their "tour guide" (e.g., "What else can you remember?" or "Tell me about what you have drawn in over here"). This interaction also helps to facilitate memory. Observations can also be shared (e.g., "It seems like you have a lot more activity in the kitchen than in the living room in this house" or "Your grandmother seems to be in there at the center of ritual making, whether it is extended family meals, birthday parties, or holidays"). These reflections can help the floor plan drawer see links and patterns.

Collecting and Sharing Stories

Another way for a therapist to inform clients and himself or herself as to the range of rituals and creative possibilities is to share stories of other families' rituals or rituals from the therapist's own family.[3] Short vignettes can help clients to recognize the role of ritual in their lives as well as stimulate ideas. For instance, Delores, the head of a single-parent family of four, was feeling disconnected from her children, that the family was always on the go, and that she was just doing things for each child all the time. The therapist described to the family a family who, every time they ate together, held hands at the table for a minute and thought about something they especially liked that had happened to them in the last couple of days. Delores decided to adapt this ritual and to ask each family member to say something they appreciated about the family in the past days. "I started doing it," said Delores, "because the kids balked at doing it at first. It's interesting how it changed my frame of mind to one much more focused on things going well in the family. I thought it would be most important

---

[3]For guidelines on when it is and is not appropriate to share stories from personal experience, see Roberts, 1997, p. 344.

to hear from the kids, and that does mean a lot. I've heard some of the things they like. But just as important, I think, is my shift to noticing what's working."

The Genogram and Rituals

If the therapist wants to look at rituals over time in a client's life, a great tool for this is the multigenerational genogram (McGoldrick & Gerson, 1985). With a basic three-generation genogram the therapist can ask questions such as the following: Who would come together for holidays, weddings, funerals, or anniversaries? What were these gatherings like? Did one side of the family predominate? How were different sides of the family similar or different regarding the kinds of rituals they liked to do and what they did for them? What emotional aura surrounded the rituals? What was passed down of your ethnic, cultural, or religious heritage in the rituals? What was *not* passed down? In what ways were the rituals important? In what ways were they difficult? How did your family ritual life change over time or with major shifts such as a death in the family, a move, or a divorce?

With the genogram, the therapist and client can look at a bigger picture of rituals over time. Shifts and changes can be tracked, multigenerational patterns examined, and different branches of the family compared and contrasted. On her genogram, Janice noticed a three-generational pattern of cutoffs from her father's side of the family around extended family gatherings. Mothers in each generation were central ritual organizers, and this had the effect of passing down more of the women's traditions as well as maintaining more contact with the maternal side of the family.

Minirituals and Therapy Sessions

Rituals often become a part of therapy sessions. Therapists may find themselves welcoming clients in particular ways or beginning sessions with certain formats. Although these kinds of rituals can be reassuring and mark the movement into a special time and place, it is important that they do not become routine and stagnant. One therapist realized that she was starting most of her sessions by asking clients what seemed most important to them from their previous session. She noted, "The beginning of my sessions often seemed flat. I needed to broaden the scope of what I asked about. I started inquiring about details of their daily life between sessions, what kinds of conversations they'd had outside of therapy that felt therapeutic. Things livened up."

Some therapists also create their own minirituals between sessions to help demarcate them. When another therapist had clients back to back, he would slip into the bathroom between sessions to rinse his face, and as he did it, he felt himself let the previous session slip away to prepare himself to be fully present for the next.

Rituals in the therapy hour can be another resource to help clients and therapists make transitions into and out of therapy time. A therapist should find ones that work for him or her and modify them if they become stale. For example, a therapist could ask his or her clients how rituals help or hinder them to get connected to therapy and to leave sessions.

These strategies are easy ways to begin work with rituals. Exploring them and learning a range of ways to bring rituals into therapy can provide a rich foundation for using rituals as an intervention.

MODIFYING AND DESIGNING RITUALS

In working with rituals, key things for the therapist to think about are fit with the client and issues they are working with, a balance of structured and open parts, simplicity and ease of doing them, and meaning for clients. Modifying or designing rituals is an organic process that grows with clients and evolves out of listening to them and their relationship issues and tapping their creativity. Rituals are not imposed on clients, but rather developed with them as opportunities to work with their beliefs and interactional patterns in new ways. Therapists should think simple, small, and creative.

An essential aspect to consider is whether to do rituals in or out of session or some combination of the two (Whiting, 1988). Location, motivation, and others present as participants or witnesses may all be reasons to decide on doing a ritual in or out of session. For instance, it may be important to have the therapist present to be part of some aspect of the ritual. When Terence brought in the Etch-a-Sketch and the lemon as symbols of why he both wanted and did not want to be in therapy, his explanation of why he chose those symbols led to an important dialogue with the therapist about how to make it safer when raw things were opened up.

Doing a ritual in the therapy room may also provide protected time and space that is not as accessible in a client's daily life. Or, there may be the possibility that strong emotions will be evoked by the ritual, and the client may want to do it within the nurturing space of therapy.

On the other hand, if the therapist is tapping into rituals already done in clients' lives outside of therapy, doing out-of-session rituals might be more salient. Also, there may be other participants who can then become a dynamic part of the process. For Nina and Ron, a couple struggling with his prostate cancer, the ritual of reassurance that they designed to share with their three children as part of their regular Shabbat dinner obviously needed to be done in their home.

Often the richest work with ritual happens when there is an in-session and out-of-session mix. Starting a ritual in session can bring the energy and focus of therapy to further expand the ritual in the client's daily life. Likewise, a ritual that is vibrant in a client's life outside of treatment can inform and expand the limited time frame of a therapy session. Therapists sometimes get a narrow view of clients because the time they spend with them is so focused on looking at dilemmas. For example, Louella, who was very saddened and depressed by her boyfriend's decision to terminate their 3-year relationship, brought her bedroom mirror into a session and shared with her therapist the self-talk monologue ritual that she had begun to start off with each day. Louella played off her image in the mirror. She was funny and able to see all kinds of irony in her situation. Her therapist was able to experience a whole new side of her, and they began to use self-talk as a strategy in sessions.

Practical logistics may also affect decisions about whether rituals should be done in or out of session. Ralph, after a 10-year relationship ended with his partner, Chico, found himself obsessively thinking about him and reading over love letters written by Chico, trying to figure out what went wrong. Ralph decided that he wanted to keep one or two of the letters to remember the specialness of the good times they had together but that he wanted to burn the others to "give those words back to the universe." Clearly, he could not do this in the therapy room. Also, Ralph wanted a supportive network with him when he did this, so he asked the five men in his men's group that had been meeting for several years to go with him on a short hike up a special hill that looked out over a valley where he found solace. There, they burned the letters.

It is important to note that rituals are also only one of many different techniques used in therapy. In working with an individual or family 10 times, for example, rituals might be used as an intervention 2 or 3 times. For instance, going back to Melanie in the opening example, in a separate couple's session exploring their ideas about why their daughter Melanie might be so anxious, the therapist found out that the father had a gambling problem and had recently gambled away a small inheritance that the mother had received when her aunt died. A whole range of other techniques were used to work with the gambling issues.

As a therapist becomes more comfortable with rituals, he or she may want to go beyond using them to gather salient information about clients and do more than just modify rituals clients already have and create new rituals. This can be especially important for clients for whom societal rituals are not necessarily available (e.g., pregnancy loss, death by suicide, adoption, foster children, and lesbian and gay marriages [Imber-Black, 1998; Imber-Black & Roberts, 1998]).

CASE EXAMPLE 1: BACK TO MELANIE AND BOBO

The case of Melanie, described at the beginning of this chapter, is presented with commentary on the previously described elements.

Case Narrative

In the second session, the therapist, Ben, asked Melanie to bring to their next meeting her least favorite stuffed animal. She brought in Bobo, her giraffe, because "he's not that cuddly."

Ben coached her and her parents on ways to pass the pain from her stomach onto the giraffe. He told Melanie, "Bobo can hold the pain easier than people can because stuffed animals don't have the same kind of nerve endings people do."

They then set up times before and after school for close, connect contact between Melanie and her parents to practice letting go of the pain and sending it into Bobo. The stomach pains rapidly diminished.

The parents continued to do the special times with Melanie, turning it into a cuddling and reading time.

Commentary

This ritual is particularly effective with preadolescent children, because they readily attribute feelings to and identify emotionally with their dolls and stuffed animals. Similar procedures can be used with older clients whenever a comparable identification with a symbol (e.g., rings representing commitment) exists.

Because this ritual was used to get Melanie and her parents reconnected in a more constructive way, the parents were included in the coaching. Ben's explanation was needed to dispel any guilt that might arise over hurting Bobo.

It was important that Ben structure these contact times between parents and Melanie *around*, rather than *in place of*, school time so that there was no "secondary gain" of missing school for Melanie to get nurturant attention from her parents.

Ben used the pain-passing ritual as an opportunity to encourage a new family ritual for Melanie and her parents to share time together.

EXPANDING RITUAL WORK

A more extensive case example is now presented to show how work with rituals may evolve over a number of sessions. For a couple, Adela and Rob, behavioral shifts in how they dealt with conflict were sustained and supported by bringing in symbols and symbolic actions. In addition, this case illustrates how use of rituals can help clients and therapists transition out of therapy.

CASE EXAMPLE 2: BEYOND FIGHTING FAIR

Adela and Rob had been married for 20 years. They found themselves becoming increasingly tense with each other and in fights in which they would "freeze" each other out for several days, two or three times a month. They were very committed to their relationship and were sure that they wanted to continue it, but with some major changes.

As the therapist, Tess, talked with them, it became clear that ways they were interacting with each other when they were upset were leading them into difficulty. Tess and Adela and Rob worked out some rules for fair fighting (e.g., not calling each other names, staying in the present with issues they were trying to work through and not globalizing, and not blaming the other person but rather looking at how to change their own behavior). In sessions, the couple found it relatively easy to follow these ground rules. At home, however, it was more emotionally charged, and they were not able to keep to them.

As Adela and Rob talked more with Tess, they each shared what came up for them when they had a disagreement or fight. As a child, Rob had felt shut out by his parents because his father had health problems and his mother was very busy holding the family together. Rob described how, when he and Adela fought, he quickly became overwhelmed with feelings from his childhood of not being cared for. He then became hopeless that he was not going to get what he wanted within the marriage.

For Adela, when Rob complained of things she had not done for him, she felt chastised, as if she were a little girl again, trying to follow what she experienced as the strict and rigid routines of her parents and always failing. She said, "It's amazing how the feelings flood me. I feel like I never do anything right—not at home, or at work—and that Rob doesn't want to be with me. So I withdraw."

Case Narrative	*Commentary*
Tess began to talk with Rob and Adela about a way each of them might calm and center themselves after a tense interchange and separate out their current feelings from some of their past experiences. Tess asked Rob if there was any place of comfort in the house where he felt particularly safe.	More needed to be done beyond the guidelines for fighting fair. Because the ground rules were not working at home Tess needed to explore what other things were being triggered.
"I have a rocking chair that my mother gave to me as an adult. It was after my dad died, and we were	

feeling more connected. It was as if she had more space for me. I go there sometimes and just sit and look out at the sky." Rob paused. "It's interesting that it came from my mother."

Tess then asked Adela, "What do you have around the house that might counteract your feelings of becoming a little girl again when you fight with Rob?"

Adela thought for a while. "I don't know. Nothing comes to my mind." "Does it feel useful as something to think about until the next session?" asked Tess.

"Yes," said Adela.

"I'd like to ask you then, as you walk around the house and see things, to think about any objects there that trigger for you feelings of competence —and of connection," said Tess.

In the next session, Adela volunteered, "I came up with two things. One is a photo album that has a lot of pictures of Rob and me in it. It's from around 8, 9 years ago when things were going pretty well between us. We had a couple of nice vacations and also moved into a new house we really loved. The other thing I did is make a stack of training manuals and brochures I put together for my company that I'm proud of."

"What's the significance of that?" asked Tess.

"Adult competence," said Adela, and she laughed. "You'd think I wouldn't need to be reminded of it. I mean, I am 52. But it's great to look at."

Tess talked to Adela and Rob about ways they could use the rocking

Tess is looking for something foundational to shift their dynamics. This choice of objects from around the house was a matter of convenience because it was winter.

A useful question, since therapists cannot assume they know their clients' values.

chair, the photo album, and "the stack," as it affectionately came to be known, as resources to calm themselves and get perspective when they got into a disagreement. Rob decided that he would like to ask for timeouts during which he could just go and sit in the chair. Adela agreed to it so long as she knew how long they were for and they set a time when they would get back to working things out. Adela decided to look at the photo album, "To flood myself with good memories rather than negative ones," and to carry "the stack" around with her in the house. She smiled and said, "My hands will be full of my work competence. Maybe I'll relax about picking up around the house so much."

Tess also suggested that when the two of them were trying to work something out that they include at the beginning of it an affirmation or appreciation of each other. "It might just change the tone of things."

Over time, as Adela and Rob incorporated these ideas, they felt like they were starting to treat each other at home more like they wanted to. "But it's still easier for us, I think, to talk about more difficult things when we are here in the therapy room," Rob said.

"Why do you think that is?" asked Tess.

"Because you're present. We have to be accountable to someone besides just ourselves."

"Humm," said Tess. "So maybe you need to set up an empty chair at home and put something in it that represents me."

Rituals do here what verbal therapy attempts to do—help restructure and reinforce boundaries.

Had they not been able to succeed at all in this, Tess would have asked them to bring their objects to the next session.

The rationale of this out-of-session intervention was to insert the therapist's presence in the clients' lives. Tess could also have asked them to write her a note. People can readily

"I know what," said Adela. "The list of ground rules we worked out with you."

Sessions were spaced out over longer periods of time. Adela and Rob had their own "mini" sessions at home in the weeks between appointments. The photo album ended up next to the rocking chair. Adela took to deliberately sitting in the rocking chair sometimes, too. The "stack" went to bed with them a few times. They felt confident that they had the skills to continue to make changes on their own, and treatment was ended.

enact such rituals because they involve concrete and structured activity full of meaning, not just behavioral tasks.

Because emotions can be overwhelming, symbols serve to ground experiences, giving clients a sense of being able to deal with feelings and interpersonal events.

This couple wanted to carry over changes they were able to implement during sessions into times at home that were emotionally charged. By connecting some of the issues and emotions evoked for them during these times to symbols and symbolic actions, Adela, Rob, and the therapist were able to construct different responses at home that activated the power of rituals. Several small rituals that built on each other but also fit into tasks they were already doing were developed. These out-of-session rituals provided a bridge to transfer skills worked on in session to day-to-day life. This enabled Adela and Rob to make a healing space in their everyday environment.

WHEN CLIENTS SEEM DISINTERESTED IN WORKING WITH RITUALS

There may be a number of factors that contribute to a lack of fit between a client and a therapist interested in action methods such as rituals. Central to motivating a client to involve himself or herself with rituals is the therapist's own comfort and energy level in working with them. If the therapist seems unsure or dubious, the client will pick up on and react to it. The connection between the therapist and client is also essential to create a safe yet stimulating environment in which new ideas can be explored. A strong, trusting relationship provides a foundation for taking risks.

In order not to appear too different or "exotic," rituals may need to be presented first as something the client is already doing. As the client sees the relevance of them in one area of his or her life, it may be easier to introduce rituals as a resource in other parts.

Also, rituals cannot feel tacked on or inserted into therapy awkwardly. They need to nestle into the rhythm and interests of the client and link up with issues and ideas discussed in treatment. Some of the most successful work I have done with rituals has occurred when clients were involved with the ins and outs of them. Planning for a ritual can be as important as the actual event because it is during this time that relationships have the potential to be reworked and new ideas explored. For instance, Rita wanted to have a healing ritual to "put to rest" her grief about her infertility. She designed it in conjunction with her pastoral counselor, her husband, and several friends. She wrote, "I found that the 6 weeks prior to the actual ceremony was a time of healing. I was able to focus my thoughts on what exactly I had lost, what I had hoped for, all of the procedures we had experienced, and what direction I wanted in my future. I had a specific time frame to work toward, as well as two people who had committed their time to hear my story and to be there with me."

Although rituals are so versatile that they can be used with anyone, they are contraindicated when their symbols are not meaningful or metaphorical. Consequently, therapists should not be too enamored of their own ideas; they need to attend closely to what clients find helpful to re-evoke hope. They should gauge the level of interest and comfort of a client and trigger his or her curiosity. The therapist needs to offer options, choices, and collaborate and develop ideas with the client. The client may then be intrigued.

RESEARCH: HOW, WHERE, WHEN, AND WHY RITUALS WORK

Researchers have looked at the efficacy of family rituals in preventing transmission of alcoholism through generations (Wolin & Bennett, 1984; Wolin, Bennett, & Jacobs, 1988); how rituals can help families with the life-cycle transition of children moving into their teenage years (Davis, 1988, 1998); the role of therapeutic rituals in separation and divorce (Copeland 1987); and how rituals can strengthen both nuclear and intergenerational family connections. Some of the earliest work was done by Bossard and Boll (1950), who systematically tracked the range and type of rituals of 186 families. They described rituals as being at the center of family culture and as key transmitters of family beliefs, goals, and worldview.

More recently, Wolin, Bennett, and Jacobs (1988), in three different studies, interviewed 137 families using their Family Ritual Interview. They talked with families in which at least one parent met the accepted criteria for alcoholic or problem drinker and matched nonalcoholic control families. They found that in those families in which there was drinking but intact familial rituals, children were somewhat protected from the transmission of alcohol problems to their generation. Also, when children from alcoholic families decided to follow a spouse's nonalcoholism-related rituals in the creation of their new family and to eliminate alcoholism-related rituals from their family of origin, this also seemed to provide some protection from alcoholism transmission.

Davis (1988, 1998) observed four Jewish families from very different backgrounds over 6 months as they planned, took part in, and then looked back on their first child's bar mitzvah. She examined the intricate ways in which the process of preparing for this ritual, the public ceremony, and the shifts in relationships that subsequently rippled through the community facilitated developmental change. Her research has many rich implications for the role of ritual in facilitating other life-cycle transitions.

Using a number of measures (e.g., Attachment Scale, Divorce Reaction Inventory, Index of Clinical Stress, and Index of Family Relations), Copeland (1987) looked at the effect of ritual as a therapeutic intervention in four different cases of separation and/or divorce. In three of the four cases, the hypotheses supporting rituals' effectiveness on personal and interpersonal functions were supported.

Women's rituals in the larger society, some of the personal and social costs involved in them, and how they then affect women in families have been looked at in depth by Laird (1988), who also raised many thoughtful questions about men's identity, roles, and rituals.

It can be difficult to research rituals in the therapy process because it is hard to pull them out as a separate intervention. Ways to do this more might include detailed work designing questions as part of outcomes studies that inquire into ritual-based interventions. A brief checklist of changes in family ritual life could also be used before and after therapy. Imber-Black (1998) has called for more study of the interaction of rituals and symptoms when the ordinary rituals of family life go awry.

More studies combining quantitative and qualitative data are needed to research rituals. Information generated from qualitative studies provides insight into the intricacies of interior shifts for people as well as the effect on relationships. Quantitative studies provide a broader database about the efficacy of rituals and ways they work or not over a wide range of families and situations.

RITUALS: THE INSIDE TRACK

A good way for a therapist to begin to learn more about how to use rituals in therapy is to access his or her own memories about their role throughout his or her life and his or her family's life. This gives the therapist scope and depth to think across a wide range of rituals and through many family transitions. He or she can modify and create therapeutic rituals in current life. This allows the therapist to intentionally experience from the inside out the power of rituals to name and mark the transitions we all experience.

After being treated for breast cancer for a year (Roberts, 1998), I gave a party of thanks for all who had helped me. My family and I fed everyone, spoke our appreciation, and threw angels carved from soap out to all in the support network. After this event, my mind felt clearer, as if I had spent enough time with the hardest memories and emotions. The ritual demarcated my life into time as a cancer patient and now as a cancer survivor. My daughter seemed happier, less watchful of me, and more easy around the house.

Sharing with others whose ritual lives may be quite different can also be a powerful learning experience. Individuals are exposed to different ritual styles, a range of types, and how they work or do not work for others. Larissa was fascinated by Dominic's explications of his family reunions. "We never had reunions in my family. There were factions that didn't get along and we were so spread out. Dominic gets together with his extended family almost every year. He and his wife plan vacation time before or after it. Different generations get together on different days—subgroups do different activities. It's usually only one day that they are all together. Hearing about how they've found ways to meet a variety of needs and relationships has inspired me to think of small ways to maybe get my family together."

Writing and reflecting on rituals in one's own life and the lives of others can add depth of analysis and the capacity to look at these lives from different perspectives. Carol's parents divorced when she was young. Her mother remarried but her father did not. It was the 1960s and there was not much emphasis on fathering and few models for divorced fathers. There was also not much support in the larger culture for the adults in divorced families to think about how to continue to parent together. As Carol wrote about her childhood and family rituals, she began to see why her father felt so left out as she realized that he got the dregs of time with her and her brother. Christmas was always celebrated with him at least several days after the fact. For Thanksgiving, her mother took them out of town to her parents' home, so they did not see their father then. Birthdays were always celebrated at her mother's, and given the tension between her parents, her father was not welcome.

For years, I have had students go into the homes of families who volunteer to be interviewed to learn more about family interactional patterns.[4] This is another good way to learn about varied rituals, especially if students make an effort to interview a family from a different cultural

---

[4]The students are encouraged to give something back to the families in return for this privilege, such as a copy of the family genogram, a night of babysitting, dinner or lunch, etc.

background than their own, or a family with children of different ages, than they are accustomed to working with, or a family with perhaps a less familiar structure (e.g., a gay or lesbian family, remarried, single parent). I encourage the students to join with the families in at least one of their rituals (e.g., a meal, children's bedtime, or a family member coming back to the house at the end of the day) so that they can see the families in action.

Yvonne, a single parent mother of a young adult son, interviewed a family of four (mother, father, and two daughters, ages 11 and 5), ate dinner with them. She observed that a place was not set at the table for the younger daughter, Ariela, and that she was not expected to sit with the rest of the family and eat. She was allowed to run around, make a lot of noise, and interrupt the others at the table at will. Yvonne found out that because Ariela did not like many of the foods the rest of the family ate her mother cooked something special for her before dinner and fed her then with some of the few things that she liked. Later that evening, when it was Ariela's bedtime, the mother remained in Ariela's bedroom with her for more than half an hour. When she came out, the mother told Yvonne, "I have to remain by her side until she falls completely asleep. If I don't, she gets up and follows me around the apartment saying she is scared." From watching these interactions, Yvonne was able to gather a lot of information about the special place Ariela held in the family and the particular closeness between Ariela and her mother. Many complex dynamics were enacted in these "simple" rituals. As Yvonne said, "I have a new appreciation after doing this, for what one can learn from rituals."

CONCLUSION

Once rituals are accepted as an intervention, there are boundless possibilities. Work with rituals pulls in the unique transitions and changes in each person's life while connecting clients and therapists through the creative meaning-making processes that are central to our humanness. Because rituals are active, people are simultaneously making and marking transitions as they occur. This can add a deep vibrancy to therapy.

REFERENCES

Bodin, A. (1989). *Stress management rituals for daily work transitions of mental health professionals*. Unpublished doctoral dissertation, University of Massachusetts, Amherst.

Boscolo, L., & Bertrando, P. (1993). *The times of time*. New York: Norton.

Bossard, J., & Boll, E. (1950). *Ritual in family living*. Philadelphia: University of Pennsylvania Press.

Combs, G., & Freedman, J. (1990). *Symbol, story, and ceremony: Using metaphor in individual and family therapy*. New York: Norton.

Copeland, M. H. (1987). *The effect of rituals as therapeutic interventions with separated or divorced persons in ongoing therapy*. Unpublished doctoral dissertation, Florida State University.

Coppersmith, E. (1980). The family floor plan: A tool for training, assessment and intervention in family therapy. *Journal of Marital and Family Therapy, 6*, 141–145.

d'Aquili, E. G., Laughlin, C. D., & McManus, J. (Eds.). (1979). *The spectrum of ritual: A biogenetic structural analysis*. New York: Columbia University Press.

Davis, J. (1988). Mazel tov: The bar mitzvah as a multigenerational ritual of change and continuity. In E. Imber-Black, J. Roberts, & R. Whiting (Eds.), *Rituals in families and family therapy* (pp. 177–208). New York: Norton.

Davis, J. (1998). *Whose bar/bat mitzvah is this, anyway? A guide for parents through a family rite of passage*. New York: St. Martin's Griffin.

Imber-Black, E. (1998). Creating meaningful rituals for new life cycle transition. In B. Carter & M. McGoldrick (Eds.), *The expanded family life cycle: Individual, family and social perspectives* (pp. 202–214). Boston: Allyn & Bacon.

Imber-Black, E., & Roberts, J. (1998). *Rituals for our times: Celebrating, healing, and changing our lives and our relationships*. San Francisco: Jason Aronson.

Kobak, R. R., & Waters, D. B. (1984). Family therapy as a rite of passage: Play's the thing. *Family Process, 23*(1), 89–100.

Laird, J. (1988). Women and ritual in family therapy. In E. Imber-Black, J. Roberts, & R. Whiting (Eds.), *Rituals in families and family therapy* (pp. 331–362). New York: Norton.

McGoldrick, M., & Gerson, R. (1985). *Genograms in family assessment*. New York: Norton.

Roberts, J. (1988a). Rituals and trainees. In E. Imber-Black, J. Roberts, & R. Whiting (Eds.), *Rituals in families and family therapy* (pp. 387–401). New York: Norton.

Roberts, J. (1988b). Setting the frame: Definition, functions, and typology of rituals. In E. Imber-Black, J. Roberts, & R. Whiting (Eds.), *Rituals in families and family therapy* (pp. 1–46). New York: Norton.

Roberts, J. (1997). Reflecting processes and "supervision": Looking at ourselves as we work with others. In T. C. Todd & C. L. Storm (Eds.), *The complete systemic supervisor* (pp. 334–348). Boston: Allyn & Bacon.

Roberts, J. (1998, July/August). Bring in the clowns: Spritzing seltzer in the face of the big C. *Family Therapy Networker*, 50–56.

Selvini Palazzoli, M. (1974). *Self starvation: From the intrapsychic to the transpersonal approach to anorexia nervosa*. London: Chaucer.

van der Hart, O. (1983). *Rituals in psychotherapy: Transition and continuity*. New York: Irvington.

van der Hart, O. (Ed.). (1988). *Coping with loss: The therapeutic use of leave-taking rituals*. New York: Irvington.

Van Gennep, A. (1960). *The rites of passage*. Chicago: University of Chicago Press.

White, M., & Epston, D. (1990). *Narrative means to therapeutic ends*. New York: Norton.

Whiting, R. (1988). Guidelines to designing therapeutic rituals. In E. Imber-Black, J. Roberts, & R. Whiting (Eds.), *Rituals in families and family therapy* (pp. 84–109). New York: Norton.

Wolin, S. J., & Bennett, L. A. (1984). Family rituals. *Family Process, 23*(3), 401–420.

Wolin, S., Bennett, L., & Jacobs, J. (1988). Assessing family rituals in alcoholic families. In E. Imber-Black, J. Roberts, & R. Whiting (Eds.), *Rituals in families and family therapy* (pp. 230–256). New York: Norton.

4

A PERSONAL VIEW OF ACTION METAPHOR: BRINGING WHAT'S INSIDE OUTSIDE

BUNNY S. DUHL

ACTION PROCESSES AND ACTION METAPHORS

A wide variety of activities can be categorized as *action processes*, a rather loose term. Many therapists consider anything that is not purely talk to be an action process, such as having a client write a letter to a relative, having couples put lists of "caring behaviors" on the refrigerator (i.e., "I feel cared about when. . . ."), or having trainees role-play an interview. There are many action methods, such as role-playing, enactment, psychodrama, simulation, sculpting, and ritual. Some of these are direct processes, such as having clients try in session a structured model of negotiation. Enactments, as in structural therapy, may include action, such as when the therapist asks family members to switch seating positions. Such a rearrangement is meant to interrupt old patterns and evoke new behaviors and new

---

Editor's Note: As noted in the Introduction, this chapter's author was not asked to adhere to the format devised for other chapters. Instead, this chapter is a first-person account of one therapist's personal experiences with action methods.

reactions and interactions on the part of family members. This type of process is a direct action intervention, and although it also can have symbolic implications, it is not metaphoric in nature. Other processes, such as sculpting and psychodrama, are more metaphoric and generative.

Action Metaphor Defined

Metaphor translates from the Greek as "carrying from one place to another." That is the sense in which I use it in this chapter: A metaphor is the transposing of an image or association from one state or arena of meaning to another, highlighting similarities, differences, and ambiguities. All people automatically carry many associations and meanings from one place to another. Metaphor, then, is the linkage of meaning—that connecting any two events, ideas, characteristics, or modes (Duhl, 1983).

Processes are action metaphors when the activity represents or sheds light on an issue, situation, theme, or set of interactions ongoing with the people in the room and when the therapist and clients or trainees physically enact the metaphor. In this sense, an action metaphor is directly indirect. It deals with a real issue indirectly, through different channels of awareness, such as in hypnosis, when attention is turned inward.

Why Action Metaphors?

There are a number of reasons to include action metaphors in clinical work, whether with individuals alone or with couples, families, or groups. Action is part of life. Interaction between people includes not only words but also gestures, voice tones, body movements, pace, energy exchanges, and all the private meanings given these behaviors by each member involved. Action methods and metaphors, unlike words alone, can capture all of these behaviors with impressive effect.

Perhaps most important, however, is that action metaphors grasp "wholes," whereas language is analytic and linear. Action metaphors allow an individual to externalize entire images of what is held in his or her mind in a form that the therapist or trainer can render safe and useful.

In the managed care reality of today's mental health care world, it is essential that therapists have quick ways to understand whole issues. Action metaphors, because they grasp whole gestalts, can cut through a morass of words, advancing clients' experiences dramatically and quickly.

Lastly, action metaphors circumvent intellectual defenses that are activated through verbal representation. Language often is used to shield what is thought, felt, sensed, or known. As a trainee stated, "We can wrap our feelings up in cognitive language to lessen their emotional intensity." An action metaphor does not allow that.

CLINICAL PRACTICES

I continually give myself permission to try new and different things, just as I offer my clients this permission. I create an environment in which it is safe to learn about, uncover, discover, add on to, and reintegrate aspects of the self in relation to the self and in interactive processes with others.

Along with action processes, I provide a variety of media for representation. I use an easel for genograms with every individual, couple, or family. This provides a visual focus and feedback process, not only during history taking but throughout therapy. (I have learned that with genograms I "see" squares, circles, lines, and words. Clients often "see" photographs, movie pictures, and storybooks.) A therapist who thinks in terms of systems can see the patterns clients are living and can, by creating action metaphors, facilitate clients' experience of these patterns with awareness.

Language Is "About"; Experience "Is"

It is well known that an individual's beliefs about his or her behavior can be very different than the actual behavior (i.e., that the "theory-as-espoused" is often not the "theory-in-action" [Argyris & Schon, 1974]). Action thus can be a mirror, as well as a route of access, to walled-in beliefs. Participants feel seen and heard through these processes. They literally are able to see and experience something differently, not just talk about it. This adds new dimensions to both their inner and outer awarenesses—their sense of how they feel, believe, and think and how they act. The covert is made overt, and a new understanding is made possible. Theories-in-action and theories-as-espoused can be explored more closely and, it is hoped, eventually aligned.

Where Action Metaphors Fit In

Action metaphors provide ways of knowing that are entirely different from those achieved through language alone. When action metaphors are used, the therapist as well as other family or group members simultaneously experience the hitherto hidden meanings of behavior. Action metaphors are always contextual. Action metaphors make manifest the unspoken and out-of-awareness images and beliefs of the person whose metaphor is being enacted. They also draw forth observers' out-of-awareness images and beliefs in response to the enactment. Such revelations, and reactions to such revelations, cannot be preplanned or predicted; nor can they be avoided. The sharing of these revelations and reactions also provides new and direct experiences simultaneously to all present.

When to Use Action Metaphors

At this point in my experience, it is difficult for me to think of action metaphors as a set of techniques to be used in certain prescribed situations, such as, "When X happens, do this." I think of action metaphors as another vocabulary that is spoken whenever it is necessary to speak in a language of impact that will communicate and be processed by those involved at a different level than their ordinary vocabulary. Because action metaphors capture whole images, they tap a symbolic level of meaning. Perhaps because they are novel, and a different language and vocabulary are being used, people remember them, like a circus bus coming down the street in the midst of ordinary traffic. Ordinary traffic is not remembered.

So, when is it necessary to use a different vocabulary? When the therapist feels that the novelty of an action metaphor can serve as a route of access to all present (e.g., when a client or the therapist is stuck in some repetitive mode). Or when the therapist wants to get across a message that has been said verbally but not received. Or when the therapist wants to communicate in a manner that is likely to be grasped at a symbolic level —easily, quickly, and without being blocked by the usual defenses. When there is great conflict concerning the "correct" view of a situation or an impasse between members, an action metaphor can illuminate that which is hidden.

Various body-in-action metaphors are very useful when people do not have a sense of themselves as making an impact on other members of a system. In sculpture, the sculptor has to describe the scene from his or her inner image and place his or her cast of characters in it, complete with gestures and movement. Most of the time, words are eliminated. The sculptor also has to put himself or herself into that cast, that scene. Feedback from other players provides their perceptions of him or her within the system. Thus, for perhaps the first time, the sculptor will experience himself or herself as an actor who makes an impact on others, who in turn affect him.

Moving Into Action Processes

Action processes are generated through a therapist's disposition, training, practice, and observation. The therapist must first allow himself or herself to think metaphorically and associatively, drawing from all experience, from everything ever known or done. A therapist gains access to action processes by giving himself or herself permission to invent, explore, experiment, and improve, by treating therapy as an art form based on theoretical principles, yet allowing for creation of new theory and processes. A therapist must summon the courage to try something that has not been done before, or not done in this new manner, as a route to new information and understanding. It is important for the therapist to realize that this process of discovery within therapy is still ongoing and, it is hoped, will never end.

ACTION PROCESSES: PERSONAL EXPERIENCE

I became introduced to and enthralled by action processes as a trainee some years ago (1969–1971) at the Boston Family Institute (BFI), where I was learning family systems therapy. I had the good fortune to be trained in a way that taught nonlinear thinking in a nonlinear way. Human systems involve the simultaneous, dynamic interactions of component members. Trainees learned systems thinking through group exercises that were basically simulations of life situations in a variety of forms—role-playing, analogic and metaphoric exercises, and family sculpting. We were the component members dynamically interacting. Didactic material followed active involvement. Thus, we had firsthand experience in animated, experiential vignettes from which to derive, learn, and attach systems theory. After we had momentarily lived it, we then stepped back to describe each part and the interaction pattern of the whole. Generic constructs were derived from multiple specific situations—from the inside out.

The action exercises drew forth the underlying dynamics and principles of how human systems operate. In this process, we became acutely aware of how people acted, felt, and thought in a variety of systemic situations. In other words, we began to read and enact body language and expressions, uniting them with spoken and unspoken thought processes, feelings, impulses, wishes, yearnings, and fears. We became actors in many scenes, later discussing the theoretical systems principles underlying our behaviors. We became comfortable moving around. Based on the personal value of this rich experience, I am convinced that this kind of training should be continued and expanded.

SCULPTURE

Key in my training was the development of the process of family sculpture by David Kantor, one of BFI's founders. In family sculpture, space is used to denote emotional closeness or distance and power or hierarchy. Kantor, a disciple of Moreno's psychodramatic work (Moreno, 1946), developed an elaborate structure and process to delve deeply into the perception and unexpressed meanings of family interactions from one member's point of view at a time (Duhl, 1983; Duhl, Kantor, & Duhl, 1973).

At BFI, trainees, in roles as family members, assumed postures, gestures, and movements suggested by the sculptor and enacted them. The pattern of movements and interactions was repeated several times to capture the pattern of the system. After the enactment, players gave feedback on what was experienced in their roles, positions, and movements. Thus, the sculptor began to get a sense of the multicentric reality—the reality from many centers—of his or her family system. When the sculpting process was experienced in a family therapy situation, from several members' points of view, family members began to see how each person was an actor in someone else's version of the same family play, and once again, the multicentric reality of each person's version of the family emerged.

SELF-DISCOVERY

As a trainee, I found the floodgates of images and imagination opened for me, in the form of myriad kinesthetic and visual images. I became a receiver and creator of mental pictures illustrative of what is happening in relationships.

In my working with simulations, role-plays, sculptures, and action metaphors as a trainee and therapist, the drama of interaction and sequences of behavior were played out as they are in real life. I began to catch the ethos of what was happening between myself and others or, when observing, between others. I discovered myself anew, and came to realize that clients are no different than trainees and therapists in this regard.

The very language of family therapy, which includes such words as *boundaries, closeness, distance, balancing,* and *triangulation,* brings up the contextual nature of definitions. In which context is someone close to or distant from another? What is the ambience of that closeness or distance? What is meant by a "boundary" between people? How can it be represented? I became aware that such abstract words often are empty vessels that we fill with our idiosyncratic images. As a trainee, I began to become aware of the "betweenness" of human interaction—that which is neither one person nor the other, but inclusive of and between them both. I began to "see" or "sense" systems as a kind of dance form, and I began to invent action metaphors that could represent that dance, those interactions, and that betweenness in ways that clients could represent their own images for which they used some abstract word. I began sharing my own mental images and encouraging clients to play with me and enact them. I also began encouraging clients to develop their own images and metaphors to try on.

Later, I became aware that the mind is populated with the auditory, visual, and kinesthetic experiences of the introjected others of one's life—a virtual cast of characters—that guide actions, reactions, beliefs, behaviors, and meanings. These can be explored and enacted through action metaphor. Over time, I also became aware that people live by their images and their unexpressed ideas of how things are supposed to be, perhaps based on past experiences, wishes, dreams, enculturation, and expectations. These images are not necessarily visual; they are multisensory, involving voice tone, body movement, facial and bodily expression, speed and rate of movement, distance, and felt interpersonal pulls or tensions. They are almost always interpersonal and interactive scenarios. The dynamics and meanings involved in such inner scenarios are not available through language alone. They are the stuff of movies, of mental images and betweenness, and are only fully accessible through action metaphor, which externalizes the felt experience and hidden meanings in a form that is comprehensible to oneself and others. They are holographically related parts of one's life, perceptions, and fantasies.

I felt at BFI as if the compartments of my mind had receded and all I had ever known was available as resource material without restrictions. I had the freedom to associate freely and to use those associations actively in joining with clients to create new routes of access to previously hidden material.

SELF-TRUST

As I began to work with clients and trainees, I became aware of my own vivid internal images, like snapshots or movies that appeared on an inner screen, as if I were daydreaming, while I was talking and working with others. It was a shock! At first, I berated myself to pay attention to what was going on in the room. However, the images persisted and repeated themselves in context. I tried to get them out of my mind but was unable to do so. So, in private practice as well as in training seminars, I began to pay attention to them. Then, one day I took the risk of offering to share one of these images with a couple with whom I was working. I did not know what this image meant, although its recurrence on my "inner screen" suggested that I was on to something. At that point, I proceeded to sculpt my inner image using the couple as the players. They entered into my action metaphor and found that it revealed at a symbolic, metaphoric level what was happening between them.

As I remember it, the image was of a pool of quicksand, with wobbly boards across it. I circumscribed the quicksand pool in the room, delineating it on the rug, walking around it, and describing it. I then described the boards around the edges, indicated the location of one or two boards stretching across the pool, and asked the couple to "walk" on them, in turn, across the quicksand. They each did so, "balancing" themselves as on a tightrope, afraid of falling in.

Each agreed that this metaphor and their participation in it captured what they had been experiencing in their marriage. They were then able to realize that the quicksand represented their mutual fears of loss and divorce, while the loose boards symbolized their tiptoeing around situations with each other, afraid to address and confront what really disturbed them.

I realized then the rich potential of my inner imagery as a therapeutic resource and that the question was not whether to pay attention to it or not, but rather when and how best to use the unconscious productions of my mind on behalf of the clients with whom I work. In this process, I always include a disclaimer such as, "I have this crazy ("weird," "funny," "peculiar," "bizarre") image. It could be 'off the wall.' However, I'd like to share it with you." Then I proceed to get up from my chair and attempt to externalize the image. I either enact it or have them enact it, depending on the situation. I have never been totally off base, though I have had people say, "No, that's not quite right." When that occurs, I am aware that they have entered into the imagery. All I need to say is, "OK, then change it"—and they do. They adjust the image metaphor and make it their own, and in doing so, they are exploring and expanding, in symbolic form, a version of their real-life issue.

BOUNDARY SCULPTURE FOR DIAGNOSIS AND INTERVENTION

When I finished my training, I had the opportunity to coteach for 2 years with David Kantor at BFI and with Jeremy Cobb at Boston State Hospital. I began to invent many other types of sculpture, both alone and in conjunction with Kantor and Cobb. In boundary sculpture (Duhl, 1983; Duhl, Kantor, & Duhl, 1973), which I developed with Jeremy Cobb, one explores the personal and interpersonal boundaries of couple, family, or group members to examine how or if boundaries are maintained and how they interface and interlace with the boundaries of others. Such questions as how people let or prevent others from entering into their space and how they then get others out of their most personal space, their social space, and their public space began to be examined through this process.

I started to use boundary sculpture with couples as a key diagnostic process. In one variation of this form of sculpture, or action metaphor, each member of the couple is invited to think of an image or metaphor for his or her ideal personal space. For some, it is the top of a mountain; for others, it is a rock by the ocean, a house in the woods, a comfortable room, a cocoon, or a steel rocket case.

These images are then explored in detail, paced out, externalized, and staged by each member. The sculptor is asked reality–fantasy questions, such as "How would I know this is your space?" "What separates it from public space?" "What are the walls made of?" "Are there windows, doors?" Or if outside, "Is there a fence around your space?" "Is it visible or invisible?" "Can you see out, can others see in?" "What is inside?" "Would I have to knock?" "What would I have to do to come in, to be invited in?" and so forth.

As the sculptor answers these questions, he or she enters more and more into the image and into trance. Sculpting is a hypnotic process. The sculptor "sees" the space as he or she walks around in it, describing it. Each element the sculptor adds allows the therapist or monitor to ask more questions and, in doing so, to flesh out the image, to externalize it, and to "see" it himself or herself.

When working with couples, after one partner as sculptor has set the scene of his or her ideal space, I then ask the other partner to begin to check or test it out—to physically enter his or her partner's space as he or she has portrayed it. In doing this, the therapist can become aware of the interpersonal dynamics of the couple in this domain: whether the partner has been paying attention, is willing to take his or her partner seriously and cooperate in the imagery, or has any tolerance for invention and play as a way of approaching an old issue in a new manner. A therapist often can discern the energy investment a couple member has in improving the relationship and closing the gaps in it. This aspect of sculpture is diagnostic.

CASE EXAMPLE 1: BOUNDARY SCULPTURE

In working with Mr. and Mrs. M early in my career, I faced a particularly troubling situation in which it was exceedingly hard for me to determine what it was that the husband was doing wrong for which the wife always felt he was to blame. Their presenting problem statements included "they just weren't happy with each other" and Mrs. M's complaint that "he is always invading my space" (i.e., that her needs for time alone and privacy were greater than Mr. M's). Mr. M said verbally that his wife's needs for time alone and privacy did not bother him. He asked that she please just tell him when she needed to be alone, and he would willingly respect it. Her answer bordered on "yes, but." I could not get a handle on this situation. Early in therapy I suggested that we do a metaphoric boundary sculpture.

Mrs. M's ideal space was a cozy cottage near the ocean, with a path leading to the front of the cottage. She paced it out in the room. Although it had a door, there were no locks and no bell. Anyone was "free to walk in," she said. I asked numerous questions about this, particularly as she felt that her husband invaded her space. I gave her permission to have a "magic, long-distance door opener" so that she would not have to move from her favorite seat by the window (her inner private space) to let someone in. I suggested a buzzer that she could control. No. She could have an invisible electric fence that only she could turn off. No. She didn't want that either.

In time, her husband was asked to come to her beach cottage. He proceeded cautiously, gently knocking and looking around the outside "door" to see if anyone was home. He entered and then looked inside the inner room door as he opened it. Mrs. M became angry and once again accused him of invading her private space! I was quite startled, as was Mr. M.

The issue on which previously both they and I had no handle became crystal clear. Mrs. M did not want a "magic door opener" because, as she said, Mr. M was supposed to have a "magic scanner" that would let him know exactly when she wanted to be alone and when she did not. She had put the guardianship of her boundaries in his hands and then accused and attacked him for not knowing and for purposely and insidiously invading her space. Her true belief was that he knew when she wanted to be alone. By not taking responsibility for her own needs and declaring them, Mrs. M made Mr. M always liable to be at fault. He in turn had felt crazy, like an oaf who bumbled along, not knowing the rules of the game of his marriage. And, indeed, he had not.

This particular metaphoric action process was both diagnostic and interventive. It cleared the air for Mr. M. He declared the game null and void. He put his wife's boundary definition back in her hands, insisting that she own her boundaries and declare them and released himself from responsibility for magically knowing what they were. Although she was unhappy with both this revelation and declaration, Mrs. M now struggled with owning herself and her boundaries. Mr. M held his resolve as well as his newfound groundedness, and their ways of relating began to change. He insisted that she state her needs, and when she did so he respected them. She began to experience trust that she could trust.

Mrs. M's revelation had not been possible in words because she was bound to deny any ulterior motives or manipulations on her part. Once her image was externalized and enacted and she was "in her space," her "real-life" expectations took over. She was in her images, deep in trance, and she was unable to pretend that Mr. M could enter her space without upsetting her. She enacted her real feelings and experience in typical fashion; the body in action did not lie.

This type of metaphoric boundary sculpture can rapidly cut through to the heart of a relationship or an issue. It provides a common experience in the presence of the therapist to which all can refer.

ROPES IN THERAPY

For many years, among other props, I have used ropes in various ways in therapy to represent boundaries physically, to represent betweenness, and to allow clients and me to see the unseeable aspects of relationship, such as the quality of that betweenness. I cannot remember if my own use of rope began before or after I witnessed Virginia Satir using rope to demonstrate how she perceived each person's loss of "the five freedoms" (Satir, Banmen, Gerber, & Gomori, 1991) to which she believed all are born and entitled. Whichever it was, I acknowledge Satir as a role model, mentor, and continued source of encouragement for creativity until her death in 1988.

CASE EXAMPLE 2: FIRST EXPERIENCE USING ROPE

My earliest work with ropes actually started with an extension cord as a metaphor of betweenness. In working with Mr. and Mrs. K, I picked up an extension cord to have them physically play out what I kinesthetically perceived as their verbal "tug-of-war" (Duhl, 1993).

That first enactment allowed the couple to see how much each was invested in the pulling although each proclaimed to hate their fights. Each, when given the instruction to "let go at a moment of your own choosing," did so, with the partner unconsciously throwing the extension cord back to the one who let go, to begin the tugging again. What they discovered was that (a) their fighting served as a way of being in energetic, involved contact with each other and (b) they needed to find other ways of drawing forth that energy with each other. They chose to resume playing tennis together.

I was impressed with how that simple action metaphor moved the therapy to a whole different level. This action metaphor, at once diagnostic and interventive, allowed them to move playfully from the content and perceived causes of their fighting to a total reframing of its causality. They could look at underlying and out-of-awareness expressions of their yearning for active contact and then take corrective actions appropriate to their own wishes and needs.

Diagramming With Ropes

After that, I brought in some pieces of clothesline and began to expand my use of rope in a wide variety of ways. (Originally, I used common cotton or nylon clothesline. After taking those to Japan with me in 1988, I was later presented with wonderful colored cords on my return trips, which I have used ever since.)

I have demonstrated boundaries with ropes on the rug in the office in many different ways, including ropes overlapped, as circles within another circle, as twisted together, as very tight and tiny, and as open arcs without a way of closing. Any depiction is used to demonstrate to individuals, couples, and family members what I hear or see them saying about their relationships with others. I use them as feedback of my understanding, not as an occasion to be "right." In turn, clients also will pick up ropes to show me what they mean. Ropes can be used to depict whatever one wants them to be. This visual feedback tends to move people to a new dimension; that is, out of their egocentric space and into a meta-awareness, a potential consciousness of the whole system.

CASE EXAMPLE 3: DIAGRAMMING BOUNDARIES

Sara argued with her partner, Jim, who had been previously married to Judy, that she did not mind his talking to Judy about Judy and Jim's children. However, Sara did mind whenever Jim shared information with Judy about Jim and Sara as a couple. She felt that he then let his ex-wife into their relationship boundaries. Jim, a very visual and kinesthetic type, could not understand what Sara was saying. It was only when I diagrammed my understanding of what she was saying with ropes that he "got it." (See Figure 4-1.) Once he understood, Jim and Sara began to discuss quite cooperatively what about them was not to be shared with Judy.

The Process

So how is the connection between the verbal and the visual made? It is helpful to consider the concept of boundaries. A boundary is some-

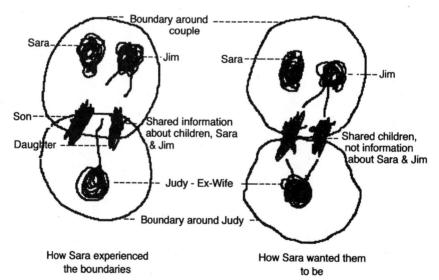

How Sara experienced the boundaries

How Sara wanted them to be

Figure 4-1. Boundary diagram.

thing that goes around, containing something, distinguishing what is inside and what is outside. It is a line or a surface that differentiates in from out.

When Sara, in the example above, stated that she felt that her partner shared information about them that let his ex-wife into their boundaries, I perceived she was talking about privacy, inclusion, and exclusion; that information about the two of them was none of Judy's business; that sharing such information with Judy was like inviting her to be in the room or in their relationship.

Jim could not "get it" in words. Yet, the word *boundary* represents a physical property. Any such physical attribute can be put into physical or active form. Thus, I put into such physical form my understanding of what Sara was saying and what I felt she was implying she wanted. This left it open for her to accept this visual interpretation of her statement or to say, "No, that is not what I mean" and to then change the visual representation of her words and feelings. Once he saw the physical diagram, Jim could understand exactly what Sara meant, could accept it, and could begin to act in accordance with it.

If therapists and trainers can pay attention not only to the meaning of words, but also to what they represent in clients' experiences, they can more easily translate them into their physical or interactive form, in ways that give clients and trainees a new handle on their struggles. And if therapists and trainers also tune into the modes of representation used by clients and trainees, they often can fit that form to their particular mode of understanding. In addition, if therapists and trainers can pay attention to the projections on their own inner screens, when they are fortunate enough for such phenomena to occur, they can externalize and share these in safe ways that can open many new doors to issues.

Rope Sculptures

In the past several years, I have begun to use ropes with clients and trainees as an expansion of various forms of sculpture—as a way of letting them perceive and illustrate (often to themselves for the first time) their multiple relationships in a family, work, or group setting. Thus, there are rope sculptures that involve other people and those that illustrate systems or ideas alone.

Sculpting With Rope With Others

The question here is, "What if people depicted their family systems and the web of relationships using rope as the metaphor of relationship between persons?" With rope used as that metaphor of betweenness, I will ask a trainee, for instance, to do a static sculpture of his or her family of origin. As the trainee positions members of his or her family one at a time, closer or more distant, hierarchically vertical or on the same power level, I ask him or her to use a rope (long or short; loose, tight, or slack) not only from him to each other person, but from each person in the family to each other member. (Although one can do this easily with clothesline, I have found that the colored cords help visually to delineate who is connected to whom and how.) When a person has to put into physical space his or her inner image of relationships, metaphorically using both physical space and rope tension to depict the essence or quality of each relationship, he or she can more easily make manifest the system in all its dimensions in his or her mind. How people see family members as connected or disconnected and how the sculptor feels about others, all come into play.

Role-players ask questions of the sculptor about their relationships and give feedback as to what it is like to be in that role, that position, and with ropes at that tension or slackness. As in sculpting, my directions for receiving feedback are as follows: "Let it come in. Create a basket to put it in and let it sit there. You don't have to accept or reject it. Feedback may or may not match what you expect and what already fits your perceptions. Your 'elves' will work on it while you are busy doing other things. Later, you may want to take out one statement at a time and consider it."

One trainee wrote of her experience:

It is easy to cover up the experience of human emotions with language. For example, I can openly and rather flatly speak about the complex dynamics in my own family of origin. However, when I physically place myself between my parents and sibling, with lines (ropes) of connection to each symbolically, it taps a dramatically different place inside of me . . . my gut and my heart.

Often, members of a family have not given careful consideration to their perceptions of how their own connections may facilitate or block others. Another recent trainee wrote of her experience sculpting her family with the addition of ropes between all members as follows:

I was taken aback at the consciousness I experienced about myself in relation to my family of origin. For instance, I came to realize that my brother's passing at such a young age (21) left an indelible impression in my life even after almost 3 decades of physical absence. . . . I realized too that the bond between my mother, my sister, and myself was much closer and stronger than I thought. I was able to see in the positioning of the ropes, as well, how my father and younger brother were in opposite directions from the three of us. The closeness we three women have had alienated the men from our inner circle, which I could see with the ropes. Apparently, we had built a wall that was not easy to permeate. To me, this was a revelation. Now, I am able to understand why my father and brother created their own inner sanctum and are much closer as a result.

I have learned that such a sculpture reverberates in the mind, body, and psyche for a very long time, involving multiple levels and modes of awareness, like fireworks going off at different times and places. Often, changes in behavior result from such a relatively quick exploration. An individual is forced to consider the total system and how it interacts, and by connecting players with ropes (whether family members, fellow trainees, or work group members), the sculptor has to put his or her deepest perceptions of the quality of relationships of members "out there." The feedback from players or family members enacting this is exceedingly powerful.

A word of caution. A therapist or trainer must be prepared to pick up all kinds of pieces when witnessing such a sculpture. The process is particularly powerful in families. If the family is in great angry turmoil or scapegoating a particular member, sculpting with ropes can become very unsafe. The actions are irreversible, and the scapegoated member will have visual and kinesthetic representations to add to what he or she already knows about being an outsider. On the other hand, when skillfully employed, this process can cut through family members' denial as to what they are doing and how they are affecting other family members.

There are times when people should work out issues while not in the presence of their natural group. In a recent workshop, a doctor chose this nonverbal method with ropes to sort out his work relationships in the hospital where he directed a department. From viewing the positioning and tension of the ropes, one woman role-player was able to say to him, "You don't want me in this job, do you?" To which he replied, "No, actually, I don't. You were hired and put there by somebody other than myself." He had been reluctant to admit to himself that he was not in charge of everything and everyone at all times. He realized also that he had treated this employee badly because he had not selected her himself.

If this doctor had created this rope sculpture in the actual work setting with his staff, all involved would have been in much more revealing and vulnerable positions, particularly as they were in a culture that fostered hierarchy. The therapist or trainer needs to be attuned to such contextual issues and the face-saving steps necessary to prevent participants' self-esteem from being injured.

Sculpting With Rope Alone

When I began using colored ropes, sculptural possibilities expanded. When working with only one person in the room, I have asked the client to sculpt on the rug his or her relationships in family of origin, work, or current living situation. I have also suggested to clients that they sculpt all the issues involved in a problem they are trying to solve, such as time commitments or career planning. I have been continually amazed at how creative people are in this domain.

Once people externalize what their internal perceptions are, they are free to interact with them as if they are separate from the self. They are free to see, to play "what if," and to make changes in perception, which can be followed by changes in action.

Ropes are particularly useful for sculpting relationships, because they are flexible and can be wound around, crossed over, knotted, twisted, used in bunches, moved, used to link several entities, and so on. Such sculptures can be small and tight, or they can use a whole room. Colored ropes can give rise to another level of symbolism, yet they do not have to. That is, some people pay no attention to the color of ropes they choose, whereas others choose particular colors and share the meaning those colors have in the representation of the system they are sculpting. They thus add yet another symbolic dimension of internal perceptions, feelings, and attributes being represented by color as well as form and connections.

THE PROCESS OF CREATING—LEARNING ALONG THE WAY

I spent about 20 years working with clay as a potter and sculptor before I began to study family systems therapy. Early in my career as a therapist, I used to joke that the creative process in pottery and in therapy was the same. That is, that it started with "What if ...?" and that the only difference was that with clay, if you did not like the result, you could smash it and start again!

Over the years, I have found that my original joke has truth to it: The initiating question still is "What if ... ?", which arises in me in context—from the tension of a stuck place, an unsolved issue, or a repeated pattern that does not resolve. I have learned to pay attention to my visceral feelings, the images, and my associations to those visceral feelings as well as to what is going on in the room. For example, with Mr. and Mrs. K and the tug-of-war, I felt pulled in both directions as the observer. Associations to those pulls led me to a feeling of obligation—that I was supposed to do something about the content when there was nothing I could do about it because it consisted of ongoing disagreements about who said what when. Another association was to a sense of futility—a feeling that I was supposed to be the judge and take sides, which I rejected.

Another way to approach this was to ask "What does this remind me of?" In such an instance, one draws on the whole of one's life experiences and imagination (for that is where metaphors come from). The image came to mind of a tug-of-war, with no one winning, yet the pulling back and forth with high energy and intensity continued endlessly. This fit with what I had learned early in family therapy: to attend to the process, not the content.

I have learned to pay attention to the staying power of an image, attending to and observing how long it remains in my mind while I continue to pay attention externally to the people in the room. It is interesting to focus on what is going on in the room and to become aware if the image then intrudes on what you think you are doing. This involves paying attention to the life of the mind while doing something else, like the dreaming mind while we sleep. Over time, I have learned to trust that the unconscious mind offers gifts and resources at a deeper level of authenticity and that it symbolically puts together elements to create new scenarios at a different level of understanding, that of process of what is happening and what it is *really* about.

And then comes the moment to grab the image (tug-of-war), allowing myself time to bring it into conscious awareness, taking the sometimes risky step of sharing the image with those who stimulated it, in a way that feels safe and inviting them to enter and participate, in an atmosphere without blame. Here, experience is the great teacher—the more a therapist or trainer takes risks in this domain, the more he or she can feel comfortable and playful with sharing such images. One of the main things I have learned is that clients and trainees will participate with me only if they feel that I am comfortable with the idea of movement and action. This means I get out of my chair first, then ask if they will join me, play with me, humor me, or whatever phrase fits. It is important to disqualify whatever it is I have in mind to render it safe for them to take the risk of entering the unknown with me. I say that the image might contain some good information or it might be off the wall and that I would like to explore it with them.

It is critical that my ego be uninvolved in whether my image is "right" or not, for my "win" can be my client's "loss." If I am way off base then I get new information that can realign me with the client or trainee.

Once people enact a metaphor such as the tug-of-war engaged in by Mr. and Mrs. K or participate as observers seeing ropes on the floor depicting boundaries, we can then discuss how the metaphor fits the situation and whether it is particular to the immediate issue or generic in the whole relationship. We talk about what it was like to do it. Often I hear that it was new and different and that they did not know what to expect. This is significant, for what is not expected cannot be defended against. We discuss options and perhaps try out new behaviors then and there.

Information from any enactment or new creative invention occurs on at least two levels. First, the client receives new information about himself or herself and his or her processes. Second, the therapist or trainer receives new information about the usefulness of the image in a particular case and its generic nature and ability to be generalized to other, similar situations. In either case, the action metaphor is a structure for exploration, a route of access to new information at different levels of awareness.

The more I take risks with my own creativity, the more I learn about myself as well as others, and the more I build associative connections within myself to be used as both verbal and enacted metaphor. I then begin to find ways of bridging to generic situations with people, creating a store-house of metaphoric processes that later someone else labels "technique." Yet, for the therapist-creator, tapping one's own resources in this fashion keeps oneself and therapy and training alive, interesting, fresh, and even fun at times. And, it invites clients and trainees to tap their own creativity, which is after all, the highest function of a human mind. It is also the goal in therapy, for people to "do something different" than what holds them prisoner to their habitual behaviors, thought patterns, and feelings.

CONCLUSION

There are endless possibilities for externalizing with action metaphors, creating new forms with which to explore new ideas and new possibilities with clients and trainees. The same prescription—to do something different—fits therapists as well as clients when caught in a routine or pattern. Therapy is never boring when the therapist's creativity is involved while tapping creative resources and strengths in clients as well. In order to try something different, you need only "pick up your courage stick" (an item in Satir's self-esteem maintenance kit [Satir et al., 1991]) and go create something new. You cannot make a mistake. You can only get new information.

REFERENCES

Argyris, C., & Schon, D. (1974). *Theory in practice: Increasing professional effectiveness.* San Francisco: Jossey-Bass.

Duhl, B. S. (1983). *From the inside out and other metaphors: Creative and integrative approaches to training in systems thinking.* New York: Brunner/Mazel. (Now available from the author at 2 Bellis Court, Cambridge, MA 02140.)

Duhl, B. S. (1993). Metaphor in action. *The Family Therapy Networker, 17*(6), 49–51.

Duhl, F. J., Kantor, D., & Duhl, B. S. (1973). Learning, space and action in family therapy: A primer of sculpture. In D. Bloch (Ed.), *Techniques of family psychotherapy* (pp. 47–63). New York: Grune & Stratton.

Moreno, J. L. (1946). *Psychodrama.* New York: Beacon Press.

Satir, V., Banmen, J., Gerber, J., & Gomori, M. (1991). *The Satir model: Family therapy and beyond.* Palo Alto, CA: Science and Behavior Books.

II

THERAPIES USING THEATRICAL FORMS

5

DRAMA THERAPY IN ACTION

RENÉE EMUNAH

Drama therapy is an active and creative approach to psychotherapy in which dramatic processes are used to facilitate therapeutic growth and change. In applying this art form to psychotherapy, clients have the opportunity to experiment with real life in a laboratorylike setting in which they can preview, rehearse, review, and revise life roles. The dramatic mode liberates clients from real-life constraints and from imbedded patterns, affording them a means of expanding their behavioral and role repertoires.

But drama therapy is not only about role expansion and behavioral change. Within an environment of play and pretence, clients' spontaneity and imagination are engaged, inhibitions dissolve, and the unconscious comes closer to the surface. According to drama therapist David Read Johnson, drama therapy is a kind of psychoanalytic free association in action (Johnson, 1991). Whatever comes to mind is played out. Even with drama therapy approaches that are more structured than Johnson's developmental transformations, play and "playing it out" (Erikson, 1950) are central components.

To some drama therapists, playing it out means being in an imaginative realm in which fantasies and images are embodied and transformed as they emerge (Johnson, 1991; Johnson, Forrester, & Dintino, 1996); to other drama therapists, playing it out means replaying actual life encounters (such encounters may have occurred recently or long ago). Between these two extremes lies a vast range of dramatic possibilities—including extended improvisation of fictional scenarios, interactive theatrical techniques, storytelling, dramatic ritual, and self-revelatory performance.

Regardless of the particular dramatic activity used, ordinary time and place are transcended. In the psychodramatic replay of real-life events, the pain from the past is brought to life, relived, and reexperienced in the body. Distance between past and present is bridged; memory comes alive, and with it, sensation and emotion. Intellectualization, or a gap between thought and feeling—a common hazard in traditional verbal therapy—is unlikely to occur in action-oriented drama therapy. As in all dynamic, action-oriented approaches to psychotherapy, the present moment is charged. Verbal processing is integrated into the dramatic action selectively; that is, when it enhances insight without inhibiting or disrupting the flow of the overall action-oriented process.

Drama therapy was established as a field in the United States in 1979 with the founding of the National Association for Drama Therapy. Like the other creative arts therapies, drama therapy emerged from the art form of drama; drama began to be applied to healing, psychotherapy, and education. However, drama therapy is profoundly connected and indebted to the older discipline of psychodrama and specifically to the brilliant visionary, Jacob L. Moreno (1946, 1959; Moreno & Moreno, 1969), who originated psychodrama in the 1920s.

How is drama therapy different from psychodrama? In my view, the two fields are far more similar than different. However, there also are clear distinctions in both concept and clinical practice. In group work, which is most typical of both psychodrama and drama therapy, psychodrama focuses on one person in the group at a time, the protagonist, who reenacts scenes that are clearly connected to his or her actual life dilemmas and unresolved issues. Although the group is involved as audience or as actors in the protagonist's drama, the therapy is nonetheless individually oriented. Drama therapy, on the other hand, is oriented more toward group process and interaction rather than focused on a single person. More important, the scenes in drama therapy are not necessarily directly related to the person's real-life experiences. Drama therapy uses more improvisation of fictional scenes, with the belief that engaging in the world of make-believe allows not only a healthy sense of freedom but also a protective disguise that actually enables self-revelation.

Drama therapists, who are required to have a theater background to become registered, use a wide array of theatrical processes—including not only psychodramatic role-playing, role reversal, and reenactment but also improvisation, adapted theater games, storytelling, puppetry, masks, mime, movement, and scripted scenes. Obviously, the decision about which of these processes to use depends on the population, age group, therapeutic needs of the individual client, stage within treatment, and theoretical approach and affinities of the drama therapist.

KEY APPROACHES WITHIN THE FIELD OF DRAMA THERAPY

One of the central debates within the field involves whether it is important to connect what emerges in the realm of play and pretence to real life. Some believe that healing takes place within the realm of metaphor and fiction and that interpretation is unnecessary and can even be contraindicated; others believe that it is in understanding the connection between one's acting and one's life that much of the therapy occurs. Along with this question is that of whether the fictional dramatic work should lead to psychodramatic work or whether it is best to sustain a client's engagement in imaginative, symbolic play and let psychodrama remain a separate discipline.

David Read Johnson developed a form of drama therapy, developmental transformations, in which "roles and scenes are constantly transformed and reshaped according to the clients' ongoing stream of consciousness and internal imagery" (Johnson, 1991, p. 11). Within this playful and dynamic method, there is no interpretation or verbal processing. The client remains in the "playspace"—generally along with the drama therapist, who engages with him or her but does not interpret the action.

Drama therapist Robert Landy works in a more structured fashion through his role method (Landy, 1990, 1993). Believing that role is the primary healing component of drama, Landy has clients invoke and identify a role, play out this role (usually within the container of a story), explore various aspects of the role, and then relate the fictional role to their real life. In contrast to Johnson's method, the drama therapist is more of a witness and director than a fellow player. One role at a time is sustained, expanded, and developed, and reflection on each role is a critical part of the therapeutic process. In Johnson's more fluid approach, the focus is more on discarding than on developing roles.

Landy's belief in the importance of working through the fictional mode and then relating the fictional to real life is similar to that of many British drama therapists, although the specific methods they use may differ. In the work of Alida Gersie (1991; Gersie & King, 1990), clients identify with classical, cross-cultural, personal, and improvised stories, and in doing so explore their own concerns and themes. Sue Jennings (1987, 1995a, 1995b), a British drama therapist and international pioneer in the field, works within a theatrical context, often using scripts. For Jennings, like Landy and Gersie, the fictional, symbolic, and metaphorical realms are central. In her current work, Jennings (1995a, 1995b) foregoes interpretation; in her view, healing takes place through the drama itself. Jennings's work, which stems from her anthropological and theatrical background, is also permeated with ritual.

My approach is based on a five-phase integrative model (Emunah, 1994, 1996) in which the therapeutic journey is paced and progressive. It offers a sense of unfolding; each phase paves the way for the next phase, gradually spiraling the series of sessions toward deeper levels of intimacy and self-revelation. The work progresses from (a) interactive dramatic play, to (b) developed theatrical (and fictional) scenework, to (c) role-playing dealing with personal situations, to (d) culminating psychodramatic enactments exploring core life themes, to (e) dramatic ritual related to closure. The fictional mode provides a protective safeguard as well as a means of expanding clients' capacities for (and range of) expression. But eventually the roles are shed and the masks unraveled, and the fictional scenarios give way to life scenes. Grotowski's (1968) comparison of acting to sculpting is relevant at these later stages: He described the acting process as one of chiseling away all that is excess and discarding roles until one arrives at the innermost form.

The shift from the fictional to the personal is dictated by the clients; it is an organic process in which the therapist is attentive to the point at which the clients naturally and spontaneously make personal connections to the fictional enactments. The first two phases afford a sense of liberation and expansion and also elicit the clients' most healthy selves as their spontaneity, creativity, and imagination are generated. The personal work that follows emerges from the fictional scenes and the individual client's associations to these scenes, thereby circumventing the danger of having preconceived notions of the client's issues when embarking on psychodramatic work.

My approach is eclectic, encompassing the wide array of processes, techniques, healing properties, and possibilities inherent in the medium of drama therapy. It occurs in a sequenced fashion, involving careful reflection and perception on the part of the drama therapist regarding the level and needs of the particular clients. The dramatic play in Phase 1 is reminiscent of aspects of Johnson's playful work, which emphasizes spontaneity. Like Johnson, I am also concerned with an overall developmental progression —from simplicity to complexity. However, Johnson's approach has a greater emphasis on free association and on freeing up the client's inner world. Johnson's Developmental Transformations is a well-developed, intricate, and innovative system unto itself.

The sustained theatrical scenes in Phase 2, involving developed roles and characters, are reminiscent of aspects of Landy's work. Like Landy, I believe that making connections to one's real life is important, although I wait for this to occur naturally rather than directing the process. Once it occurs, I know that before long we will be entering Phase 3. In Landy's role method, the process is typically one of beginning with a role, making connections to that role, and then playing another role, and so on. In contrast, in the five-phase integrative model, clients will play many roles over time, without making personal connections. The lack of processing is intended to decrease inhibition and expand clients' sense of freedom and possibility. But at a certain point, connections are made spontaneously. This generally occurs when the fictional scenes have become more emotionally evocative and intense and when the relationships between therapist and client and among group members have become more solidified. After a period of time in which clients play out scenes and discuss their personal associations and responses to these enactments, the fictional mode dissolves, and the dramatic enactment of real-life material takes its place.

Phases 3 and 4 are psychodramatic in nature, although there also are distinctions between the drama therapy work occurring at these stages and classical psychodrama (see Emunah, 1994). There are an increasing number of psychodramatists whose works are similar to drama therapy and begin to bridge the gap between the two disciplines. Key among them are Adam Blatner (1991; Blatner & Blatner, 1988), who stresses the therapeutic significance of play and also advances theory regarding role-playing and role dynamics, and Jonathan Fox (1981, 1994), who developed playback theater. Playback is a blend of psychodrama, drama therapy, and community theater, in which audience members tell personal stories that are then played back by a troupe of actors who dramatically and aesthetically convey the essence of the story. Playback theater is one of the many ways in which dramatic methods can be used outside the therapy office and within the larger community.

A BEGINNING METHOD: LINE REPETITION

Drama therapy uses numerous and diverse processes and techniques, and the variations on these methods are endless (Emunah, 1994). This chapter offers only a peek at what might take place in a particular drama therapy session. The reader should keep in mind that he or she is glimpsing only a small fraction—from a single angle—of a very broad field. It is also important to note that the drama therapist constantly modifies and adapts given techniques to meet particular clinical needs.

One of the action methods I use most in drama therapy is what I refer to as *line repetition* (Emunah, 1994). This method can be used, with different objectives and outcomes, with any age group or population. The method involves breaking the group into pairs (or in individual therapy, the therapist partnering with the client). Each pair engages in a conversation using only two lines. The most commonly used lines are "I want it" and "You can't have it!" The lines can be said in numerous ways, according to a wide array of emotional attitudes and strategies and with a range of intonations and voices (from whispering to screaming), but participants are instructed to use only these words.

Despite the initial verbal aspect of this method, line repetition progresses into action and enactment. The method is an ideal warm-up to theatrical improvisation because it immediately alleviates clients' anxieties about acting and improvising. The focus is on expression, communication, and emotion rather than on about what lines to say next. The structure and simplicity of the method, in conjunction with its emphasis on a basic emotional conflict, easily engages clients and elicits their dramatic skills. The repetition of conflictual lines tends to invite powerful and evocative moments of theater.

On a therapeutic level, the method addresses one of the most central objectives in drama therapy: the expression and containment of emotion (Emunah, 1983, 1995). Dramatic acting that is therapeutically oriented enables clients to identify, acknowledge, express, and release strong emotion. Equally important in drama therapy is helping clients achieve a sense of distance from—and mastery over—their emotions. Obviously, clients who have lost contact with their emotional lives or who have difficulty communicating feelings (i.e., overdistanced) will require more help with expression; clients who are overwhelmed by feeling or lose control when they become emotional (i.e., underdistanced) will need more help with containment. For the majority of clients, however, the therapeutic focus is on the dynamic interplay between the two edges of the emotional expression–containment continuum. The experience of simultaneous expression of strong feeling and containment of (or mastery over) these feelings can bring about a sense of catharsis and inner strength.

In using line repetition over many years of work with adult psychiatric clients, I have been impressed by how clients who typically manifest very minimal affect will become quite expressive during this exercise. In this playful, nonthreatening context, these clients begin to experience emotional expression in safe, paced doses. Equally impressive is the extent to which acting-out adolescents who typically have little sense of control over their feelings will maintain full control even as they unabashedly emote feelings within this exercise. The structure of the exercise provides natural boundaries and limits.

I most often incorporate line repetition at the start of Phase 2—that is, once an atmosphere of play and spontaneity as well as a degree of trust and rapport have been established. Clients generally are not yet comfortable or skilled at improvising and developing scenes, but they have become accustomed to engaging in dramatic play and are ready for more emotionally evocative dramatic activity.

Any lines or words may be used, from a basic "Yes!"–"No!" to a more complex "Help me."–"I can't." Combinations of lines can be devised to address specific individual or group issues. A set of lines that I initiated to facilitate exploration of issues related to separation, autonomy, dependency, and loss is "I want to go."–"I need you to stay." Such evocative lines are best used only when the group has reached some level of trust and readiness to explore personal themes. The more basic "Yes"–"No" words allow for greater distance and are therefore more appropriate for a group or client that needs more emotional containment. The therapist also may choose to use lines that are more geared toward helping clients practice new behavioral stances rather than emphasizing emotional expression. An example of lines aimed at self-assertion is "I can do it."–"No you can't."

It is important to lead into all dramatic processes gradually and gracefully, so that participants are properly warmed up. Line repetition is best preceded by a physical warm-up that relates to the nature of the conflict to follow. For example, as a lead-in to the lines "I want it."–"You can't have it.", each pair stands back-to-back and push against each other as if their backs are engaged in an argument and one person is attempting to get the other moving forward while the other resists.

During line repetition, directions entailing physical action may be added to develop and dramatically intensify the interaction. Such an instruction might be as follows: "If you're saying 'You can't have it,' try to run away from your partner, to get rid of him or her. But if you want it, don't let your partner get out of your sight!" The reversal of roles when participants seem to come to a spontaneous ending point is a natural way of extending the exercise. The therapist-director simply states, "Switch roles," intentionally avoiding any lengthy verbal instructions that would break the theatrical momentum.

In group work, each pair may be asked to perform an interaction in front of the other group members. Such miniperformances tend to elicit a series of unique vignettes, each one displaying the actors' humor, playfulness, and dramatic expressiveness. Improvisational scene work can be initiated by asking clients to spontaneously incorporate other lines as the impulse arises. Gradually, a particular relationship between the two actors is established, and the nature of the conflict is clarified. Another way of developing scenes is for the clients to decide in advance on a situation in which two characters would be saying these lines or to ask the audience to prescribe the specific situation to be played out.

Discussion following line repetition generally revolves around emotional responses and associations to the lines. A helpful way of initiating discussion and self-reflection is to ask participants which side of the conflict felt more comfortable or familiar and whether any particular relationships came to mind. Dramatic scene work that follows a discussion that has been self-revealing tends to be more personal and often psychodramatic in nature.

Examples Using Line Repetition

Each client and group brings to line repetition their own unique styles and themes. The following are examples drawn from the use of the lines "I want it."–"You can't have it.":

Andy, a frightened 3-year-old boy in individual therapy, has had little sense of control in his chaotic life. He is also undergoing developmentally appropriate issues related to assertion and autonomy. He relishes repeating "No! You can't have it!" He clutches the basketball with which we had just been playing and delights in hearing me plead for it (and also in watching me "break role" intermittently to remind him that in our game he has permission to keep telling me "No!"). His voice and gestures become increasingly animated as he fervently restates his lines.

Adolescents in a residential treatment program devise scenes related to the lines they have just been dramatically repeating. In one scene, a 16-year-old boy wants the keys to the car, but his father refuses because the last time the car was borrowed, the boy damaged it. A 15-year-old girl asks for permission to go to a party, but her parents forbid her because they do not trust that she will stay sober. The teens enact these scenes with impressive realism. The ensuing role reversal enables them to gain some understanding of the perspective of the parents and serves as a catalyst for a dynamic group discussion.

With a group of female creative arts therapy students in Israel, I notice the participants' tendency to rapidly focus improvisational interactions on something concrete. Two women are performing line repetition in front of the group. One of the women, Dorit, is religious and is wearing a hat. When invited to add new words, the other woman, Gila, immediately exclaims, "I want your hat!" Dorit responds emphatically, "I can't give it to you. I need to be wearing it always." The animated exchange provokes much laughter in the audience as the tension related to religious and political differences is playfully addressed and diffused.

Annette, a 40-year-old woman in a group of recovering addicts, becomes very emotional as she cries out, "I want it. . . ." Her voice becomes childlike, and soon there is a faint tremor, accompanied by a sense of deep longing and pain. Now there is a wail, stemming from some primal place, as she repeats the words that clearly evoke intense wounding; she has reentered her child self, who is craving love. The group has been meeting for some time, and I know there is enough support among the members to tolerate and contain this expression of emotional pain. Later, another group member assumes the role of the child Annette, as adult Annette reaches out to her with compassion and nurturance.

At the session following the one mentioned above, the group divides into pairs. One person is to once again repeat "I want it," but this time the partner responds with "You *can* have it." Many clients become tearful, later claiming that it felt rare and unfamiliar both to ask for something and to receive an affirmative response. I then add an exercise in which each person begins with the words "I want" and then finishes the sentence with something he or she actually wants (e.g., love, peace of mind, to be able to soothe myself, hope).

AN ADVANCED METHOD: SELF-SCULPTURES

The following method, which I refer to as *self-sculptures* (Emunah, 1994), is a means of aesthetically (both visually and dramatically) externalizing internal feelings and states, thereby facilitating self-examination and helping clients achieve clarity and mastery. Depending on how the method develops and the kinds of interventions used, the method also can evoke the expression of intense emotions and result in a powerful experience of catharsis.

Self-sculptures is most often used in group therapy, but it can be adapted to individual or family therapy. It is best used with adult or adolescent clients who are at a mid to high level of functioning and possess a fair amount of insight—or who are at least capable of self-examination. The method is optimal at a later stage of therapeutic work, when a group has already achieved a high level of intimacy and self-disclosure as well as sufficient dramatic skills and ease so that roles are played with the authenticity and complexity they warrant. (In the five-phase model, this method usually is used at the beginning of Phase 4.) It can be incorporated at earlier phases of a group's development, but the ensuing work will then be less emotionally rich and revealing.

There are a number of developmental stages within the five-phase model, and each one can stand on its own, with the therapist stopping at any point:

1. One person is asked to sculpt or mold three others of the group to represent various aspects of himself or herself. The persons selected to be in the protagonist's sculpture respond like clay, allowing their bodies to be positioned according to the protagonist's wishes. The protagonist intentionally places the three parts in relation to one another (e.g., a psychically dominant part may be placed in front of, or blocking, the others). Although three is the usual number, any number of parts/people may be selected.
2. Once the sculpture is complete, the protagonist is asked to stand by each part and verbally identify it (e.g., "I'm the part

of Diana that is very critical—of myself and of everyone else."). The protagonist then gives each part a representative line to say. He or she stands back and watches as the sculpture "comes alive," with each role-player not only stating the given line but also embodying in tone, gesture, and movement the part he or she represents. After a few minutes, the miniscene is frozen in action, becoming a sculpture once again. The protagonist-director may wish to modify or redirect the actors to refine the representation of his or her internal self-image.

3. The protagonist then is asked to take over one of the roles. The dramatic interaction becomes an open-ended improvisation, with each player moving and speaking freely. The emotional and dramatic tension is heightened by the protagonist's action in the scene, as he or she best knows the intricacies of each part of himself or herself and the way they interface with the other parts. After some time, the protagonist is asked to embody another of the roles, until he or she has had the experience of assuming all of the roles. The last role usually is the most emotionally challenging and intense; this is the role the protagonist may have intentionally avoided playing earlier.

At this point, the drama therapist can intervene in various ways, according to the issues that are evoked. Possible interventions include directing the protagonist to (a) step outside the scene and make revisions that symbolize his or her hopes for inner change or psychic integration (sometimes entailing the addition of a new part); (b) address each of the parts from the vantage point of the self-observing ego that can witness and guide himself or herself or offer self-acceptance; (c) focus on two parts only, thereby intensifying the examination of aspects of the self that seem to be at the heart of the protagonist's struggle; (d) take on the role of a double for a part that seems to be holding back information or expression.

CASE EXAMPLE: SELF-SCULPTURES

The following example is taken from an outpatient group of high-functioning adults. Wendy is a 28-year-old woman who is pursuing a master's degree in sociology. She works part-time as a receptionist for a social action organization. She has intermittently been involved in sociopolitical work and also in dance. Wendy is often critical and angry or self-critical and depressed. She suffered a major loss in her childhood: Her older brother died of leukemia when Wendy was 12 years old. It is our 15th session, and I have introduced self-sculptures.

Case Narrative

Using three members of the group, Wendy creates a sculpture depicting parts of herself.

Tom is placed in a standing position, with one arm behind his back with a clenched fist; the other arm is outstretched, pointing a finger accusingly toward Karen. Karen is half-kneeling, also with an arm outstretched, but the hand is open, beseeching, as if asking for help or forgiveness. Janice is placed in a seated position between them, with her back facing the group/audience. Her legs are crossed, as are her arms, which rest with palms upward in her lap.

I ask Wendy to stand behind each part and tell the audience something about it.

"This is the part of me that is critical and angry, at the world and at myself."

She then moves slowly to the seated player in the center. "This part is meditating, trying to stay centered."

Hesitantly, she goes over to the kneeling figure. She looks at her sadly. "This is the part that is needy and wants to be accepted."

"Can you give each of them a line?" I ask.

She comes up with lines for the first two roles easily. For the critical part, "You screwed up again!" And for the other, "Om...."

Commentary

There is a both a tension and an aesthetic balance to this sculpture, which speaks for itself, showing graphically more than words could easily express about what goes on inside Wendy.

Now that the work has been registered visually and aesthetically, I want Wendy to communicate in words—to the group and to herself —what these parts represent.

I note her hesitation again before the kneeler.

"I'm sorry, forgive me."

I am struck by these words, and I realize that the scene we are about to see will likely be emotional and painful. I glance at the group, our audience. Their faces are attentive and their expressions compassionate.

"Come back here and look at the sculpture," I say softly. I stand next to her. "That's about right," she says.

"Are you willing to see the sculpture come alive?"

"Yeah."

I note her nonverbal language as well, to assess her readiness.

"You can say "Action," and then say "Cut" whenever you want to. You can let it go on for just a few seconds or let it roll for a few minutes."

I want her to feel in command so that she is not overwhelmed by witnessing the enactment of her internal psyche.

She says, "Action." After about a minute she says, "Freeze." I ask what she thinks and feels and whether the depiction seems accurate.

Her choice of words is interesting—*freeze* instead of *cut*—perhaps implying her willingness to continue the work.

In response to the latter part of my question, she says that the accusatory part needs to be much stronger and fiercer and that the meditator should also be louder, to block out the rest. She goes to the sculpture and places the meditator's hands over her ears and also sets her further in the background. Remolding the part seeking forgiveness, she bends Karen's knees more, which results in a shakier, less stable position and a more vulnerable, childlike stance.

It is becoming clear that the meditator is attempting to block out or deny feelings and conflict.
I feel for the pain of this part of Wendy.

The sculpture comes alive again. The actors play their roles with greater energy and emotional commitment. Wendy looks mesmerized. After a few minutes, she says, "Cut."

I look at her, waiting for her words.

"Yes, that's it. It's hard to watch."

"What are you feeling?"

"It's sad to see what I'm dealing with internally all the time, the pain of it."

"Yes, I know." [Pause.] "Are you willing to enter it?"

"Yeah. I'm in it anyway," she says with the faintest grin.

I want to develop this work further, toward some healing (or insight or integration); yet I also want Wendy to feel empowered along the way— to choose whether or how far to move into yet more emotional terrain. For sculptures with this kind of intensity, I believe it is fruitless to ask the sculptor at this point to simply revise the sculpture according to how he or she would like his or her internal dynamics to be modified. The protagonist needs to enter the drama—and the emotional territory —more fully before being able to create some distance and new perspective. I trust that the dramatic process we are embarking on will lead the way toward some healing.

Wendy becomes the meditator. Her chants are louder and louder, with a frantic edge.

Next, she becomes the accusatory part. She begins by denouncing politicians and social ills.

"And what about her?" I ask from "off-stage," glancing at the childlike part.

"And you, you keep screwing up," she responds in role. "You're no good. You're late on your assignments, you blew your last relationship, and there you are just groveling. You look pitiful. Stop groveling." Her partner, improvising, mutters, "But forgive me, accept me."

"How can I, you disgust me!" she aggressively retorts. After these words, she breaks out of her role to tell me that this accusatory part is actually much more intense than she can portray.

I note the part she chose to play first. Clients often select the least emotionally threatening part first.

I ask Tom and another group member to join her in this role. They repeat and add to her critical accusations. I ask Janice as the meditator to sit in silence. In the midst of the fiery accusations, Wendy suddenly exclaims, "You should have been like your brother." When I ask her to repeat this line, she shouts, "You should have been your brother."

Wendy is trembling and crying. I go over to her. Gently, I ask her if these are thoughts she has been aware of, if these are familiar lines coming from the critical part of herself. She softly responds, "No, but I guess this is what I think my father thought. I guess I felt guilty . . . for not being more like my brother and for not being the one to die."

I suggest that Wendy now assume the role of the beseeching part. She makes this transition naturally. "Please forgive me for not being him," she pleads. "For not being good enough."

She is silent.

I motion to Karen to assume this role again, and I ask Wendy to stand behind Karen, becoming the double who voices internal feelings or thoughts of the beseeching part. Wendy speaks quietly, almost as though she were talking to herself. "I feel guilty." [Long pause.] "I'm so lonely. For my brother, and for myself. For who I was before we lost him. My parents are thinking of him, missing him all the time. I feel so alone."

I want to help her portray this part in all its intensity and to offer her support as this takes place. This part, now magnified, becomes much more forceful, intense, and chilling.

I notice that Wendy's voice seems to have taken on a deeper, masculine tone.

I want to soothe her pain, but I know that we need to get more fully into this drama—with all its pain—before coming out of it and that the soothing will need to come from Wendy. While moving through it, I can serve as her ally, witness, and guide.

I sense that she has suddenly pulled back, become slightly more distanced from the drama. I wonder whether there are some feelings or thoughts she is struggling to keep at bay.

I am hoping the role of the double will enable Wendy to access and express more.

I notice that her voice sounds younger.

I motion to the three remaining group members—those who have been the audience—to join her. They echo her words and her feelings of loss, guilt, and loneliness. As if buoyed by their support, she says, in role, "I'm not my brother. I never was like him, can never be like him, can never replace him. But what happened wasn't my fault. And who I am has to be good enough."

I am conscious of wanting to actively engage those who have been witnessing one person's scene for some time. I also want Wendy to feel supported and accompanied at this point of loneliness. These group members seem eager to transition from witnesses to participants in the drama.

Still standing near her, I softly tell her to repeat the words "You're good enough."

I want to underscore and to have Wendy hear herself say these important words.

As she says these words, the tears come again. I mention to her that in saying these words, she seems to be embodying another part of herself. I ask her to identify this part. "It's the nurturing part of me," she responds. I ask her to continue the scene, saying the same words, and any others that come, but to now direct these words to the beseeching part of herself. I remove everyone else from the scene.

I feel it is important for Wendy to identify (and ultimately foster) this part of herself.

I want the entire focus to be on Wendy's nurturing self addressing the part of her that craves forgiveness.

Wendy repeats, "You're good enough," and then simply, "You're enough." In a genuinely gentle manner, she adds, "I'm here with you. I'll be with you always." Spontaneously, she puts her arm around Karen. Karen leans on her, and soon Wendy is holding her as she tearfully comforts her.

I am moved, especially by the sense of healing that I feel is taking place.

Wendy briefly looks up, stating she needs the meditator to now come. Janice reenters the scene. "Tell her what you need from her," I interject. Wendy says, "I need you to be with me, not over there on your own. Your meditation cannot be used to block us out. You have to embrace and contain us."

I feel that Wendy is now ready to consider and move toward behavior changes.

I suggest that the three of them, who
are now huddled together, address
the accusatory part. Tom reenters the
scene, reiterating his critical accusations. Wendy, along with her
now-soothed beseecher and her
more authentically grounded meditator, asserts her needs for acceptance,
and he softens his stance. Wendy
tells him to direct passionate,
critical energy outward, toward
social ills that require committed action.

I now ask Wendy to step outside of
the revised scene and to watch it
from a distance. She does this literally, by standing on a chair and looking down at the scene. Again, she
looks engrossed by the dramatic display of her churning and changing
internal dynamics.

I want to see what else may occur to
her as she gains some distance. I also
want to begin working toward closure of the scene.

Suddenly, she says, "There is another
part. She wants to move." I ask her
to show us this new part by assuming
it. She crouches close to the meditator and then gracefully emerges, as
though out of a cocoon, and begins
to dance. Her eyes are closed,
and her movements are slow and
fluid.

There is an impulse within her, and I
do not want to curtail it by having
her direct or explain.

As she dances, I encourage her to relate to each of her parts. Over the
vulnerable beseeching part of her,
her arms gently flutter, as though
sprinkling something cleansing. She
does a powerful energized dance
around the accusatory part, thrusting
loud breaths and movements outward. Beside the nurturing, accepting
part, her movements seem to convey
graciousness and love. Before the
meditating part she becomes still,
with her hands clasped in a prayerful
pose. Then she opens her arms wide,
encompassing the whole of the sculpture.

Her dance indeed seems to be an
outgrowth of a meditation.

"Freeze," I say softly. It is here that the scene ends, and after a few silent minutes the group comes together, seated in a circle.

I end the scene here so that this poignant moment can be held, highlighted, and remembered.

Through self-sculptures, Wendy was able to identify internal facets of herself, express and embody conflicting emotions, explore and gain insight into underlying sources of her pain, and achieve a sense of mastery and internal strength along with hope for her future.

RESISTANCE

Drama therapy is not composed of isolated techniques, but rather involves a developmental process comprising smooth transitions and interconnected methods (Emunah, 1994). Resistance is minimized when the work is paced, with each step leading organically to the next (Emunah, 1985, 1996). The therapist should carefully choose methods that will ease clients' entrance into both the dramatic language and self-revelatory experience. The therapist should be keenly aware of clients' fears and anxieties related to the process and help to both ensure the safety of the experience as well as challenge clients in accordance with their level of capacity.

Clients often are apprehensive that drama therapy will involve childish play, acting other than how they feel or who they are, or humiliating performance. It is important that the therapist immediately dispel these fears by choosing age-appropriate and process-oriented methods (rather than performance-oriented techniques) that make use of clients' actual state of being rather than asking them to play characters.

Over the years, I have worked with very resistant groups, including acting-out adolescents and severely depressed adults. In drama therapy, clients are first invited to enact actual feelings and emotional states, rather than ones that are foreign. For example, acting-out clients may enact—in the context of a dramatic game—rebelliousness or hostility, thereby immediately experiencing an acknowledgment of who they are and how they feel at the same time that they experience success at the activity. The exaggeration of actual behavior promotes humor and perspective on the behavior (Emunah, 1983) and gradually enables clients to experiment with alternate behaviors. The activation—as opposed to the suppression—of the resistance releases energy that can be channeled constructively and creatively.

Similarly, the passive and depressed states in which I find many adult psychiatric clients are incorporated into the dramatic activity. In a game in which one person leaves the room while the others decide on a mood that the whole group will display when the person returns (and then tries to guess the group mood), clients frequently suggest enacting "depressed," "tired," or "lonely." These feeling states are thus acknowledged and actively expressed; paradoxically, the clients gain a degree of distance from the enacted mood. Additionally, I find that methods geared toward a high level of nonthreatening interaction reduce resistance with this population. Breaking through the isolation many of these patients experience creates a shift in their depressive state, releases some energy, and transforms passivity into activity within the session.

Little resistance is encountered in drama therapy with younger children, for whom play (including dramatic play) is part of their natural mode of self-expression. However, in work with children whose childhoods have been interrupted by traumatic or painful experiences, embodied role-playing can be threatening. Beginning with more distanced play involving the use of objects (e.g., puppets or dolls) rather than a child's own body reduces resistance.

The relationship between therapist and client is always at the heart of therapeutic work, and it is the primary factor that diminishes clients' resistance to action-oriented work. In group work, the relationships among group members are also crucial in sustaining participants' involvement and commitment to the treatment process. The interactive nature of dramatic activity helps to promote interrelationships within the group and also fosters a playful, flexible, and trusting relationship between the therapist and individual clients.

FROM DRAMA TO REAL LIFE

The dramatic mode is powerful, and the therapist may be surprised by the degree of transformation that can occur within a single session. However, the degree to which the changes experienced within the dramatic setting are integrated into a client's life hinges largely on the length of treatment. Often the dramas played out in session are one step ahead of a client's real-life capabilities. But these dramas are drawn from a client's potentialities, and the ongoing playing out of the dramas strengthens the client's belief in and assimilation of these potentialities. Over time, the client experiences an increasing connection between what is possible in drama and what is possible in life.

New facets of the self emerge in role and become precursors of real-life roles and relationships. Sometimes a client consciously uses drama to preview real life, whereas at other times the playing out is not conscious. Recently discarded parts also reemerge in role-plays. As the client changes and lets go of undesired parts of his or her self, these parts occasionally find a place for themselves within the dramatic arena, as though needing to take a break from dormancy. The dramatic arena serves as an outlet and forum for the new and the old, the intolerable and the hoped for, shadow and shame, dreams and aspirations.

The dramatic arena not only embraces past and future but also magnifies the present. Clients bring issues from daily life into the dramatic mode, and in the replay there is time and space for reexamination, retrospection, and new insight. Clients also take dramas from sessions into real life, trying out in life what has been rehearsed through therapeutic acting. Dramatic actions instill courage for related real-life actions. These may not be literal transpositions from dramatic to real-life scenes, but rather may involve using skills acquired through dramatic processes. For example, after engaging in line repetition, a client may act more assertively. After identifying and externalizing parts of the self in self-sculptures, a client may be able to identify (and have the necessary distance from) self-destructive or obstructive parts as they emerge in his or her life.

Drama becomes a catalyst for real-life change, and real life becomes material for drama. Clients have spontaneously halted moments of real life by jotting something down, such as a script of internal berating voices, and brought these to a therapy session as material for scene work (i.e., a dialogue with such voices). One client described the process as "turning pain into art."

The methods described in this chapter are but two of innumerable methods and techniques that can be used in drama therapy. More important than particular methods, however, are the interventions that are made in the course of the dramatic work and the developmental progression of processes within the session, which creates an aesthetic flow, if not a work of art of the session itself.

EFFICACY AND RESEARCH DIRECTIONS

In the past several decades, there has been a growing body of literature supporting the efficacy of drama therapy. Most of the literature is descriptive in nature (Emunah, 1983, 1994, 1995; Jennings, 1987; Johnson, 1982; Jones, 1996; Landy, 1994). Although most studies involve qualitative reports, there also have been a small number of quantitative studies (Irwin, Levy, & Shapiro 1972; Johnson & Quinlan, 1985; Landy, 1984). More recently, there has been a surge of case materials (Cattanach, 1994; Emunah, 1994; Landy, 1993, 1996; Mitchell, 1996; Schnee, 1996). Students in the two approved American master's-level drama therapy programs are required to write a thesis, and some of this research is methodologically based. However, the field is still young, and further research is sorely needed. I agree with Landy's suggestion of encouraging research "firmly based in theory that is, itself, dramatic in nature and applying new research paradigms such as heuristic and hermeneutical methodologies" (Landy, 1997, p. 11). Areas that I particularly hope to see develop in the future include assessment, prevention, expansion of current methods and models, and attention not only to various psychological arenas but to ways drama therapy can address critical social issues such as racism, violence, and AIDS.

THE DRAMA THERAPIST IN ACTION

The drama therapist's own playfulness and ease with dramatic processes are essential; his or her energy is contagious, particularly in group work. The drama therapist is not a bystander, but an active player who serves as a role model and catalyst for clients' engagement in the action-oriented treatment process. The drama therapist must also be able to access his or her own creativity, particularly in designing and devising appropriate methods, as there are no formulas in this work. Spontaneity and perceptivity are key; without these characteristics the therapist will have difficulty deciphering and then discovering ways of working with what clients present at a given moment.

Once clients are engaged in scene work, the therapist with an aesthetic sensibility will be more adept at pacing and directing such scenes. Theatrical directions tend to coincide with therapeutic ones (Emunah, 1994; Emunah & Johnson, 1983). That is, directions that develop and enhance the scene on a theatrical level are also likely to deepen its therapeutic content. The therapist's own skills in acting are also important because at times he or she will play roles within a client's scene. The more authentically these roles are played, the more believable and potentially therapeutic the scene will be. But more important than acting skills is empathy. The empathic and intuitive therapist will be able to enter the world of the client, playing in and witnessing the client's dramas with sensitivity. Whether the therapist is in the position of audience, director, or coactor in a client's dramas, he or she must be able to tolerate and support deep expressions of feeling, including pain and rage, that may be more palpable within this action-oriented therapeutic mode as clients relive evocative and, at times, traumatic scenes from their lives.

TRAINING REQUIREMENTS

Many drama therapy techniques can be used in conjunction with verbal psychotherapy without the therapist having had formal training as a drama therapist. Certainly, role-playing and other action-oriented methods have long been incorporated in various traditional, verbal, group, and family therapies. Drama therapy techniques can serve as a catalyst for facilitating beginning interaction in groups or to deepen the level of self-exploration of particular themes or issues. The skillful therapist can interweave these action-oriented methods with verbal therapy. However, because drama therapy does not involve the use of isolated techniques, but is a complex, multifaceted form of treatment involving the systematic and intentional use of dramatic processes, training is necessary to work responsibly and efficaciously when it is the primary therapeutic medium being used. Learning and practicing the subtle and intricate interventions necessary in the dramatic mode and understanding the theoretical underpinnings of the interface between theater and psychotherapy are some of the critical aspects of the training and development of a drama therapist.

Registered drama therapists are required to have a background in theater. This is logical; drama is the art form that is used in the treatment process. In addition, a master's degree from an approved drama therapy training program is required. Experience in the field must be accumulated before a therapist may apply to become a registered drama therapist. The master's program in drama therapy entails a broad background in psychology and psychotherapy, as well as specialized training in drama therapy. Required practicum experiences include supervised work in two different clinical settings. Alternative ways of pursuing drama therapy training and registry, primarily designed for already licensed clinicians, are also available. (See the Additional Resources section at the end of the chapter.)

CONCLUSION

Through the action-oriented, creative process of drama therapy, clients confront and explore limitations (often manifested by repetitive and predictable scripts) and constraints based on history at the same time that they experiment with aspirations. In the realm of drama, everything is possible. Through drama therapy, a new relationship between limitation and aspiration develops as clients encounter the multifaceted nature of identity and the human capacity to review and renew their way of being in the world throughout the life cycle.

REFERENCES

Blatner, A. (1991). Role dynamics: A comprehensive theory of psychology. *Journal of Group Psychotherapy, Psychodrama, and Sociometry, 44*, 33–40.

Blatner, A., & Blatner, A. (1988). *The art of play: An adult's guide to reclaiming imagination and spontaneity*. New York: Human Sciences Library.

Cattanach, A. (1994). *Playtherapy—Where the sky meets the underworld*. London: Jessica Kingsley.

Emunah, R. (1983). Drama therapy with adult psychiatric patients. *The Arts in Psychotherapy, 10*, 77–84.

Emunah, R. (1985). Drama therapy and adolescent resistance. *The Arts in Psychotherapy, 12*, 71–80.

Emunah, R. (1994). *Acting for real: Drama therapy process, technique and performance*. New York: Brunner/Mazel.

Emunah, R. (1995). From adolescent trauma to adolescent drama: Group drama therapy with emotionally disturbed youth. In S. Jennings (Ed.), *Dramatherapy with children and adolescents* (pp. 150–168). New York: Routledge.

Emunah, R. (1996). Five progressive phases in drama therapy and their implications for brief dramatherapy. In A. Gersie (Ed.), *Dramatic approaches to brief therapy* (pp. 29–44). London: Jessica Kingsley.

Emunah, R., & Johnson, D. (1983). The impact of theatrical performance on the self images of psychiatric patients. *The Arts in Psychotherapy, 10*, 233–239.

Erikson, E. (1950). *Childhood and society*. New York: Norton.

Fox, J. (1981). *Playback theatre: The community sees itself*. In G. Schattner & R. Courtney (Eds.), *Drama in therapy* (Vol. 2, pp. 295–306). New York: Drama Book Specialists.

Fox, J. (1994). *Acts of service: Spontaneity, commitment, tradition in the nonscripted theatre*. New Paltz, NY: Tusitala Publishing.

Gersie, A. (1991). *Storymaking in bereavement: Dragons fight in the meadow*. London: Jessica Kingsley.

Gersie, A., & King, N. (1990). *Storymaking in education and therapy*. London: Jessica Kingsley.

Grotowski, J. (1968). *Towards a poor theatre*. New York: Simon & Schuster.

Irwin, E., Levy, P., & Shapiro, M. (1972). Assessment of drama therapy in a child guidance center. *Group Psychotherapy and Psychodrama, 25*, 105–116.

Jennings, S. (1987). *Dramatherapy: Theory and practice for teachers and clinicians*. Cambridge, MA: Brookline Books.

Jennings, S. (Ed.). (1995a). *Dramatherapy with children and adolescents*. New York: Routledge.

Jennings, S. (1995b). *Theatre, ritual, and transformations*. New York: Routledge.

Johnson, D. R. (1982). Principles and techniques of drama therapy. *The Arts in Psychotherapy, 9*, 83–90.

Johnson, D. R. (1991). The theory and technique of transformations in drama therapy. *The Arts in Psychotherapy, 18*, 285–300.

Johnson, D. R., & Quinlan, D. (1985). Representational boundaries in role portrayals among paranoid and nonparanoid schizophrenic patients. *Journal of Abnormal Psychology, 94,* 498–506.

Johnson, D. R., Forrester, A., Dintino, C., & James, M. (1996). Towards a poor drama therapy. *The Arts in Psychotherapy, 23,* 293–306.

Jones, P. (1996). *Drama as therapy, theatre as living.* London: Routledge.

Landy, R. (1984). Conceptual and methodological issues of research in drama therapy. *The Arts in Psychotherapy, 11,* 89–100.

Landy, R. (1990). The concept of role in drama therapy. *The Arts in Psychotherapy, 17,* 223–230.

Landy, R. (1993). *Persona and performance: The meaning of role in drama, therapy, and everyday life.* New York: Guilford.

Landy, R. (1994). *Drama therapy: Concepts, theories, and practices* (2nd ed.). Springfield, IL: Charles C Thomas.

Landy, R. (1996). *Essays in drama therapy: The double life.* London: Jessica Kingsley.

Landy, R. (1997). Drama therapy—The state of the art. *The Arts in Psychotherapy, 24,* 5–15.

Mitchell, S. (Ed.). (1996). *Dramatherapy—Clinical studies.* London: Jessica Kingsley.

Moreno, J. L. (1946). *Psychodrama: Vol. 1.* Beacon, NY: Beacon House.

Moreno, J. L., & Moreno, Z. T. (1959). *Psychodrama: Vol. 2.* Beacon, NY: Beacon House.

Moreno, J. L., & Moreno, Z. T. (1969). *Psychodrama: Vol. 3.* Beacon, NY: Beacon House.

Schnee, G. (1996). Drama therapy in the treatment of the homeless mentally ill. *The Arts in Psychotherapy, 23,* 53–60.

ADDITIONAL RESOURCES

Journals

International Journal of Action Methods: Psychodrama, Skill Training, and Role Playing
Heldref Publications
1319 18th Street, NW
Washington, DC 20036-1802
(202) 296-6267 (telephone)
(202) 296-5149 (fax)

The International Journal of Arts in Psychotherapy
Elsevier Science Inc.
655 Avenue of the Americas
New York, NY 10010

(888) 437-4635 (telephone)
(212) 633-3680 (fax)
E-mail: esuk.usa@elsevier.com

Professional Associations and Organizations

The British Association for Dramatherapists
The Old Mill
Tolpuddle, Dorchester
Dorset DT27EX England

The National Association for Drama Therapy
5055 Connecticut Avenue, NW, #280
Washington, DC 20015
(202) 966-7409 (telephone)
(202) 966-2283 (fax)
E-mail: nadt@danielgrp.com

Nonprofit association designed to uphold high standards of professional competence and ethics among drama therapists, develop criteria for training and registration, sponsor publications and conferences, and promote the profession through information and advocacy.

Training Programs

Approved U.S. Master's Degree Training Programs in Drama Therapy:

California Institute of Integral Studies
9 Peter Yorke Way
San Francisco, CA 94109

Master's degree in counseling psychology—concentration in drama therapy. In addition to certification as a registered drama therapist, graduates are eligible to pursue licensure as a marriage, family, and child counselor. Founder/director: Renée Emunah

New York University
35 West 4th Street, #675B
New York, NY 10012

Master's degree in drama therapy
Founder/director: Robert Landy

Training Programs in Nonacademic Settings (No Degrees Offered):

Drama Therapy Institute of Los Angeles
1315 Westwood Boulevard
Los Angeles, CA 10024

The Institute for the Arts in Psychotherapy
Chelsea Arts Building, Suite 309
526 West 26th Street
New York, NY 10001

The New Haven Drama Therapy Institute
19 Edwards Street
New Haven, CT 06511

6

PSYCHODRAMATIC METHODS IN PSYCHOTHERAPY

ADAM BLATNER

Psychodrama is an especially rich approach to psychotherapy that combines imagery, imagination, physical action, group dynamics, and a mixture of art, play, emotional sensitivity, and clear thinking. Historically, it was the first real "action" method that was proposed as a more holistic alternative to psychoanalysis by its creator, Jacob L. Moreno (1889–1974), who developed this application of improvisational drama as a therapeutic approach in the mid-1930s. Moreno, who was raised in Vienna and came to the United States in 1925, was also a significant pioneer in the field of group psychotherapy, social role theory, and applied sociology (Marineau, 1989). At the root of Moreno's work, however, there is a philosophical foundation that has as a core value the creative process, especially in its spontaneous expression.

In general, psychodrama involves having clients *enact* specific scenes related to their life problems instead of merely talking about them. These scenes are set up as small dramas, with a special area in the room assigned for the "stage," in contrast to the rest of the room, which is where the group, as "audience," remains. The main player, the "protagonist," is facilitated in presenting his or her experience by a "director," usually played by the therapist. Other group members or cotherapists are assigned specific roles of figures in the protagonist's scene, and while they are playing these roles they are called "auxiliary egos," or more often, simply "auxiliaries." These elements, of course, may be found in most dramas.

The point of the enactment is to help the client to experience his or her own feelings more vividly, develop insight into underlying assumptions and associated memories, and consider or even practice new, alternative responses. Many other therapeutic goals are also possible using this approach. Scenes may represent events that happened in the past or are anticipated in the future, and they can include not only actual events, but also those that express the "truth" of the client's inner world. To achieve these goals, a number of dramatic techniques are used, including role reversal, replay, doubling, the empty chair, the mirror, soliloquy, and scores of others. (Indeed, most of the action techniques now used in various other approaches were first developed by Moreno; Blatner, 1996, p. 181.)

Psychodrama is the basis of most role-playing practices. Although it has been described as a form of group therapy, it, in fact, involves a complex of techniques and principles that may be adapted for use in counseling with individuals, couples, and families, and in other settings as well.

RATIONALE

There are numerous benefits from integrating psychodramatic action within psychotherapy:

1. Although putting feelings and images into words helps bring them into more explicit consciousness, and various imagery-evoking techniques can intensify this, the process of actually physically enacting a situation generates the most vivid experience and sharpest insight into previously repressed ideations. Physically moving and depicting the protagonist's inner experience in association with the remembered actual interaction brings the associated feelings and thoughts into a more explicit awareness, from which it then cannot be so easily avoided. (Verbal expression is preferable to keeping feelings and thoughts inside, but such statements are nevertheless more vulnerable to rerepression.)

   Also, the more such experiences are expressed in the interpersonal sphere, the more the individual feels that he or she really exist—in contrast to the feeling that he or she might just be illusions of no consequence. Thus, he or she has a greater capacity to feel a kind of "ownership" for those experiences. Also, action adds the dimension of physical feelings, the kinesthetic mode, to what might otherwise be more intellectual insights.

2. Drama offers clients a sense of direct encounter—talking "to" the other rather than "about" the relationship. This adds a relational dimension to the previously mentioned process. In other words, dialogue is better than narrative in reinforcing the sense of ownership for statements made.

3. Psychodrama more fully uses the mind's capacity for imagination and speculation—that is, the ability to wonder "What if . . . ?" Moreno assigned a category for consciously exploring this realm, "surplus reality" (Moreno, 1971, p. 483). In many ways, psychodrama is a method for using and exploring surplus reality to more effectively cope with ordinary reality. Using the context of drama, various possibilities can be considered, played out, revised, and replayed, all of which permit a more thorough process of addressing complex personal issues while witnessed by others, thus evoking a sharper form of self-reflection.

4. Enactment reframes experience as a part of the human condition so that there is a greater sense of sharing with others. For example, experiences of shame, grief, and vulnerability are less personally overwhelming when framed as part of the human condition, and drama creates that somewhat transpersonal context. Everyone shares in such dramas, and such sharing adds a collective and so-called existential dimension to what can be an otherwise very lonely and personal struggle.

5. Playing out a more satisfactory response to a situation offers a psychological experience of completion, or what in Gestalt psychology is called *closure*. Actions such as speaking up when previously one had stifled one's self-assertion or more vigorously expressing anger, fear, or grief can result in a measure of symbolic gratification.

DIFFERENCES IN APPROACH

The main method of psychodrama, in its classical format, involves a process that generally requires at least an hour; is held in a group setting; and includes a warm-up phase, an action phase, and a sharing phase that serves as closure.

In the warm-up phase, the group leader as director helps the group choose someone whose problem will become the focus of the group (i.e., the protagonist). The problem chosen should express a concern that is relevant to the dynamics of a significant number of people in the group at the time. This process includes the use of activities that strengthen group cohesion and foster a sense of safety and trust.

In the action phase, the problem is explored using a series of scenes that allow for a variety of points of view. For example, a scene in the present might be followed by one in the more recent past in which a similar event occurred. This might then be followed by a scene in the more distant past in which some of the reaction patterns shown in the first two scenes may have been established. Various techniques are used to bring out the underlying attitudes and feelings that may have shaped those beliefs. As the protagonist re-encounters aspects of his or her deeper feelings that may have been repressed, a catharsis often occurs. Although psychodrama has often been characterized as a cathartic process, its aim is not simply the expression of emotion itself, but rather the deeper dynamic of integration of dissociated elements within the psyche that releases those emotions (Bemak & Young, 1998; Blatner, 1985).

Further scenes follow in which the insights become integrated into the present and as preparation for the future. New reaction patterns are explored and practiced (i.e., role-training) so the protagonist can feel some sense of direction toward the working through of the problem.

Finally, a natural sense of closing occurs, and the director has the group shift from the protagonist's enactment to everyone being able to share what may have been evoked in the group members. This is not a time for group members to make interpretations, but rather a time to speak about their own lives and situations.

This classical approach can be very emotionally powerful, so a full enactment should be managed only by a therapist adequately trained in psychodrama. However, far wider use is being made of various psychodramatic techniques that can be woven into group therapy (Corey, 1995), family therapy (Blatner, 1994), and even individual therapy. Various role-playing procedures can be modified for nonclinical settings such as education and business. Sociodrama, in which the group works with a general social issue of concern to everyone involved, uses modified psychodramatic methods to explore these more collective themes.

Drama therapy is a related approach that often uses principles and techniques derived from psychodrama. However, drama therapy tends to use the playing of scenes from actual theatrical pieces or assigned character roles, whereas psychodrama improvises scenes based on some aspects of the protagonist's own life. In fact, though, there has been some overlap between the two fields, drama therapy deriving more from people whose background was originally in the theater, psychodrama from psychotherapists who have learned Moreno's approach. Drama therapy is rich in warm-up techniques and also ways to ritualize closure. It often is more helpful than psychodrama for those protagonists who cannot tolerate acknowledging the depth of their own problems. Psychodrama often is used at certain points in the drama therapy process as a fairly direct extension of the work and a powerful method for problem exploration, insight, and catharsis (Emunah, 1994).

Other variations of psychodrama include modifications made in South America and Spain that include more imaginal, surrealistic approaches. These integrate such symbolic devices as masks, fabrics, and ritual (Hug, 1997). In the late 1950s, some French psychoanalysts began to use psychodrama, modifying the classical approach to work with clients along more Freudian lines. Another modification has developed in response to the recent trend toward briefer psychiatric hospital stays. Sachnoff (1995), for instance, has described ways to shorten and focus psychodrama sessions in inpatient units. These more intense sessions can become a rich source of shared experience and discussion in other group settings or in individual therapy.

BRINGING OUT THE INNER DRAMA

Psychodrama may be better understood by recognizing that people not only play many different social roles, but they also play different roles within their own minds. In that role-playing, they also imagine how the other significant people in their lives (e.g., mother, teacher, or friends at school) are reacting to them. Psychodynamics may similarly be better understood as being the various interactions of these inner roles. This view has been stated well by a psychoanalyst:

> Psychic life is now seen not as an apparatus of control over impersonal instinctual drives, but as a complex and highly personal drama throughout its inner nature. This personal drama of aspects of the ego and of objects in constant interaction constitutes the complex structure of the psychic individual (Guntrip, 1957, p. 59).

Psychodrama, then, introduces the idea of thinking of the mind and relations among people as if life were a kind of play. Shakespeare, of course, articulated this well in having one of his characters give the famous monologue sometimes called "The Seven Ages of Man," which begins with the following: "All the world's a stage, and all the men and women in it, merely players." (As You Like It, act II, scene vii).

But Moreno added a dimension. People are not merely players; they also can use their capacity for self-reflection to play what I have termed the *meta-roles* of director, playwright, audience, and critic. From these stances that operate outside of the action, the roles may be reconsidered and revised and the scripts figuratively rewritten. Participants can pause and change the way they approach a situation. This is the liberating factor and the element that makes psychodrama an agent of insight, change, and healing.

Thinking of the mind and its relationships as a kind of drama makes psychology more accessible and more understandable to nonprofessionals who are not familiar with its jargon. The dramatic metaphor also implicitly suggests that there is flexibility in the ways situations may be played. Actors, after all, are not only the parts they play, but also the actor who is not really that part, but just someone playing the role. And this suggests that people also can figuratively stand back from the roles they play to get a bit of psychological distance so as to reevaluate their performance, or perhaps, determine whether or not they even want to play that role. All of this is taken for granted in thinking of life as drama. Psychodrama thus makes self-reflection easier by offering relatively concrete images and a context of interaction—the stage, players, and action—instead of having to process psychological insights through the abstract realm of language.

CASE EXAMPLE 1: PARTS OF SELF TECHNIQUE

For example, the experience of confusion can be reframed as a conflict between parts of the self who interrupt each other so noisily that one cannot think out the problem. Using what is called the parts of self technique, the director has the protagonist represent each part of a conflict in a separate chair, thus externalizing the inner dialogue and concretizing each point of view as a role with a position in space on the stage. The protagonist then presents each role in turn, switching parts. It is also possible that an auxiliary may take one of the parts to intensify the dialogue. The protagonist is also helped by taking a meta-role of mediator, who is helped to vigorously stop the confusing tendency of each role to interrupt and overpower the other. People tend to overwhelm themselves with ongoing qualifications and disqualifications of feelings and ideas, paralyzing clear thinking. The protagonist as mediator insists that each role take turns and even draws them out, allowing the issues to be presented more completely and also suggesting to the subconscious a deep respect and inclusion of all facets of the psyche. Moreover, the warring parts are pressed to talk directly "to" each other, which tends to bring out feelings more effectively. This concretized process of self-reflection then moves from some degree of insight into the nature of the confusion to a process of negotiation. Through negotiation the director helps the protagonist, who shifts among the roles of the various parts of the self and the mediator, to work toward a synthesis that can resolve the conflict.

Here is an example of this technique. A professional woman in a group was conflicted regarding a situation at work. Her employer had changed the organization's benefits package and the nature of the work so that disadvantages were beginning to outweigh advantages. She was helped to position two chairs and then asked to name each position.[1]

Case Narrative	Commentary
D: You seem to be having a conflict. [Protagonist, identified as P, nods.] One way to clarify a conflict is to bring out the two different sides of the question by having you play each side as if it were a distinct role. And in psychodrama, we actually assign the roles to different positions—in this case, let there be two chairs. What are the two sides of the question?	The director in this example, identified as D, is the functional role played by the therapist facilitating the psychodrama.
	Clarifies and instructs as to how the problem may be approached to foster a more mutual treatment alliance.
P: This chair is the part who is the "victim," and that chair is . . . the part who will not put up with it.	
D: Just one or two words for that second part.	If a role is described in a wordy fashion, the director-therapist can ask the protagonist to try to give it a more compact "name."
P: Fight back.	
D: Who starts first?	
P: The victim. [Sits in the victim's chair.] It isn't fair. They have cleverly designed a benefits package so that if we get hurt or disabled, there's a cap on the total amount. If I am hurt, and so is someone else, I could be left vulnerable! And there are other aspects of the package that are subtle but really disadvantage the workers . . . [goes on about other problems].	
D: Change parts.	It is important that the director-therapist direct assertively, not letting talking drag on. It is important to get both sides identified and presented—and, indeed, any other relevant sides as well.

---

[1]*Editor's note:* Compare this to the empty-chair technique described in chapter 1.

P: [Gets up and goes to the other chair.] Well, you don't have to put up with it. You can leave. [Spontaneously, then, the last statement motivates her to jump up and go back to the first chair.]

P: [As victim] It's not so easy to get another job. I like having a dependable salary. My "inner bag lady" gets scared.

Some protagonists are warmed-up enough or experienced enough to engage in some self-directed action without the director suggesting a change of parts.

At this point, the director might pause and, as mentioned above, help the protagonist establish the further role of mediator, thus objectifying the observing and managerial functions of the self-reflective self. This meta-role is more alert to the potentialities of the moment—less driven by the illusions, memories, and transferences of the past—and also led by the goal of seeking a creative breakthrough rather than a more role-dependent fixation on having one's own way within the frame of reference of that role. The mediator role can comment on both of the other roles, engage in a reflective discussion, and access the support of the director and the group. The mediator may then be helped to "talk" with both the other roles, challenging their tendencies to polarize (i.e., engage in either/or thinking or portraying situations in their extreme terms). More discriminations may be introduced to the categories of the protagonist's thinking—akin to cognitive therapy—and also supportive and encouraging statements made to the more vulnerable and threatened subparts of the psyche.

ADDITIONAL TECHNIQUES

A related technique in psychodrama that can deepen the encounter among parts of the self is that of the *double*, which brings out into the open those thoughts that tend to flit through the mind but tend not to be expressed because they are embarrassing or uncomfortable.[2] One aspect of most psychotherapies is the fostering of disclosure, from the preconscious to the explicitly conscious, and from there into the social sphere—that is, spoken out loud knowing that others are listening. When expressed, thoughts take on a greater clarity, whereas in unexpressed form they are vulnerable to a variety of subtle mental mechanisms that compartmentalize them and in other ways keep them out of conscious awareness.

Doubling involves having someone else speak those thoughts that may be ignored or suppressed. Because the client is encouraged to correct

2*Editor's note*: Compare the use of doubling described here with its use as described in chapter 7.

the double, the process differs somewhat from the more loaded challenge of questioning the therapist's interpretation, with all the transferential load it carries.

Applied to the parts of self technique, group members may be asked to come up and stand behind the two chairs that are facing each other. They can then imagine what feelings each position might be having. Indeed, a given position may have more than one double; there can be more than two viewpoints in a given encounter. With the double technique the therapist can more fully help the protagonist bypass tendencies to become superficial or defensive and instead bring into consciousness underlying attitudes, feelings, and beliefs. In turn, those assumptions can then be questioned or worked with.

The inner-dialogue technique is appropriate for almost any population that can express itself verbally with any degree of competence. However, this leaves out those with less than the mental ability of about a 12-year-old. The inner-dialogue technique may be useful whenever a client complains of conflictual feelings or mixed reactions to a given situation. Moreover, many other problems, after some discussion, become more usefully framed as inner conflicts, at which time the inner-dialogue technique can then be applied.

Another commonly used technique is action sociometry, the most commonly recognized derivative of which is family sculpture (Duhl, 1983). The protagonist is helped to create his or her most relevant social network as if it were a sculpture of people standing in various positions and distances from each other—as a kind of living diorama. This staging of relationships using gesture or other nonverbal cues often expresses more vividly than can words the protagonist's perception of the relationships in a family or other social network.

Sociometry is a method of surveying and then portraying concretely, in diagrammatic form or in action, the interpersonal preferences among the various people in a social system. It is another invention of Moreno's that continues to offer promise as an aid in clarifying group dynamics (Blatner, 1988). The following example shows a variation of action sociometry—an approach that combines the techniques of empty chair, auxiliary world, and concretization.

CASE EXAMPLE 2: INTRAPSYCHIC ACTION SOCIOMETRY

A woman in her 30s who was fighting chronic mild depression spoke about the many losses in her life. To help her experience the full range of all the losses, the (male) director decided to have the protagonist present all the lost figures at once on the stage to circumvent her tendencies toward denial or minimization of the losses. The protagonist was instructed to bring empty chairs onto the stage to represent her inner social network. Group members were then assigned as auxiliaries to play the roles of all the lost figures. The director invited the woman to become the protagonist and, on the stage, he began to gently draw her out, helping her name and stage the various lost people.

The protagonist began with an uncle, and as his chair was drawn forward, the director posed some identifying questions aimed at specific memories. As a few came to the protagonist's mind, the director had her reverse roles and become the uncle. She sat in the chair and said, "Uncle Ottie."

New associations then formed to other uncles, and as the protagonist qualified the closeness of the relationship, the director interrupted the explanations and focused on the action. "Would you go get a chair for him?" he asked. The protagonist nodded and went to the edge of the stage area and brought back a chair.

Case Narrative	Commentary
D: This is . . . ?	Leading phrase
P: Uncle Wesley.	
D: What do you remember about him that describes him in just a few words?	
P: A real cowboy. He broke horses. [She went on to describe a few details.]	Identify role briefly.
D: Good. Now, you mentioned your dog.	Pets as well as people may be part of a person's inner social network.
P: Oh yes. Gee, she is, I mean, was . . . just a dog.	
D: Dogs can be here too.	

The scene continued to unfold, with the protagonist portraying the various figures. The childhood home and its "special places" also were assigned to a chair.

As the protagonist seemed to be warming up, speaking more spontaneously about the characters, the director decided to portray all the losses and deepen the portrayal by having her begin to experience the lost others in encounters. He had the protagonist go back and name all the chairs so far. He then asked the audience to bring up to the stage some more chairs that represented, for example, a cousin who died in an auto accident when the protagonist was 12 years old; another uncle who committed suicide about a year later; several old friends who moved away, leaving her especially lonely (she was raised in a somewhat isolated, semirural area); and several others.

The protagonist protested that there were getting to be too many chairs, and the director decided that this was less a true statement of overload and more her being worried about confusing the audience. So, to communicate the innate generosity of the method, the value of allowing the "truth" of the protagonist to be fully expressed, he pushed even further—he invited even more losses to be presented, more chairs to be placed on stage. The point is to have the protagonist experience the fullness of the actual complexity of his or her life experience and the multiplicity of internal object relations.

Then, to deepen the enactment, the director then invited the protagonist to engage in a dialogue with several of the key figures. To further vivify this dialogue, auxiliaries were brought in to play those significant lost others. The director had the protagonist choose various group members to serve as auxiliaries. Then the encounters were played out.

Case Narrative	*Commentary*
P: Uncle Dan, when you committed suicide, it really tore me up.	Begins a dialogue.
Auxiliary [as Uncle Dan]: I—Uh, I'm sorry	Auxiliaries sometimes need to be helped to warm up to their role, and one use of the technique of role reversal is to demonstrate the correct way (according to the protagonist's inner world) to play that role.
P: No, that's not what he'd say.	
D: Change parts and show us what he'd say.	
P: [Changes positions and, now in the role of Uncle Dan, says to the place where she was standing.] Well, Papoosie, it wasn't about you. My stomach just couldn't take the foods I liked to eat!	

The director recognized that this was the beginning of a need for some grief work, and the technique for facilitating that involves the gentle guidance of the dialogue toward addressing three general questions: (a) What are the specific memories we (the protagonist and lost other) shared? (This makes the loss very concrete in the imagery rather than remaining abstract, and it draws out evocative details and helps the client-protagonist break through tendencies toward isolation of affect and intellectualization.) (b) What have you (the lost other) meant to me? (c) What have I meant to you? This last question is answered by having the protagonist reverse roles, with the auxiliary playing the lost other or sitting in the empty chair. From the role of the other, the protagonist can open his or her mind to how the lost other may have been affected by the protagonist in the past. Thus, a technique of structured questions can sometimes evoke a deeper encounter than might otherwise occur.

After going through this kind of dialogue with a few of the protagonist's more significant others, some of the tension began to dissipate. It became clear to the director that an encounter with every lost other was not necessary, because beyond a certain amount of catharsis, the energy for work lags and the insights and experiences tend to adequately generalize to the other relationships. If further encounters were needed, they could be pursued on other occasions.

TIMING

When should action methods be used? There are many opportunities for the use of action techniques or structured experiences. First, they may be applied as warm-ups, to promote interaction, group cohesion, self-disclosure, and deeper involvement in themes of personal or group development. Second, they may be used to clarify the dynamics of what is being said to a group. Sometimes words may be used to disguise or distance the speaker from what is being discussed, and action approaches tend to rebalance tendencies toward becoming too abstract or intellectualized by offering more concrete experiences.

However, action alone cannot suffice. There are times when more verbal, nonaction approaches are appropriate. Often, even after the sharing portion of an enactment, the group needs to discuss a number of issues, such as feelings about the group leadership or reactions to other group members. Many such group processes cannot be reduced to mere technique, although when impasses occur, the leader may choose to draw on a broad range of action methods to catalyze new insights or exchanges. Group leaders must be alert to the needs of group members as individuals and of the group as a whole, and this must take precedence over any wish to generate action.

There are some groups in which certain participants are eager for more intensive action experiences, yet such desires may not always be in keeping with the needs of the group as a whole. And, having noted that psychodrama is a tool, it should not be the sole theme of a group devoted to the holistic development of both individual and group dynamics. Thus, the timing of the use of psychodrama depends on scores of variables in the complex process of group formation and work.

RESISTANCE

There are two common types of resistance to the use of action methods. One is that the approach is unusual, that it differs from the cultural stereotype of counseling as primarily a verbal interchange, either as classical psychoanalysis (on the couch) or simply a conversation in a therapist's office. The other is that becoming actively involved in self-expression is (validly) sensed as making one unusually vulnerable. People often wish to distance themselves from their problems, either by hardly owning that they even have a problem or by minimizing their own responsibility in the situation. Enactment makes them more sharply aware that it is indeed they who are the actors rather than just the passive victims of circumstances.

Overcoming these types of resistance is part of the art of therapy. For the first, that psychodrama seems unusual, what is needed is a brief "sales talk," a way of presenting the method so that it seems simple and ordinary. I usually emphasize the way role-playing is used by astronauts and other professionals to explore the subtleties and complexities of situations that cannot be anticipated or described in textbooks. People recognize this intuitively, and it even supports their suspicions about the limitations of book-based learning.

Related to both types of resistance is the gradual development in group settings of group trust and cohesion through helping people to become acquainted. Using action methods or guided or structured experiences gradually introduces group members to the dimension of physical activity while fostering a climate of mutual and symmetrical self-disclosure; that is, the feeling that one is not alone and "on the spot," but rather that everyone is sharing or expressing himself or herself or making themselves vulnerable to the same degree.

If the therapist assumes a dramatic mode of discourse, as if the situation is like a rehearsal in a play, then even the ordinary mode of talking with the therapist becomes reframed as a type of experiment. Whatever is spoken by the client, instead of being responded to at the level of content and verbal exchange, can instead be "staged." That is, the client's or group member's communications can be considered to be a form of role-playing, which can in turn be amplified, exaggerated, answered, doubled, or in other ways worked with as a spoken text capable of dramatic elaboration.

The dramatic mode is heightened by the way a skilled director or therapist moves into and out of it. It is almost like interspersing poetry with explanatory prose. The ordinary, nondramatized, discussionlike mode of discourse is used to ground, orient, and suggest a "breaking of set," as if to say, "OK, now, outside of the scene, here's our commentary" or "If we were to replay this scene, how else might we want to write the script or otherwise stage the action?" These shifts in modes of dramatic and nondramatic discourse also heighten or reflect the corresponding shifts between the person as actor-in-role and the person as observer and director/playwright of his or her life. Such shifts are, in theater and social psychological role theory, called *role distance*.

The psychodramatic approach, when handled in this fashion, draws most clients in. For those who still resist, that reaction too can be made even more explicit and concretized as action. The refusal to enact may be explored as having its own related issues (e.g., a refusal to own any problem or any involvement in a problem-solving or problem-exploring process). This is a not-uncommon situation in many settings in which clients are expected to participate in counseling as part of receiving other services or where counseling is mandated rather than elective.

FURTHER USES

I frame psychotherapy as a type of skill building, which tends to demystify the process and shifts the contract from a more passive expectation of idealized (or suspected) "treatment" to a more participatory, collaborative, quasi-educational approach. Clients who come for therapy often benefit from a certain amount of orientation as to how best use the procedure.

The skills developed in psychotherapy involve such general themes as promoting and integrating more effective communication, interpersonal problem solving, and self-awareness. Such skills must be individualized to be applied according to the levels of understanding, ability, cognitive style, and experience of the client. The kinds of skills described cannot be learned simply through lectures, books, or other ways of acquiring information. They involve a "knack" and must be learned experientially, and so, experiential, action approaches are logically appropriate for their practice.

With experience using psychodrama as the method for rehearsal and experimentation, the skills acquired may then be practiced in between sessions or after therapy ends. Role reversal, for example, offers a method for being more accurately empathic and sensitizes and encourages people to consider more actively the viewpoints of the others in their lives. The technique of doubling fosters psychological mindedness; that is, considering deeper levels of self-disclosure and becoming more explicitly aware of ideas, impulses, and feelings that may have previously remained out of awareness.

One technique I often use is to invite significant others to a session targeted for teaching them how to interact most effectively with a client. The client becomes a codirector and is challenged with reframing tendencies to blame or complain into constructive requests for specific behaviors, agreements on codelike phrases, or strategies for addressing tensions. This makes the therapy a cross between family therapy and role-training, and the approach then can be refined in later sessions after the skills are tried out as homework (Blatner, 1994).

EMPIRICAL SUPPORT

Psychodrama is one of the oldest of psychotherapies, having been developed in the 1930s, and over one thousand journal articles describing its use and value have been published. It is used internationally by thousands of practitioners. There are numerous articles in which role-playing or psychodrama has been evaluated scientifically, but on the whole, the research is not up to current standards of rigor, partly because it is difficult to assess any psychotherapy that does not follow a fairly predictable path. Nevertheless, Kipper (1978) and Kellermann (1987) produced reviews of a number of studies that offered some empirical evidence supporting the use of psychodrama as an effective psychotherapy method. For example, Schramski, Feldman, Harvey, and Holiman (1984) used symptom ratings that changed in the course of treatment, and Carpenter and Sandberg (1985) found that psychodrama was effective in improving ego strength and in developing socialization skills in a small group of delinquent adolescents.

Part of the problem is that psychodrama is rarely used as the sole method of treatment, with no other adjunctive approaches. Rather, it is generally used—as it should be—synergistically with other, more general approaches (i.e., family therapy, group therapy, couples therapy, and even individual therapy). Its principles and techniques may be modified and applied in the treatment of children, in which case it is often more like play therapy or drama therapy, or with the developmentally disabled, in which case it is often closer to role-playing for skills training. Psychodrama also has been applied to education, at spiritual retreats, and in business. In all these various settings the method must be modified and adapted to the situation and the population, making it difficult to assess its unique value. If I were to suggest an experimental approach to studying the efficacy of psychodrama, it would be one comparing group or family therapy that integrates action methods with similar therapies that do not. Looked at in another way, however, the widespread adoption of psychodramatic methods attests to their value.

TRAINING

Psychodramatic methods can be emotionally powerful and therefore should be used only by those who have had sufficient training in the approach. Unfortunately, the method looks as if one could apply it without much training, which has led to psychodrama being used widely by relatively untrained therapists and even by those who are not therapists. Because of this, a professional certification process has been established, and those who would work with anyone claiming to be a psychodramatist should first check to see if that person is in fact certified by the American Board of Examiners in Psychodrama, Sociometry and Group Psychotherapy.[3] For the practitioner relatively new to psychodrama and interested in applying its methods, it is valuable to know about its underlying principles and other techniques so that using psychodramatic methods can be rationally integrated as part of a holistic treatment plan.

Training in psychodramatic techniques involves both theoretical and experiential learning processes and a good deal of personal work in groups. Those using the method as a form of psychotherapy must have a master's degree in one of the psychologically oriented helping professions as well as over 780 hours of training. Psychodramatists need to develop in several areas: the director as dramaturge, the ability to stage a situation in some ways like a theatrical director; as a group therapist, sensitive to the issues that come up in group dynamics; as a diagnostician analyzing the somato-psychic, intrapsychic, interpersonal, and group and cultural levels of the protagonist's problem; and as an authentic person who can use his or her own self as an instrument of sensitive engagement, warmth, support, and, at times, confrontation.

CONCLUSION

Psychodrama involves a complex array of methods and ideas that offer a valuable theoretical and practical contribution to psychotherapy, education, community building, spiritual development, personal growth, conflict resolution, social action, and other consciousness-enhancing endeavors. Although neither psychodrama nor any other single approach is fully comprehensive or sufficient to accomplish all therapeutic objectives, it serves as an important addition to the applied behavioral sciences. It may best be appreciated as a kind of "laboratory" for psychosocial experimentation (Moreno, 1956, pp. 327–331). It is a natural setting in which the component techniques and the underlying principles combine so that people can explore more creative alternatives to human problems. I view it as a major tool for what may be the real challenge of the next millennium: the conscious transformation of consciousness itself.

---

[3]See Blatner, 1996, for a fuller discussion of training.

REFERENCES

Bemak, F., & Young, M. (1998). Role of catharsis in group psychotherapy. *International Journal of Action Methods, 50*(4), 166–184.

Blatner, A. (1985). The dynamics of catharsis. *Journal of Group Psychotherapy, Psychodrama, and Sociometry, 37*(4), 157–166.

Blatner, A. (1988). *Foundations of psychodrama: History, theory, and practice.* New York: Springer. A complement and amplification of the theoretical material in *Acting-in* (Blatner, 1996), with extensive references. (A significantly revised edition is set to be published in 2000.)

Blatner, A. (1994). Psychodramatic methods in family therapy. In C. E. Schaefer & L. Carey (Eds.), *Family play therapy* (pp. 235–246). Northvale, NJ: Jason Aronson.

Blatner, A. (1996). *Acting-in: Practical applications of psychodramatic methods* (3rd ed.). New York: Springer. The best general introduction to the method, with extensive, updated references.

Carpenter, P., & Sandberg, S. (1985). Further psychodrama with delinquent adolescents. *Adolescence, 20,* 599–604.

Corey, G. (1995). *Theory and practice of group counseling* (4th ed.). Pacific Grove, CA: Brooks/Cole.

Duhl, B. (1983). *From the inside out and other metaphors.* New York: Brunner/Mazel.

Emunah, R. (1994). *Acting for real: Drama therapy process, technique, and performance.* New York: Brunner/Mazel.

Guntrip, H. (1957). *Psychotherapy and religion.* New York: Harper.

Hug, E. (1997). Current trends in psychodrama: Eclectic and analytic dimensions. *The Arts in Psychotherapy, 24*(1), 31–35.

Kellermann, P. F. (1987). Outcome research in classical psychodrama. *Small Group Behavior, 18*(4), 459–469.

Kipper, D. A. (1978). Trends in the research on the effectiveness of psychodrama. *Group Psychotherapy, Psychodrama, and Sociometry, 31,* 5–18.

Marineau, R. F. (1989). *Jacob Levi Moreno, 1889–1974.* New York: Routledge.

Moreno, J. L. (1956). Psychotherapy: Present and future. In F. Fromm-Reichmann & J. L. Moreno (Eds.), *Progress in psychotherapy: Vol I.* New York: Grune & Stratton.

Moreno, J. L. (1971). Psychodrama. In H. I. Kaplan & B. J. Sadock (Eds.), *Comprehensive group psychotherapy* (pp. 460–500). Baltimore: Williams & Wilkins.

Sachnoff, E. A. (1995). Managed care and inpatient psychodrama—short sessions within short stays. *Journal of Group Psychotherapy, Psychodrama, and Sociometry, 48,* 117–120.

Schramski, T. G., Feldman, C. A., Harvey, D. R., & Holiman, M. A. (1984). A comparative evaluation of group treatment in an adult correctional facility. *Journal of Group Psychotherapy, Psychodrama, and Sociometry, 36,* 133–147.

ADDITIONAL RESOURCES

Books

Blatner, A. (1995). Psychodrama. In R. J. Corsini & D. Wedding (Eds.), *Current psychotherapies* (5th ed., pp. 399–408). Itasca, IL: Peacock. A good, relatively succinct overview.

Blatner, A., & Blatner, A. (1997). *The art of play: An adult's guide to reclaiming imagination and spontaneity* (2nd ed.). New York: Brunner/Mazel. Offers both a psychological and cultural analysis of improvisational play and offers a technique for enjoying it with more mature participants; its middle section is a useful guide to developing role-playing skills.

Dayton, T. (1994). *The drama within: Psychodrama and experiential therapy.* Deerfield Beach, FL: Health Communications.

Fox, J. (Ed.). (1987). *The essential Moreno: Writings on psychodrama, group method, and spontaneity.* New York: Springer.

Holmes, P. (1992). *The inner world outside: Object relations therapy and psychodrama.* New York: Routledge.

Holmes, P., Karp, M., & Watson, M. (Eds.). (1994). *Psychodrama since Moreno: Innovations in theory and practice.* New York: Routledge.

Karp, M., Holmes, P., & Bradshaw-Tauvon, K. (Eds.). (1998). *Handbook of psychodrama.* New York: Routledge.

Kellermann, P. F. (1992). *Focus on psychodrama: The therapeutic aspects of psychodrama.* London: Jessica Kingsley.

Kipper, D. A. (1986). *Psychotherapy through clinical role playing.* New York: Brunner/ Mazel.

Leveton, E. (1992). *A clinician's guide to psychodrama.* New York: Springer.

Moreno, J. L. (1946). *Psychodrama: Vol. 1* (Rev. ed.). Beacon, NY: Beacon House. Available from the American Society of Group Psychotherapy and Psychodrama, 301 North Harrison Street, Suite 508, Princeton, NJ 08540; (609) 452-1339; E-mail: asgpp@asgpp.org.

Moreno, J. L. (1959). Psychodrama. In S. Arieti (Ed.), *American handbook of psychiatry* (Vol. 2, pp. 1375–1396). New York: Basic Books.

Moreno, J. L., & Moreno, Z. T. (1959). *Psychodrama: Vol. 2.* Beacon, NY: Beacon House.

Moreno, J. L., & Moreno, Z. T. (1969). *Psychodrama: Vol. 3.* Beacon, NY: Beacon House.

Sacks, J. M. (1993). Psychodrama. In H. I. Kaplan & B. J. Sadock (Eds.), *Comprehensive group psychotherapy* (3rd ed., pp. 214–228). Baltimore: Williams & Wilkins.

Sacks, J. M., Bilaniuk, M., & Gendron, J. M. (1995). *Bibliography of psychodrama: Inception to date.* New York: James M. Sacks. Listing of over 2,000 items on 130 pages with an extensive, 30-page index. Also available on either Macintosh or IBM-compatible computer diskette. Available for $35 from Dr.

James M. Sacks, Psychodrama Center of New York, 71 Washington Place, New York, NY 10011-9184.

Williams, A. (1989). *The passionate technique: Strategic psychodrama with individuals, families, and groups*. New York: Tavistock/Routledge.

Yablonsky, L. (1992). *Psychodrama: Resolving emotional problems through role-playing*. New York: Brunner/Mazel.

Journals

Blatner, A. (1991a). Role dynamics: A comprehensive theory of psychology. *Journal of Group Psychotherapy, Psychodrama and Sociometry, 44*(1), 33–40.

Blatner, A. (1991b). Theoretical principles underlying creative arts therapies. *The Arts in Psychotherapy, 18*(5), 405–409.

Blatner, A. (1997). Psychodrama: The state of the art. *The Arts in Psychotherapy, 24*(1), 23–30.

International Journal of Action Methods. Washington, DC: Heldref. (Formerly Journal of Group Psychotherapy, Psychodrama, and Sociometry.)

Professional Associations and Organizations

American Board of Examiners in Psychodrama, Sociometry and
  Group Psychotherapy
PO Box 15572
Washington, DC 20003-0572
(202) 483-0514

Establishes criteria for certification and examination procedures in the United States and publishes a directory of certified psychodramatists.[4]

American Society of Group Psychotherapy and Psychodrama (ASGPP)
301 North Harrison Street, Suite 508
Princeton, NJ 08540
(609) 452-1339 (telephone)
(609) 936-1659 (fax)
E-mail: asgpp@asgpp.org
Web site: www.asgpp.org

---

[4]For a directory of trainers in psychodrama in other countries, see appendix in the British third edition of Blatner's *Acting-In: Practical Applications of Psychodramatic Methods* (London: Free Association Books).

7

GROUP THERAPY FOR PEOPLE WITH MENTAL RETARDATION: THE INTERACTIVE–BEHAVIORAL THERAPY MODEL

DANIEL J. TOMASULO

A person who is severely impaired never knows his hidden sources of strength until he is treated like a normal human being and encouraged to shape his own life.

—Helen Keller

Despite evidence of its effectiveness, group psychotherapy (with or without action methods) for people with mental retardation is seldom considered a viable therapeutic modality. Historically, the research on this issue showed that people with mental retardation could not profit from insight-oriented interactive therapy because they lacked the specific cognitive abilities thought necessary for therapeutic change. Although many clinicians have not regarded people with mental retardation as suitable candidates for any form of psychotherapy (see Hurley, 1989; Hurley, Pfadt, Tomasulo, & Gardner, 1996), there are many case reports on the effectiveness of individual psychotherapy (Hurley, 1989) as well as group psychotherapy (Pfadt, 1991). Psychotherapy for people with mental retardation has been most effective when a directive style with structured sessions is used (Fletcher, 1984; Hingsburger, 1987; Hurley, 1989; Hurley & Hurley, 1986, 1988; Hurley, Pfadt, Tomasulo, & Gardner, 1996; Hurley, Tomasulo, & Pfadt, 1998; Tomasulo, 1992; Tomasulo, Keller, & Pfadt, 1995). Although lack of cognitive abilities may be the primary reason that psychotherapy is overlooked as a treatment modality for people with mental retardation, there have been a number of erroneous assumptions on the part of practitioners, including the following:

- Because many developmentally disabled people are not verbal (or have difficulty verbalizing) they are thought to be unable to produce clues to regulating their behavior.
- The secondary disabilities that often accompany mental retardation (e.g., short attention span, auditory and visual handicaps, and seizure activity) are thought to be insurmountable obstacles to interactive group therapy.
- People with mental retardation are thought to lack the cognitive ability to profit from insight into the causes and consequences of their behavior.
- Many practitioners understand the emotional disorders displayed by people with mental retardation as a side effect of a biochemical brain dysfunction. For this reason, they feel there is little that psychotherapy can offer people with mental retardation.
- Alternatively, the emotional and behavioral problems of people with mental retardation are widely felt to be the result of either mental illness *or* behavior disorders. Hence, only psychopharmacological or behavioral treatments alone are attempted. The use of psychotherapy to help ameliorate these problems is rarely considered.

THE INTERACTIVE–BEHAVIORAL THERAPY MODEL

Traditional psychodrama group action methods generally consist of three components: (a) a warm-up, (b) an enactment, and (c) a sharing. The warm-up allows participants to prepare for the enactment stage by having them identify what they want to work on. The enactment phase allows action methods to be used to explore the problem, and the sharing phase allows each member to reflect on his or her experiences within the group. In pilot studies, this traditional process was only marginally effective with people with mental retardation. As a result, the interactive–behavioral therapy (IBT) model was constructed (Tomasulo, 1998). It was designed specifically to assist people whose cognitive skills are diminished in some way to benefit from interaction with their peers in a therapeutic setting. The IBT model of group therapy offers a format for using action methods from the field of psychodrama with people who have a primary diagnosis of mild or moderate mental retardation (IQ scores between 40 and 69) and who often have a secondary psychiatric diagnosis. Specific modifications made to accommodate people with mental retardation include the following:

- shortening the session time to between 45 and 60 minutes (the more typical timetable is 90–120 minutes);
- describing the process and mechanics of the action to members during the enactment stage;
- dividing the process into four distinct stages (i.e., orientation, warm-up and sharing, enactment, and affirmation; see Figure 7-1) as a way of readying members for using action methods and ending their group experience in a positive fashion; and
- identifying therapeutic factors displayed by members during the process and reinforcing them when they occur as well as in the affirmation stage.

These modifications have been adopted for the following reasons:

INTERACTIVE BEHAVIORAL GROUP PROCESS

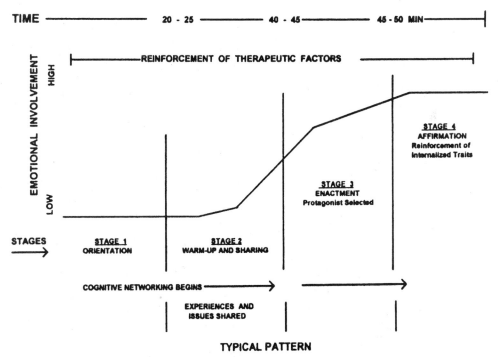

Figure 7-1. A typical pattern of the interactive–behavioral therapy group process.

- The condensed time increases the possibility that members will remain physically and emotionally present.
- The time frame and four-stage model keeps the facilitator or facilitators more focused on the necessary tasks to be accomplished in each stage. In addition, facilitators are better able to attend to the process of the group rather than the content.
- The shorter time frame more readily fits into the schedules of most hospitals, agencies, residences, vocational settings, and schools; that is, IBT groups can easily replace social-skills training groups.

Psychodrama and sociodramatic theory (Blatner & Blatner, 1988; Steinberg & Garcia, 1989) offer the most widely accepted format for facilitating role-playing techniques within a group setting.

During the enactment stage, participants are provided with a greater awareness of the mechanics of the action than are nondisabled members of traditional psychodrama groups. This awareness requires that the facilitator or facilitators ensure that participants can follow the action, identify the roles played by auxiliaries, know who is supposed to be occupying the empty chair, and recognize what role is being played during role reversals. Additionally, the use of active and interactive techniques often is preferred because they stimulate more sensory and affective modes of learning than verbal therapy alone (Hurley, Pfadt, Tomasulo, & Gardner, 1996; Tomasulo, 1994).

INTERACTIVE–BEHAVIORAL THERAPY STAGES

Stage 1: Orientation and Cognitive Networking

In a group of individuals with mental retardation, many secondary disabilities (e.g., poor eye contact, difficulty with short-term recognition or memory, impaired hearing, delayed responding, confusion, echolalia, inattention, distractibility, speech impediments, and hyperactivity), as well as primary cognitive deficits, inhibit interaction among members. For this reason, the facilitator needs to work to engage the members in cognitive networking during the initial orientation stage and throughout the group process. Having members repeat what was said to them, turn toward the person speaking, acknowledge what was said, and in some way participate in the group process through interaction are the goals of this first stage. If group members fail to attend to each other, their ability to successfully use action methods in the enactment stage will be severely impaired, or not even possible. Indeed, without orientation among group members, no therapeutic, corrective, or instructional goals within the group will be realized.

Stage 2: Warm-Up and Sharing

In the warm-up and sharing stage, the facilitator invites group members to speak about themselves within the group. Since this is a process-driven exercise, the content of members' presentations is of lesser importance than the process itself. In other words, the facilitator's concern is with the dynamics of the group, not necessarily with what is being said by the participants. The facilitator's job is to pay attention to the nature of the interactions between the various members. During this second stage, group members take turns making their self-disclosures, and the cognitive networking begun in the orientation stage is continued. Following this, the facilitator then asks group members if any of them has a problem to work on in the group. It is during this deeper level of sharing that the members experience a greater sense of emotional involvement within the group (see Figure 7-1). The group becomes more cohesive, and the stage is set for action to take place.

Stage 3: Enactment

During the enactment stage, psychodramatic action techniques such as empty-chair work, various forms of doubling, auxiliaries, and role reversal are used. The issues presented in the warm-up and sharing stage are developed into an enactment with the help of the facilitator. Although only certain group members may take part in the enactment, the entire group's focus is on the action taking place.

Stage 4: Affirmation

Finally, in the affirmation stage, the facilitator validates the participation of each group member. This is done with specific attention to individual therapeutic factors involved (Bloch & Crouch, 1985; Yalom, 1995). Each member is verbally acknowledged for his or her interactive contributions to the group. Specifically, any displayed trait that is interactive and reflective of a therapeutic factor should be reinforced.

TECHNIQUES

Within the enactment stage, a number of techniques are used to stimulate interaction among group members. One of the most useful techniques is that of the double (Tomasulo, 1994). Broadly stated, a *double* is a role played by one or more group members that gives voice to the feelings and thoughts of another member who is struggling with a given problem. The use of the double can be a tremendous asset in groups of people with mental retardation, chronic psychiatric illness, and dual diagnoses (mental retardation/mental health; MR/MH).[1] Role-playing has been used widely in working with people with mental retardation. However, the primary use of role-playing has been for role-training. More specifically, these techniques are used almost exclusively for social-skills training rather than for the purpose of counseling; teaching and training rather than facilitating therapeutic interactions are the aims of social-skills training groups.

In these groups, trainers foster interaction between themselves and the participants rather than between and among the participants. The emphasis of IBT is on increasing interaction among participants for the purpose of creating a therapeutic environment in which selective behaviors are reinforced as a way of strengthening therapeutic group processes. The use of a double provides a clear vehicle for generating support in an IBT group.

Doubles may be single, in pairs (to allow for contrast or amplification or restatement), or in multiples (usually done to help the protagonist experience such therapeutic factors as acceptance and universality with fellow members). The emergence of a protagonist within the group indicates that one person has presented a problem that is significant enough for exploration within the group. There are many parameters that determine the selection of the protagonist. These have been discussed elsewhere (Blatner, 1996; Tomasulo, 1992). In most cases, the protagonist presents a situation that reflects a deficiency or an interpersonal or intrapsychic conflict. This deficiency or conflict often is the central issue of the drama.

CASE EXAMPLE 1: AN ELEMENTARY ACTION METHOD— THE SINGLE DOUBLE

Following is a partial transcript of an initial IBT session. This session was the first of a series of five done for the purpose of making a training video. The videotape, which demonstrates IBT principles and identifies its stages, is used to train staff to use the IBT model. It includes a manual (Tomasulo, 1992).

None of the six people in this group were known to the facilitator before the taping or had ever taken part in an IBT group. However, they were somewhat familiar with role-playing and lived together in a group home. With other groups, when members do not know one another well initially, more orientation to other members is needed, and members have less opportunity to apply their new awareness socially. In either case, however, members must transfer the skills they learn in group therapy to people they encounter in other settings. All of the members of this group were classified as dually diagnosed, meaning they had both mild or moderate

---

[1]*Editor's note:* Compare the use of the double here with that described in chapter 6.

mental retardation and a psychiatric diagnosis. The group also had a co-facilitator, Catrina.

The principles of the IBT model are demonstrated in this initial group. Each of the stages of the group are identified. The facilitator takes a highly active, directive approach to running the group. Each interaction is encouraged and facilitated by involvement of the group leader. This type of involvement lessens as the group matures. Indeed, in studies conducted on the model (Keller, 1995), greater and greater involvement was found among group members over sessions as the interaction between the facilitator and members lessened. We offered the members a pizza dinner before the group session each week. Their inclusion in the group was voluntary, and permission for us to record the group was obtained. The group is representative of the IBT model and accurately characterizes an initial group interaction. However, there is one thing that makes this particular group unique. First is the fact that all are residents of the same group home. This means that they perhaps will need less orientation to each other. The work done in these types of groups usually has a tremendous effect on the members. They get to work in a more direct way on the issues that develop during the course of group meetings. Groups whose members do not live together have less opportunity to put their new awareness into effect with each other. Instead, they must transfer the skills they learn in group therapy to work with people they encounter in other settings.

The group in this example has already moved through Stage 1 (orientation) and is in the latter part of Stage 2 (warm-up and sharing). In this particular session, the group has its attention on Gretta, who explains that she is going to have an operation. The example reflects a shift from horizontal self-disclosure (less emotionally charged information) toward vertical self-disclosure as Gretta discusses her deeper feelings.

Case Narrative	Commentary
Gretta: On Thursday . . . after 15 years, I'm having surgery. I never had surgery in the residence before.	
Facilitator: OK.	
Gretta: So . . . and Catrina knows about it because she was with me last week.	
Facilitator: OK. So you're a little bit frightened about going in for some surgery.	The facilitator acknowledges Gretta's fear with a comment about its intensity. This allows her the opportunity to clarify or correct the facilitator's statement of how she is feeling.

Gretta: And also because I don't
. . . . I like doing this thing. I like to
be on tape! [Everyone laughs.] And I
feel I have to go because I scheduled
it already.

The depth of Gretta's sharing shows
the greater emotional involvement
characteristic of the second part
of Stage 2. This allows for self-
disclosure from others while moving
the whole group toward the central
feature of the IBT method: Stage 3,
the enactment.

Facilitator: OK. So you're a little nervous. I have a way we could work on
this.

Cindy: How?

Facilitator [To Cindy]: I know you
want to help. Gretta, would you be
willing to do this, to. . . . I'll show
you how it works.

Gretta: Yeah, but . . . , I was going to
say, How is this going to help my
problem?

Facilitator: Let's see how it works. I
want to hear more about your problem.

Gretta: Why? What are you, a doctor? [The group laughs.]

Facilitator: I am a doctor, as a matter
of fact. [The facilitator motions for
Gretta to come out, to bring her
chair to the center.]

David: Dr. Ben Casey. [Everybody
makes jokes about doctors from tele-
vision programs.]

The facilitator chooses the protagonist
in this instance because the issue is
concrete, the protagonist is ready, and
the group is interested. Gretta is an
easy choice in this example. There are
other ways of choosing a protagonist,
however. For example, the protagonist
can ask to work in the group and the
group can agree, or the group can
choose who works. A question like
"Who do you think needs our help?"
may prompt group members to select a
person whom they feel needs the
group's attention. It is important to
choose a protagonist with the support
of the group. The group must both
understand and be in sympathy, or at
least tolerant, with the protagonist.

Facilitator: We're going to do a different kind of role-playing than you've
probably done before. What I am going to do is ask people to think about
what Gretta said about going into the
hospital. Right. The spot right behind
Gretta here is where you would stand,
and you say how you think she feels
about going into the hospital. As an
example, I'm going to say, "I feel
scared." [Turns to see Gretta's face.]
Does that sound right?

This is an example of the single double. The facilitator demonstrates
both the position and the words that
are appropriate.

Gretta: Yes.

Facilitator: And when I do that, when I stand here, do you know what they call this spot?

Gretta: Role-playing?

Facilitator: Right. But they call this spot "the double." [Everyone repeats the phrase "the double."]

David: Yeah, that means you're going to stand in for her . . .

Facilitator: Yeah!!!

David: . . . on the operating table!!!

Facilitator: Well, not on the operation! And because Cindy knows you so well, Gretta, why don't we have her stand behind you here. [Gretta is seated in a chair in the middle of the group, and Cindy moves to stand behind the chair Gretta is seated in.] Now Cindy is in the "double" role. Cindy, say how you think Gretta feels. Say "I feel. . . ."

Cindy: Errrrr. . . . Gretta, how do you feel?

Facilitator: Now, you say how you *think* she feels.

Cindy: Well, she's. . . . I know she's scared about having surgery done.

Facilitator: OK, so say "I'm scared."

Cindy: You want me to say "I'm scared"?

Facilitator: Yes, because you're trying to be her feelings. You just try and take it in, Gretta. You just wait there. [To Cindy] Say "I'm scared."

Cindy: I'm scared.

Facilitator: Does that sound right, Gretta?

Gretta: Yes, it does.

Cindy was chosen because it was obvious that she was a friend of Gretta's and cared a great deal for her.

People with mental retardation suffer from cognitive limitations that often require them to need concrete examples and descriptions to benefit from therapeutic encounters. The use of various types of doubles during group therapy can meet this need through a graphic demonstration of support. People usually will stand behind and slightly to one side of the protagonist. During the doubling it is not uncommon for the double to show his or her support by placing his or her hand on the protagonist's shoulder. These gestures make doubling a natural technique for use with people with mental retardation. Modifications that aid in the use of the double for this population are as follows: (a) The double typically may only say a single word or perhaps a single

Facilitator: OK, Cindy, say some more, but say it as though you are Gretta.

Cindy: I'm scared.

Facilitator: . . . AND . . .

Cindy: . . . about having the surgery done.

Facilitator: Does that sound right, Gretta?

Gretta: Yes.

Facilitator: All right! Let's give Cindy a hand! Wasn't that great? [The group applauds.]

noise to express how the protagonist feels. (b) The protagonist usually does not repeat the phrase of the double as is done in traditional groups. Rather, the protagonist simply agrees or disagrees with what was said. (c) Protagonists with secondary psychiatric conditions (e.g., paranoia or extreme anxiety) as well as traumatic histories (physical, sexual, or emotional) may be too uncomfortable to allow the double to stand behind him or her. In these situations, the double may need to stand to the side of the protagonist or a "double chair" placed beside and in full view of the protagonist may be used. (d) Doubling for profound losses (e.g., death of a parent) is not encouraged, as the effect of the doubling on group members may prove to be overwhelming, creating a downward spiral.

CASE EXAMPLE 2: AN ADVANCED ACTION METHOD— MULTIPLE DOUBLING

Once a single double has been used successfully, it sets the stage for a more comprehensive type of doubling. What follows is an example of the use of *multiple doubling*. Multiple doubling is used specifically to enhance the feelings of support and evoke the therapeutic factors of belongingness, acceptance, and universality.

Case Narrative

Facilitator: Cindy, you did a good job. [She returns to her seat.] Now that Cindy did a good job of that, Lenore, how about you?

Lenore: I can't get up. I have a bad back.

Facilitator: OK, Dave, how about you?

Lenore: David!

Commentary

There must always be an invitation to participate. Group members must know that they are free to participate or not. Rather than seeing members' lack of participation as resistance, it may be more fruitful for the facilitator or facilitators to think of it as a need for a different warm-up.

David: [Gets up to go stand behind Gretta's chair, which is still in the middle of the group.] Not David, Regis!

Facilitator: Regis . . . Regis! [David is now standing behind Gretta.] Say "I feel. . . ."

David: I feel. . . .

Facilitator: How do you think she feels?

David: [In a very high-pitched voice] I feel beautiful!

Facilitator: Yes, she feels beautiful, but how do you think she feels about the operation?

David: [Loving the attention] Happy? [A number of group members say David's name with a note of admonishment for not doing the enactment the right way.]

David: Nervous. I feel nervous.

Cindy: Scared.

Facilitator: Very good. And good, Cindy, that you said that. Let's give David a hand. All right, excellent. [Group members applaud.] So, Gretta, it was good that people know a little bit about how you feel. Who else wants to try? Leah, how about you?

Leah: You want me up there?

Facilitator: Yeah, how about we give it a try. [David returns to his seat, and Leah makes her way to the space behind Gretta's chair.]

Facilitator: That's very good. [Helps Leah into the spot.] And now, say "I feel. . . ."

David had requested at the beginning of the taping that he be referred to as talk-show host Regis Philbin. He was jovial and oppositional at the same time.

The group apparently is used to David's antics and lets him know about it. This may be considered a therapeutic example of interpersonal learning, as David immediately responds with an on-target response.

Leah [Looking to see Gretta's face]: How do you feel?

Facilitator: Now, how do you think she feels?

Leah [Repeating her question to Gretta]: How do you feel?

Gretta: Nervous.

Facilitator [To Leah]: What are you going to say?

Cindy: Scared.

Leah: Scared.

Facilitator: She said, "I feel nervous."

Leah: I feel nervous.

Facilitator: ". . . and scared."

Leah: And scared.

Gretta: And I feel scared!!!

Facilitator: OK, good. All right, let's give Leah a hand. [Everyone claps and is quite happy with themselves. Gretta brings her chair back into the group.]

Facilitator: Let's give Gretta a hand for doing that. Let's give her a hand for coming out. That was terrific. [Everyone claps.] What was good about what Gretta just did? What did you like about it?

David: She brought all of her emotions out.

Facilitator: Yes, David. That's very good. Cindy, what was good about what Gretta did? David said it was good that she got her emotions out. What was good. . . ?

For people with mental retardation as a primary disability, egocentricity often is so great that speaking in first-person as if another person can be very difficult. Although this is the way doubling is done in traditional psychodrama, it is often necessary to modify and accept the double's comments as observations about the protagonist rather than requiring people with mental retardation to make first-person descriptions.

This begins the affirmation of the protagonist. This happens at the end of the enactment stage and just before the affirmation stage. It is sometimes referred to as the postencounter affirmation. Here, members are affirmed for their participation in the group process and particularly for their involvement in any action that took place. The multiple-double process allows many members of the group to receive such affirmation.

Note that this statement is from the same man who has been so oppositional in the group!

Cindy: It's good she brought her feelings out.

Facilitator: Yes, Cindy, good. Leah, how about you? What did you like about what Gretta did?

Leah [Pointing to the center of the group]: She walked out.

Facilitator: Yes.

Gretta: I didn't walk out.

Facilitator [To Gretta]: Well, you walked out to the middle.

Gretta: Oh. Oh, sorry.

Facilitator [To Leah]: Right.

Leah: Yeah.

Facilitator: That was good. OK, and you liked that she took a little space for herself.

Leah: Yeah.

Facilitator: Very good. Lenore, what did you like about it?

Lenore: She was honest.

Facilitator: Yes. She was honest. Lenore, very good! And Hollis, how about you? What did you like about what Gretta did?

Hollis: It's all right.

Facilitator: It's all right. She did good, huh?

Leah was very excited about having to take part in the group and was particularly drawn to the use of the center of the group. When she used the phrase "walked out," she made a slight hand movement, and the facilitator realized that she was pointing toward the center. In this context, it was the fact that Gretta was using the chair in the middle of the group to do her work that Leah liked so much. Gretta's concrete interpretation of Leah's comment is an example of a common problem that facilitators need to be conscious of.

Hollis was the lowest-functioning member of the group and needed the most direction from the facilitator. In the postencounter affirmation of the protagonist, the feedback is directed by the facilitator from the group members to the protagonist. As this is the first group, it is particularly important to impress on group members that the feedback to the protagonist be positive. The reason for this is that the protagonist is vulnerable after the vertical self-disclosure usually displayed as part of the enactment. The emphasis on positive affirmation for the protagonist strengthens efforts toward self-disclosure while sanctioning the protagonist's participation. Other members can then learn from the protagonist that it is safe to participate with self-disclosure and action methods in the group.

This group was typical of those depicted in Figure 7-1. Group members' readiness to take part in the enactment portion of the process (Stage 3) allowed them to have greater concentration, presence, and emotional involvement. In this way, the format and process of the IBT model lends itself to creating an opportunity for such "teachable moments"; that is, when participants are able to take part in a way that allows learning to take place.

RESISTANCE

Two types of resistance are observed in people who are invited to play a double. David's and Lenore's comments above may be referred to for greater clarity. In the first, Lenore is asked to take part. This invitation to participate is offered without prejudice or criticism toward the participant. Rather, Lenore is asked if she would be willing to double for someone else. This willingness is entirely a matter of readiness on the part of the participant and does not interrupt the flow or process of the group. When using action methods, a lack of willingness to participate can be better understood as a need for the individual to have more warm-up and readiness. Rather than resistance, it is better to see this inhibition as an indication to the facilitator or facilitators that another way to warm up this person is needed. In Lenore's case, respecting her choice not to take part in the work allowed her to enter the process later, at the end of the enactment stage, when group members affirmed the protagonist. Although Lenore did not participate in the action method, she was nevertheless able to help affirm Gretta and interact with the group at this level.

David was more of a challenge. He deliberately said the wrong things when in role as the double. (But, as with most oppositional people, he had to know exactly the right answer so he could give exactly the wrong one!) Again, rather than seeing this as a form of resistance, the facilitator viewed it as a challenge to find a way to help David interact more helpfully. The facilitator coached David through the doubling, and David's attention-getting actions were reduced. By avoiding a contest with him, the facilitator allowed David to reenter the group process in a more helpful way later on, such as when he first affirmed Gretta for her work.

There are four general principles that can be used when working with resistance to action methods with people with mental retardation:

1. See the resistance as an indication of the need for a different warm-up for the individual.
2. Respect an individual's right to make a decision not to act or to stop acting if they have started and want to quit.
3. Provide opportunities for people to make other contributions to the group that do not involve action.
4. Allow people to benefit from the group through the audience role. Watching action can be a powerful way to stimulate therapeutic changes.

VALUE OF SUCCESSIVE USES

The four-stage IBT model allows group members to anticipate a format that has predictability and structure. The security that evolves from regular exposure to this method allows for trust between group members, which adds to the therapeutic foundation of the group. Members are in a state of readiness when the group is held at a regular time, in a regular place, with regular stages. For individuals whose cognitive abilities are diminished, the highly structured sequencing of the stages in a familiar place at an expected time also can be very comforting. Members know when it is time to act and when it is time to affirm. Perhaps most important, however, is that group members realize when they need to bring an issue to the group, when they want something from the group, and when they need to give something to the group. The structure of the sessions and the regular use of action methods to convey the work of the group thus help to establish a viable forum for therapeutic change.

As a rule, there is no out-of-session homework assigned for group members. However, if there are specific issues or incidents worked on (e.g., being assertive), there usually will be encouragement to the individual from the group to attempt to engage in these behaviors before the next meeting.

EMPIRICAL SUPPORT

A 1995 article by Tomasulo, Keller, and Pfadt summarized a study conducted by Ellen Keller (1995) using the IBT model. Keller's study reported that the number of interactions between group members increased as the number of interactions between members and the leader decreased. Simply put, during IBT, group members, over time, will interact more with each other than with the facilitator. Figure 7-2 shows how, over 12 sessions, a distinct pattern emerged.

In the same study (Keller, 1995), raters were briefed in the stage format of the model and were asked to note which interactions in the group could be considered examples of therapeutic factors. Eight factors

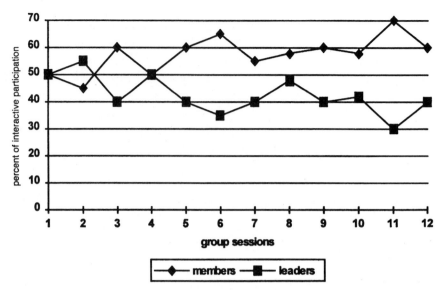

Figure 7-2. Group member identification with other as a function of group duration.

were chosen for observation: acceptance/cohesion, universality, altruism, installation of hope, guidance, vicarious learning/modeling, catharsis, and imparting of information. Two groups (a high-functioning group [mild mental retardation] and a low-functioning group [moderate mental retardation]) used IBT over 12 weekly sessions. Analysis revealed the presence of all eight therapeutic factors (see Table 7-1).

THERAPIST CHARACTERISTICS AND TRAINING

Although it may be self-evident, a therapist wishing to successfully employ action methods in a group setting with people with mental retar-

TABLE 7-1
Therapeutic Factors Observed in Combined Groups with
Corresponding Interrater Reliability Coefficients

Therapeutic factor	Reliability rating
Acceptance/cohesion	.86
Universality	.90
Altruism	.76
Installation of hope	.86
Guidance	1.00
Vicarious learning/modeling	.45
Catharsis	.96
Imparting of information	.91

Note: The ratings were provided by independent observers who watched videotapes of the IBT session. The closer the agreement of the raters to each other the higher the score. Perfect agreement that a factor had taken place is represented by a score of 1.00.

dation must possess three basic interests: (a) in working with people with mental retardation; (b) in group work in general; and (c) in using action methods in a therapeutic setting. It follows that to prepare for this type of work, therapists should, at a minimum, have prior experience in working with people with mental retardation; have training in group work; and have been a participant in an action method training program such as psychodrama.[2]

Specific materials to aid in facilitating IBT groups are listed in the Additional Resources section at the end of the chapter. Also, some of the references contain information that should provide sufficient information for beginning and maintaining a group. It is important that the therapist have supervision by someone more experienced in the field. Also, forming a peer supervision group with others can help develop skills and increase feelings of support. Suggestions for how to start and maintain a group are included in an article by Tomasulo (1997).

Perhaps one of the most common errors an IBT group facilitator makes when first using action techniques is having the protagonist engage in an encounter or rehearsal at the onset of the action. Although it is certainly appropriate for a group facilitator to use role-playing to rehearse a new behavior or to act out an encounter, it often is not the best place to start. Although such role-playing may, on the surface, seem reasonable, it may actually have the result of distancing the protagonist from the group (if he or she is not ready for such an event) or alienating those members of the group who cannot relate to the encounter. Additionally, the protagonist may be able to change his or her behavior in the group, but, if not adequately supported, he or she is unlikely to carry over the newly learned behaviors into his or her environment. The solution to this dilemma may come from using the double as a means of support. Creating an atmosphere of support is probably the most important condition the facilitator can help create. It is best to err on the side of having too much support rather than too little; trust and safety are the cornerstones of a well-functioning group.

CONCLUSION

As noted earlier, the shift to group counseling from social-skills training groups may require that the content of the group become secondary to its process. The IBT model has enjoyed wide usage, due in large measure to the fact that it describes a process taken from well-established principles in group psychotherapy that have been modified to address the needs of

---

[2]Additional readings as well as specific references regarding IBT training are included in Tomasulo (1998).

people with mental retardation. Additionally, the IBT model is being used in anger management, AIDS awareness training, relationship counseling, sexual abuse avoidance training, therapy for offenders and victims of sexual abuse (Razza & Tomasulo, 1996a, 1996b, 1996c), mental health counseling, chronic psychiatric patients (Daniels, 1998), vocational training, behavior management training, travel training, independent living training, sex education, socialization, educational readiness development, parent–child education, birth control education, and advocacy training, among others. Such broad use of the model would seem to indicate that the four-stage process of the group is more essential to the functioning of the group than its content. The presence of therapeutic factors within the group sets the stage for corrective work to be done. Future research should focus on outcomes studies measuring behavioral and attitude changes of group members. Several studies are now under way using the IBT model in comparison with other models with respect to differences in outcomes among participants. It is in this area of differential outcomes research (i.e., comparing the IBT model with other models of group therapy not involving action methods) in which the greatest gains in validating the model can be made.

In conclusion, using action methods in group counseling with people with mental retardation is a methodology whose time has come. There are both the need and desire for a therapeutic format in which learning can occur. There is a need for peer support groups, both with or without a particular curriculum attached to them. There is also the need for counseling groups designed for members to change not only their behaviors but also their feelings about themselves. As more clinicians are willing to develop the skills necessary to facilitate IBT groups, more participants will experience the positive life changes that can be attained through this process.

REFERENCES

Blatner, A. (1996). *Acting-in: Practical application of psychodramatic methods* (2nd ed.). New York: Springer.

Blatner, A., & Blatner, A. (1988). *Foundations of psychodrama: History, theory, and practice*. New York: Springer.

Bloch, S., & Crouch, E. (1985). *Therapeutic factors in group psychotherapy*. New York: Oxford University Press.

Daniels, L. (1998). A cognitive–behavioral and process oriented approach to treating the social impairment and negative symptoms associated with chronic mental illness. *Journal of Psychotherapy Practice and Research, 7*, 167–176.

Fletcher, R. (1984). Group therapy with mentally retarded persons with emotional disorders. *Psychiatric Aspects of Mental Retardation Reviews, 3*, 21–24.

Hingsburger, D. (1987). Sex counseling with the developmentally handicapped:

The assessment and management of seven critical problems. *Psychiatric Aspects of Mental Retardation Reviews*, 6, 41–46.

Hurley, A. D. (1989). Individual psychotherapy with mentally retarded individuals: A review and call for research. *Research in Developmental Disabilities*, 10, 261–275.

Hurley, A. D., & Hurley, F. J. (1986). Counseling and psychotherapy with mentally retarded clients: I. The initial interview. *Psychiatric Aspects of Mental Retardation Reviews*, 5, 22–26.

Hurley, A. D., & Hurley, F. J. (1988). Counseling and psychotherapy with mentally retarded clients: II. Establishing a relationship. *Psychiatric Aspects of Mental Retardation Reviews*, 6, 15–20.

Hurley, A., Pfadt, A., Tomasulo, D., & Gardner, W. (1996). Counseling and psychotherapy. In J. Jacobson & J. Mulick (Eds.), *Manual of diagnosis and professional practice in mental retardation*. Washington, DC: American Psychological Association.

Hurley, A., Tomasulo, D., & Pfadt, A. (1998). Individual and group psychotherapy approaches for persons with mental retardation and developmental disabilities. *Journal of Developmental and Physical Disabilities*, 10, 365–386.

Keller, E. (1995). *Process and outcomes in interactive–behavioral groups with adults who have both mental illness and mental retardation*. Unpublished doctoral dissertation, Long Island University, C. W. Post Campus, Longvale, NY.

Pfadt, A. (1991). Group psychotherapy with mentally retarded adults: Issues related to design, implementation and evaluation. *Research on Developmental Disabilities*, 12, 261–285.

Razza, N., & Tomasulo, D. (1996a). The sexual abuse continuum: Therapeutic interventions with individuals with mental retardation. *The Habilitative Mental Healthcare Newsletter*, 15, 19–22.

Razza, N., & Tomasulo, D. (1996b). The sexual abuse continuum: Part 2. Therapeutic interventions with individuals with mental retardation. *The Habilitative Mental Healthcare Newsletter*, 15, 84–86.

Razza, N., & Tomasulo, D. (1996c). The sexual abuse continuum: Part 3. Therapeutic interventions with individuals with mental retardation. *The Habilitative Mental Healthcare Newsletter*, 15, 116–119.

Steinberg, P., & Garcia, A. (1989). *Sociodrama: Who's in your shoes?* New York: Praeger.

Tomasulo, D. (1992). *Interactive–behavioral group counseling for people with mild to moderate mental retardation* [Two videotapes]. New York: Young Adult Institute.

Tomasulo, D. (1994). Action techniques in group counseling: The double. *The Habilitative Mental Healthcare Newsletter*, 13, 41–45.

Tomasulo, D. (1997). Beginning and maintaining a group. *The Habilitative Mental Healthcare Newsletter*, 16, 41–48.

Tomasulo, D. (1998). *Action methods in group psychotherapy: Practical aspects*. Philadelphia: Taylor & Francis.

Tomasulo, D., Keller, E., & Pfadt, A. (1995). The healing crowd. *The Habilitative Mental Healthcare Newsletter, 14*, 43–50.

Yalom, I. (1995). *Group psychotherapy* (4th ed.). New York: Basic Books.

ADDITIONAL RESOURCES

Journals

The International Journal of Action Methods: Psychodrama, Skill Training and Role-Playing. Washington, DC: Heldref Publications. (Formerly *Journal of Group Psychotherapy, Psychodrama, and Sociometry.*)

Professional Associations and Organizations

American Society for Group Psychotherapy and Psychodrama
301 North Harrison Street, Suite 508
Princeton, NJ 08540
(609) 452-1339

Division 49, Group Psychotherapy
American Psychological Association
750 First Street, NE
Washington, DC 20002-4242
(800) 374-2721

National Registry of Certified Group Psychotherapists
25 East 21st Street, 6th Floor
New York, NY 10010
(212) 477-1600
Fax: (212) 979-6627

8

REHEARSALS FOR GROWTH: APPLYING IMPROVISATIONAL THEATER GAMES TO RELATIONSHIP THERAPY

DANIEL J. WIENER

In life, people improvise whenever they respond purposefully to situations in a way that is not routine or fully planned. Ordinary social conversation, for example, is improvisational in that each speaker has to adapt continually in the moment to the utterances and reactions of the other or others without knowing where the conversation will lead. Most human activities, to varying degrees, draw on people's ability to improvise; that is, to make things up as they go along. Theater improvisation (*improv*), in contrast to scripted performance, is the stage use of improvisation-as-performance, particularly the use of playful and interactive theatrical games (Spolin, 1983).

Two major figures made significant therapeutic use of theater improvisation—Vladimir Iljine and Jacob L. Moreno. Iljine, who was most active from 1908 to 1917, used improvisation training, impromptu performances, and scenarios around which improvisation would occur in working with long-term groups of psychiatric clients, university students, or actors (Jones, 1996, pp. 57–61). Moreno created improvisational theater performances in his earliest work in the 1920s that he called "theater of spontaneity," which later led to psychodrama as "therapeutic theater, or theater of catharsis" (Moreno, 1983, p. 38). Currently, a number of drama therapists use improvisational methods (see chapter 5). Characteristic of all these approaches is the use of improvisation within groups to achieve therapeutic goals for individuals.

Improv provides therapists with a powerful resource to address three broad tasks in the successful therapy of relationships: (a) changing dysfunctional yet stable transactional patterns; (b) broadening the range of displayed identities that clients present to significant others; and (c) altering overly serious and negative affective interpersonal climates. Since 1985 I have applied improvisational theater games to the practice of relationship therapy with groups, couples, and families. Since 1989 I have called my method Rehearsals for Growth (RfG; Wiener, 1994a). RfG is not itself a complete therapy or theory, but an action approach that can be used to supplement therapies and psychoeducational approaches that aim to improve relationships and develop relationship skills.

REHEARSALS FOR GROWTH METHODS

RfG methods consist of offering client dyads or groups the opportunity to enact brief tasks and scenes (games) that involve unusual conditions or rules or the playing of characters different from those that the clients ordinarily identify as themselves. Such offers, made in the spirit of invitations to play or experiment, may serve as therapeutic tools for both assessment and intervention (Waters, 1992). Numerous theater games have been adapted, modified, or invented to serve therapeutic ends (Wiener, 1991, 1994a, 1994b, 1995, 1996, 1997a, 1997b, 1998).

Competent stage improvisation shares a number of characteristics with good interpersonal relationship functioning: (a) attentiveness to others' words and actions; (b) flexibility in both initiating and accepting others' directions and suggestions (i.e., giving up overcontrol); and (c) validation of others' reality, thereby supporting them (i.e., making others "right"). In addition to those benefits common to all action methods, such as broadening sensory, emotive, and movement expressiveness, there are additional therapeutic advantages to RfG, such as (a) encouraging novelty and playfulness; (b) experiencing spontaneity and taking risks; (c) building and expanding personal trust; and (d) cocreating new realities with others.

Encouraging Novelty and Playfulness

RfG games involve pretense and are clearly identified as nonrealistic adventures. They shift the context of therapeutic reality to a more playful and fantastic mode, thus lessening fear of real-life consequences of change and empowering exploratory behavior. They also provide opportunities for clients to access playfulness (which is unavailable to many adults and even some children) and a safe, nonjudgmental context in which to "face fear through fun" (Wiener, 1994a, p. xii).

Experiencing Spontaneity and Taking Risks

When clients are engaged in theatrical enactment they are referred to as *players*. Effective improvisation requires that players give up their conception, expectation, or script concerning what is supposed to be and attend to what is happening in the here and now, both intra- and interpersonally. Improvising thus entails spontaneity, which is defined as "an ability to experience fully, express without inhibition, and respond to new situations in an immediate, creative, and appropriate manner" (Wiener, 1994a, p. xviii).

The major obstacle to being fully present in the moment is the overriding tendency of the human mind to prepare for the future. Because improv requires people to respond spontaneously without knowing what will come next, the mind interprets the situation as dangerous; the improviser feels anxious and at risk of failing. Keith Johnstone, founder of the theatrical form of improv that gave rise to RfG, observed that spontaneity is socially threatening because it reveals one's natural self rather than the self one has been trained to present to others (Johnstone, 1981). Anxiety and defensive behavior, then, are likely responses to improv, even when there are no real-life consequences. When clients are encouraged successfully to overcome their fears of failing and looking foolish by improvising playfully they awaken to an enjoyable and expanded use of the self. Paradoxically, the spontaneous use of pretense also leads to the discovery and expression of therapeutically useful truths.

Building and Expanding Interpersonal Trust

RfG games are constructed so that their tasks can be accomplished only when client-players put aside their willfulness, defensive overcontrolling, and competitiveness to attend fully and receptively to their partners. Because of the previously noted sense of being in danger when improvising, people who improvise together share an adventure. This provides a social bonding experience that permits enjoyment, friendship, and trust for further adventuring.

Cocreating New Realities With Others

RfG provides opportunities for clients to stretch themselves by incorporating other roles into their social identities and to rehearse possible roles by enacting them dramatically. Such dramatic role rehearsals also provide relationship partners with opportunities to try on complementary identities in scenes that bring forth novel patterns of interaction. In this way, established relationships can be expanded safely beyond their existing, habitual limits. RfG games also can be used to promote the restorying and performance of individual and relationship narratives. Improv does not provide an escape from reality but rather gives clients permission to create and explore new realities, to experience imagined truth as present truth.

When applied to the assessment of couples, RfG games reveal and locate relational rigidity manifested by difficulty in entering or leaving the play context; players ignoring or undermining the choices made by their partners; long hesitations indicative of overcontrol and risk avoidance instead of spontaneity; emotionality that is inhibited or contextually unjustified; breaking of character or breaking off of dramatic action; and incapacity to play together in a way that both partners experience as satisfying. Also, how clients interpret instructions is as much a part of assessment as the content, style, skill level, or outcome of the enactment itself.

DIFFERENCES IN THE THERAPEUTIC USE OF IMPROVISATION

Improvisation occurs whenever therapists encourage role-taking, whether in the realistic simulation of social-skills role-playing or in the exploration of fantasy. Since its inception, drama therapy has made therapeutic use of improvisation in a variety of ways. Drama therapists, as noted above, focus their work on individuals, usually in a group setting, and typically have clients engage in relatively lengthy explorations of roles, punctuated by therapeutic conversation. In contrast, RfG games are brief interludes to the conduct of mostly verbal psychotherapy that focuses therapeutic attention on how the improv enactment reveals or alters relationships among the players.

Emunah (1994) describes three levels of improvisation used in drama therapy (presented in descending order of structure): (a) *planned* (roles are assigned, and the scenario is given before enactment); (b) *extemporaneous* (only role relationships are given); and (c) *impromptu* (nothing is given; everything is discovered in the moment). RfG games can be either planned or extemporaneous improvisations. RfG games have the following characteristics:

- *They are voluntary.* Participation is always based on informed consent; that is, the game or exercise is explained first and the potential players are asked whether they are willing to participate.
- *The future is unknown.* There are always aspects of the nar-

rative or performance that are unknown to the players at the outset and are created during enactment.

- *There are explicit forms and rules.* There are rules that distinguish one game from another in the form of limiting conditions that determine how scenes are to be played.

RfG games are designed and selected to explore or demonstrate some specific, therapeutically relevant point. However, RfG therapists are encouraged to vary any game to fit the exigencies of the case at hand—after all, therapy itself is an improvisation.

STEPS IN INTRODUCING REHEARSALS FOR GROWTH GAMES

Therapists directing RfG enactments should adhere to the following guiding principles:

- Create a safe, playful atmosphere that facilitates exploration and spontaneity (remembering and reminding clients that the enactment is a rehearsal, not a performance.
- Accept whatever players do in enactments within the bounds of physical and emotional safety while encouraging further stretching of their comfort boundaries through repetition and selective coaching.
- Remain open to the creative impulses of the self and clients that may lead to novel observations and insights or new enactments.

CASE EXAMPLES

For simplicity of presentation, this chapter describes only examples of dyadic enactment with adults. (For a description of the minor differences in implementing RfG with larger relationship systems and with children, see chapters 9 and 11 of Wiener, 1994a.)

CASE EXAMPLE 1: AN ELEMENTARY GAME—PRESENTS

Jon and Mimi, married 12 years and in their late 40s, had begun marital therapy after Jon's discovery of Mimi's 3-month affair. Although the crisis in their relationship had subsided and both were apparently committed to making the marriage work, there remained a climate of wariness, particularly Jon's holding back of warmth from Mimi. Mimi previously had complained of Jon's reserved manner and had offered it as a contributing factor to her having begun the affair. Jon disputed her characterization of him as reserved, countering that she was "rejecting." These underlying judgments threatened to undermine the reparative process begun during the three couples therapy sessions before the one outlined below.

Case Narrative	Commentary
"Let's try something different," I suggested. "Let's have the two of you exchange some imaginary gifts. Stand over here," I said as I motioned for them to stand facing each other a yard apart. "Now, Jon, hold your hands out, palms up, toward Mimi. You don't know what you're giving her, only that it's a wonderful present. Mimi, look at his hands and wait for your imagination to make the present appear. Then, mime picking it up and using it and show your appreciation to Jon for giving you this gift."	*Presents* is a simple game that I use often in conjoint therapy. It stages the universal social transaction of gift-giving, facilitating the emergence of intra- and interpersonal issues. When staged between persons with minimal relationship history, intrapersonal issues and generalized social responses emerge; when staged between persons having a significant relationship, responses are shaped by sentiment toward and history with the other. The purpose here was to assess and facilitate discussion of feelings and attitudes that emerged during and following the enactment. Given Jon and Mimi's previous quarreling, I was doubtful that they would have a mutually positive experience from their initial enactment.
Mimi looked intently at Jon's outstretched hands, hesitantly reached over, and mimed picking up what appeared to be a necklace. She mimed putting it over her head and holding it on her chest with one hand. She smiled brightly at Jon.	
"Don't forget to thank him for it," I reminded Mimi. She started, and then her smile faded. In a small, trembling voice she said, "Thanks." Jon appeared expressionless and tense.	The acknowledgment of the giver is an essential part of this game, as it transforms personal wish fulfillment into an interpersonal transaction.
"How was getting the present from him?" I asked Mimi. "I really liked getting that pendant, but [she looked at Jon] you know, I had trouble feeling like he wanted to give it to me," she reported, rather surprised. "And for you, Jon, how was receiving her thanks?" I asked. Glaring at Mimi, Jon snapped, "What thanks? She only wanted the pendant, not a gift from me at all."	

In presents, unlike some other improv games, players need not assume fictional roles. Consequently, partners are more likely to enact actual interpersonal issues during the game than when they are in role as characters. Here, the game's outcome was diagnostic of Mimi's conflict between wanting to receive Jon's generosity (i.e., forgiveness for the affair) and her vulnerability to guilt and rejection from someone whom she had wronged. Jon became reactive to Mimi's change of affect when I reminded her to thank him. He took it that she was begrudging him the credit for having given her the present she wanted, which activated his hurt and anger.

"Let's discuss this some more," I said, motioning for them to return to their seats.

I chose not to have Jon receive a present from Mimi at this time, as we had uncovered a central dynamic of their relationship (i.e., that Mimi could not take from Jon, which activated his punitiveness) that I judged needed immediate processing.

As is typical in the use of RfG games, the therapist moves the client-players off stage to process the enactment whenever he or she believes the on-stage action has produced a meaningful learning experience. In this case, Jon and Mimi had experienced a powerful demonstration of the extent of their mutual mistrust and negative interpretation of each other's actions.

Other choices include following up the present enactment with one that flows from what was just learned. With Jon and Mimi, for example, it would have been possible to invite them to repeat the exercise with different instructions, such as to receive an undesirable present, with the receiver acting, or overacting, out his or her displeasure. Although that choice might exacerbate feelings of failure, hurt, and hostility, it often can detoxify the atmosphere through catharsis or (paradoxically) implode tensions through taking expressiveness to a level experienced as absurd.

After eight more biweekly sessions during which other RfG games were used successfully to build trust and mutuality, I felt we were ready for Jon and Mimi to have an experience of accepting each other's benevolence.

I again invited Jon and Mimi to play presents. I gave the same instructions as before, but this time with Jon as the first receiver.

Case Narrative	Commentary
Mimi held her hands out, palms up, to Jon, leaning her body slightly away from him and holding quite still.	Mimi's body language suggested some trepidation about proceeding; she later confirmed that she had been re-calling the emotionally disagreeable experience of playing the game 4 months earlier.
Jon, appearing at ease, immediately received a fishing rod with which he mimed casting lines to different corners of the room. "Thanks, sweetie!" he said in a slightly surprised but happy tone.	Jon's initial ease and rapid accep-tance of his imaginary present sug-gested an eagerness to get a gift from Mimi. The fishing rod was also an indication that Jon now saw himself as having Mimi's blessing to go away on a fishing trip, a topic that had previously been a source of friction for the couple.
Mimi visibly relaxed, smiled, and leaned forward.	Jon's unqualified pleasure at getting the fishing rod from her was, psycho-logically, a real present from him to Mimi.
"Now, let's have Jon give the next present," I instructed.	
Jon hesitated, putting his hand to his chin. I reminded him that he did not have to think of what he wanted to give, that he was just to hold out his hands and Mimi would "see" the present.	The assumption that the giver has to determine the specific present is a fairly common mistake, reflecting the way real-life gifts are selected. Occa-sionally, this is an indication of over-control, the anxiety-based unwilling-ness to allow another to influence oneself.
As he put his hands out, Mimi hesi-tated, then grinned and tenderly lifted a small animal from his hands, cuddling and petting it against her shoulder. It was the fox terrier puppy they had been discussing getting. Mimi blew Jon a kiss (forgetting to hold the imaginary dog!). Jon lit up when he "saw" the puppy.	By making the present something that they both wanted, Mimi strengthened the feeling of "we-ness" in their relationship. As with Jon's enthusiastic acceptance of Mimi's present, Mimi made him look good for giving such a wonderful present.
"Let's discuss what has happened," I said, motioning them back to the couch. They sat nearer one another	Clearly, this round of the game had reinforced this couple's mutual posi-tive feelings and allowed them to

| than before; Jon slid his arm along the back edge of the couch, then around Mimi's shoulder. | contrast favorably their present on-stage achievement with their earlier performance. |

In the emotionally receptive afterglow of this enactment I encouraged Jon and Mimi to reminisce about other times they had cocreated this tender atmosphere rather than dissipate the mood through analyzing their performances. After stressing that they had it in their power to give themselves the present of these feelings, I contracted with them to use the presents game before their next financial discussion. They later reported that they had done so and attributed the cooperative and productive meeting to the game. In the successful therapy that continued for five more sessions, we made use of the presents game twice more.

CASE EXAMPLE 2: A MORE ADVANCED GAME—PUPPETS

Rick and Sondra, a married couple in their early 30s, entered brief couples therapy with the presenting problem of mutually competitive interaction over nearly everything. Although affectionate and devoid of persistent negative feelings or judgments toward one another, they were worried about the enormous amounts of time and energy each expended to "win" at the expense of the other. They also were aware of how seldom they reached agreement over even minor decisions, a frustrating and demoralizing state of affairs. Because they both appeared eager to break their impasse I gave them some preliminary RfG games in the second and third sessions that began shifting their process toward playfulness and cooperation.

In the fifth session, I placed an armless chair opposite mine and motioned for Rick to sit in it. "This game is called *puppets*," I said to both of them. "Rick, you're the puppet, and, Sondra, you're the puppeteer (I motioned for her to stand behind Rick's chair). "Together, you play the part of an expert lecturing me on a topic I will supply in a moment. First, let's practice how the puppeteer moves the puppet." I instructed Sondra to move Rick's limbs and head; she was to let go each time she placed Rick's body in a new position. Whenever she moved Rick repetitively he was to continue the motion until Sondra stopped or changed it. Sondra was told to move Rick's body frequently but not continuously and to be gentle when moving his neck and head. Rick was to accept Sondra's movements and to refrain from moving his body on his own.

| *Case Narrative* | *Commentary* |

| After they had practiced the instructions for about 90 seconds, I said, | The practice period allows the couple to familiarize themselves both |

"Remember, the two of you together make one character. Rick, you can speak but not move, and Sondra, you can move but not speak. You are an expert on the subject of" I paused, "the value of manicuring cows." Rick looked startled; Sondra tittered. I added, "Remember, your *character* considers himself an expert on this topic. Start with movement from the puppeteer." Smiling, I sat back in my chair, in role as an expectant audience.

[Sondra placed Rick's right arm out at shoulder level and turned his open hand palm down.]

Rick: Notice how my manicure gives me confidence to speak here tonight? Well, think about how ashamed of their appearance most cows are.

[Sondra placed both of Rick's hands behind his back.]

Rick: That's right! If *your* hooves were rough, dull, and dirty, you'd have trouble looking people in the eye, too!

[Sondra placed Rick's hands in front of his eyes, then made them into fists.]

Rick [Getting excited]: Folks, it's a disgrace!

[Sondra shaped Rick's extended right hand into an index finger, jabbing repeatedly at me. When she released his hand, Rick held it still and began to speak. I interrupted him to direct, "Keep the movement going!" and jabbed with my own index finger to illustrate.

Rick [Now jabbing rhythmically]: If we expect cows to have dignity, they MUST have manicures! [Sondra turned Rick's pointing finger down toward his left foot. She then leaned

with the unusual instructions and with cocreating one character as interdependent parts or faculties.

The topic I made up can be anything so long as it is absurd, relieving the couple from the burden of trying to be sensible or actually knowledgeable.

My role as audience establishes their actions as performance.

Rick accepts Sondra's physical offer, building on it for his speech, which also accepts my offer of the cow-manicure topic.

Sondra in turn picks up on Rick's offer by giving Rick a gesture consistent with what he is saying. I notice that they are accomplishing the cocreation of the character of the expert quite well; throughout the game they attend to one another and support the other's offers.

My choice here is to remind Rick of the rules, not to interrupt the on-stage action, which is going well.

over to lift Rick's lower leg straight out from the hip and adjusted his finger to point at the extended foot.)

Rick [Now "selling" to the crowd]: All right, friends, a manicure, . . . no, a "hoof-i-cure," to cure cattle shyness. [Sondra started laughing and Rick began wagging his left foot on his own. I grinned broadly and gestured for him to stop, which he did not see. Sondra lifted his left leg from under the knee and moved his foot up and down. Then she moved Rick's right arm straight up along his head and made his right hand into a fist.]

Sondra takes care of Rick's departure from the rules and makes him look good by rendering his movement "lawful."

Rick: Power to the cows! Cows proud to hold their heads high! [Rick's head and eyes are turned upward toward his fist. He stopped wagging his foot. By this time, all three of us are laughing. I gestured for them to "bring down the curtain" and applauded. Clearly pleased with themselves, Rick and Sondra returned to the couch.]

It is important to signal clearly the end of the scene and to have the players leave the stage and return to their conventional identities before reviewing their experiences of the enactment.

This enactment provided Rick and Sondra with a vivid example of their capacity to play cooperatively. In animated discussion immediately following the enactment, they came to see how this capacity could be an asset in their marital partnership, an insight that I referred to productively in the remaining three sessions of couples therapy.

Puppets may be used with dyadic client partners and with family members of all ages. In particular, children typically are fascinated with the opportunity to move their parents' bodies. The only contraindications are active hostility between the partners and touch–boundary issues (e.g., physical or sexual abuse) between the partners.

RESISTANCE

Resistance of Therapists to Allow Client Play

Although therapists ordinarily are not judgmental or insensitive to the feelings, strivings, and vulnerabilities of their clients, they are occasionally unprepared for the unpredictable range of behaviors and affective displays that can come from initiating play. In some cases, the therapist may have a more restrictive agenda for play and become intolerant of the exuberance or egocentrism of the playing client, thus getting anxious and displaying disapproval or even punitive overcontrol. Although RfG therapists need to be clear and explicit in setting boundaries for any therapeutic play experience, they must then be prepared and willing to support whatever happens within those boundaries.

Client Play As Acting Out

Antisocial or competitive behavior can be explored or contained constructively with RfG by limiting its expression to on-stage (in-role) behavior. Maintaining role and physical stage boundaries supports the therapeutic safety of engaging in pretense. Afterward, however, some clients may not readily or willingly drop the role. It is important that the therapist not ignore, nor even appear permissive of, any such boundary violations. I establish in advance a time of debriefing and reflecting on the completed enactment and always use a fictitious name for the player's character to clearly differentiate between character and client so that the client may be held accountable for off-stage social behavior.

Overcoming Client Reluctance to Play

Before offering any games, the RfG therapist needs to establish a context within the session that is safe enough to support experimentation while encouraging risk taking. Indeed, unless the therapist establishes a play context and is personally prepared to model playful interaction, these games will be of limited clinical value. Many adult clients are reluctant to initiate play or play timidly. I usually wait for clients to be familiar with their social role as therapy clients and for a point when humor, boredom, or stuckness signals receptivity to novelty and play before introducing RfG games. Clients worried that they might look foolish or do poorly can be reassured by the therapist's reminder that the enactment "is just a rehearsal"—a reframing that distinguishes the enactment from some real-life performance. It can be counterproductive to urge players to "do their best" or to coax them to participate with statements such as "This will be easy" or "This is going to be fun." These statements can set up expectations that undermine spontaneity.[1]

---

[1]For further, detailed practical suggestions, see Wiener, 1994a, especially chapter 9.

SEQUENCING AND REPEATING IMPROVISATIONS

Although improv games may be presented as isolated interventions, more benefit results from using them sequentially and repeatedly. Sequences of improv exercises can be used to build up play skills, usually by adding exercises that are successively more challenging or that increase the degree of complexity. Repetition of improvs reduces the need to focus on instructions and allows clients to explore different choices. Repetitions with different partners are particularly valuable in group and family therapy. In couples therapy, the therapist can compare a dyadic improv conducted between the spouses with one in which the therapist participates with each partner separately.

In improv, each scene is a new performance that allows players to assume new characters. However, when repeating improvs, players often recreate recognizable and stable characters that possess memory of their appearances in previous improvs and who resist offers that define them in other than established ways. Most often, other members of such a player's relational system recognize these characters and can be encouraged to relate to them playfully and in novel ways. In my work, I make intentional use of such emerging parts (Schwartz, 1995) as formative characters in further improvs in which these characters are given at the outset, or I work with them through other action modalities such as drama therapy or psychodrama.

Additionally, when clients are encouraged to perform improvs that they have enacted in session as homework it is helpful to have them establish a stage area (e.g., their living room, backyard, or a public beach) in advance of enactment.

RESEARCH AND EMPIRICAL SUPPORT

In the only attempt to gather data on the real-life effects of stage improvising of which I am aware, Wiener (1994a, pp. 237–238) interviewed 42 experienced stage improvisers. Questions focused on comparing clients' current lives with their lives before they performed stage improvisation (time between improvisation and questioning, average 3½ years). Content analysis of responses revealed that nearly all reported improvement in certain social skills and greater confidence in dealing with interpersonal situations in their off-stage lives.

A modest psychometric literature exists on assessment approaches to both individual personality and interpersonal relationship functioning involving improvisation (McReynolds & DeVoge, 1977). In particular, McReynolds and his colleagues (McReynolds & DeVoge, 1977; Osborne & Pither, 1977) have developed and empirically validated two personality assessment protocols, the Improvisation Test for Individuals (Impro-I) and the Improvisation Test for Couples (Impro-C) that involve structured role-play scenarios requiring clients to improvise. The Impro-C has been used as an assessment tool with couples to observe interpersonal process regarding emotionally congruent expression, mutual acknowledgment, and listening skills (B. Pither, personal communication, February 26, 1998).

Outcomes research to demonstrate the clinical effectiveness of RfG would appear to require that a protocol be compared with that of other methods; however, because of the highly variable and spontaneous nature of therapeutic improv, such research would be difficult to design. It might, however, be feasible to compare the outcomes of therapy that included RfG games with therapy that was exclusively verbal.

THERAPIST CHARACTERISTICS

Therapists who use RfG games effectively are those who can access their own playfulness and who are willing to lose their professional "mask" when the situation calls for it. Training and experience are also needed. Although RfG games are easily learned, therapists need some personal experience with stage improvisation to apply them successfully as clinical techniques. This is so for the following three reasons:

1. Only the experience of playing these games can give the therapist an appreciation of their impact, particularly the discomfort that players typically encounter at first. A therapist, however knowledgeable, who has not experienced the process of improv will tend to make interpretations reflecting an outside, judgmental viewpoint. As noted above, clients need the safety of being free from the consequences of being judged to take therapeutic risks.
2. Many clients need to see the therapist struggle—and even fail occasionally—to be sufficiently reassured to attempt improv. For this reason, therapists need to be able to model playful, failure-risking, crazy, silly, or immature behavior while in role, thus offsetting such clients' tendencies to project onto a passive observer-therapist "professional" qualities of being aloof, power retaining, and judgmental.
3. The therapist must be available to demonstrate, model, and —in many instances—even enter the enactment to achieve therapeutic goals.

When the RfG therapist gets involved as an improviser there can be the problem of who is left in charge while everyone is playing. In therapy groups and workshops I work with a cotherapist when possible; when working solo, I clearly delineate my moving in and out of any player role. In this solo position, however, part of my attention needs to remain "on duty," so I am not free to immerse myself fully in the playfulness of the improv.

TRAINING

The RfG trainer certification program consists of 50 hours of direct training in nonintroductory workshops plus demonstration of skill in application and teaching of the method's principles and techniques. Additionally, I encourage therapists interested in developing proficiency in RfG techniques to form peer play/study groups to explore and experiment with improv games and exercises. Another way to benefit from improv training is to learn from actors who improvise on stage. I recommend Theatre-Sports©, a copyrighted form of team improvisational comedy (Johnstone, 1994), because these improvisers work according to Keith Johnstone's principles, something not always true for other performance improvisers.

CONCLUSION

The safety of the psychotherapy context offers a near-unique opportunity for clients to discover, explore, struggle, and grow by unleashing their capacity for play and pretense. RfG games provide structured, teachable methods to test and develop an expanded repertoire of interpersonal roles, skills, emotional expressiveness, and use of imagination. Above all, improvisation is itself a paradigm for change, as it propels its players into spontaneity; that is, into the present moment in which any choice influences the immediate future. Finally, the therapist using RfG will experience how the immediacy of these methods enhances the possibility of bringing forth the novel and unexpected from self and clients alike.

REFERENCES

Emunah, R. (1994). *Acting for real: Drama therapy, process, technique, and performance.* New York: Brunner/Mazel.

Johnstone, K. (1981). *Impro: Improvisation and the theatre.* London: Methuen.

Johnstone, K. (1994). *Don't be prepared: TheatreSports© for teachers.* Calgary, Alberta, Canada: Loose Moose Theatre Company.

Jones, P. (1996). *Drama as therapy: Theatre as living.* London: Routledge.

McReynolds, P., & DeVoge, S. (1977). Use of improvisational techniques in assessment. In P. McReynolds (Ed.), *Advances in psychological assessment, Vol. 4* (pp. 222–277). San Francisco: Jossey-Bass.

Moreno, J. L. (Ed.). (1983). *The theater of spontaneity*. New York: Beacon.

Osborne, S., & Pither, B. (1977). *The Improvisation Test for Couples (Impro-C): A preliminary manual*. Unpublished manuscript, University of Nevada, Reno.

Schwartz, R. C. (1995). *Internal family systems therapy*. New York: Guilford Press.

Spolin, V. (1983). *Improvisation for the theatre: A handbook of teaching and directing techniques*. Evanston, IL: Northwestern University Press.

Waters, D. (1992, September/October). Family therapy as an excellent adventure: Learning to lighten up. *Family Therapy Networker, 16,* 38–41, 43–45.

Wiener, D. J. (1991). You wanna play? Using enactments in couples therapy. In T. J. Goodrich (Ed.), *Women and power: Perspectives for therapy*. New York: Norton.

Wiener, D. J. (1994a). *Rehearsals for growth: Theater improvisation for psychotherapists*. New York: Norton.

Wiener, D. J. (1994b). Rehearsing for growth: Improvisational group therapy. *Tele, 5*(1), 3–4.

Wiener, D. J. (1995). The gift of play. *Family Therapy Networker, 19*(1), 65–70.

Wiener, D. J. (1996). Tug-of-war: A theatrical technique for marital therapy. *Dialog, 27*(2), 37–43.

Wiener, D. J. (1997a). Presents of mind. *Journal of Family Psychotherapy, 8*(2), 85–93.

Wiener, D. J. (1997b). Rehearsals for growth: A methodology for using theater improvisation in MFT. *The Family Journal, 5*(4), 309–314.

Wiener, D. J. (1998). Mirroring movement for increasing family cooperation. In T. S. Nelson & T. Trepper (Eds.), *101 more interventions in family therapy* (pp. 5–8). New York: Haworth Press.

ADDITIONAL RESOURCES

Theatresports, Keith Johnstone, Loose Moose Theatre Company, 1129 9th Avenue, SE, Calgary, Alberta, Canada T2G-0F9, (403) 269-1444, E-mail: mail@loosemoose.com. Irregularly published newsletter on Theatresports techniques and principles. An annual, two-week Loose Moose International Summer School trains actors, professional and amateur, in stage improvisation.

The RfG Newsletter, % Daniel J. Wiener, Department of Health and Human Service Professions, Central Connecticut State University, 1615 Stanley Street, New Britain, CT 06050-4010, (860) 832-2121-telephone, (860) 832-2109-fax, E-mail: wienerd@ccsu.edu. Semiannual newsletter containing feature articles on RfG games applied to therapy and education, book reviews, and a calendar of RfG training events.

III

BODY PSYCHOTHERAPIES

9

CORE ENERGETICS: A THERAPY OF BODILY ENERGY AND CONSCIOUSNESS

KARYNE B. WILNER

Core Energetics is based on an integrated vision of the human being: The physical, emotional, intellectual, and spiritual aspects are unified. Through work with the body using physical exercises, deep breathing, cathartic experiences, and self-massage, energy blockages are released, feelings are expressed, and contact with one's essence is established, enabling the client to integrate the many aspects of his or her self. Core Energetic therapists work with overt psychological dynamics as well as unconscious processes, using the body as an instrument of diagnosis and treatment. Powerful, out-of-awareness dynamics, stemming from relationships with parents, heredity, the environment, and the culture, mold the body and create an individual's character structure and personality.

People begin their lives with the capacity for beauty, creative potential, honesty, and love. This is the essence of the higher self or *core*. However, early in life, people discover that true, instinctual, emotional responses to threatening events (e.g., anger, rage, fear, and terror), called the *lower self*, are not tolerated by society. Children are punished, violated, chastised, or shamed for expressing these emotions. In reaction to the lack of acceptance by the outside world, strong affect is hidden, even from the self, and repressed in the body. Lower-self emotions become distorted in their frozen state and are replaced in the personality by the socially acceptable mask self, which is composed of chronic tensions, projections, rationalizations, and diminished feeling states. This character defense system, in one sense, allows the child to survive, but in another, causes energy dysfunction, a hardening of the musculature, a suppression of natural sensation and feeling, and a distortion in thought processes and behavior. Therefore, children grow into adulthood acting and reacting from their defenses, separated from the truth and beauty of their natural essence (Pierrakos, 1987).

Core Energetics was created by John C. Pierrakos in the 1970s. The theory developed from his therapeutic studies with Wilhelm Reich, Pierrakos's mentor, and his work with Alexander Lowen, with whom he developed bioenergetics. Core Energetics was also inspired by the spiritual studies of Carl Jung and Eva Pierrakos, the leader of the Pathwork Community (Pierrakos, 1986). Core Energetic therapists are trained to help clients work with energetic blocks and physical dysfunctions to break through the mask to express and transform lower-self emotions and connect with their deepest truth and beauty. The two major components of Core Energetic theory are energy and consciousness.

For mental health to occur, energy must flow through five levels of being: body, emotion, mind, will, and spirit. If the emotional level is energized, people identify and communicate their feelings, whereas emotions that are repressed or somaticized lead to energetic dysfunction. When the mental level is energized, the mind is flexible and reasonable; when its energy is blocked, negative thoughts such as judgments, statements of blame, rationalizations, and rigid belief systems take over. The will, which is used to initiate activity, is also affected by energetic dysfunction. It can be overused in attempts to control others, or it can be underused, leading to passive and submissive behavior. A balanced will, the result of a healthy energy flow, leads to assertive behavior that does not usurp the power of others and to the integration of the masculine and feminine forces within the individual. Finally, the highest level, spirituality, pervades the entire being with love and energy. People who are cut off from their spiritual centers live too much in the material realm. Those with too much spirituality may lose touch with reality and fail to function in a healthy way.

Energy, the main focus of Core Energetics, is considered analogous to the life force. It is called "chi" by the Chinese, "prana" by the Indians, "libido" by Freud, "animal magnetism" by Mesmer, and "orgone" by Reich (Pierrakos, 1974). Healers, shamans, and mystics from many cultures see or sense energy and describe it as an aura surrounding the human body. This was often depicted as a golden circle around the heads of figures in early religious paintings. Energy is an absolutely neutral force and is not, in and of itself, sufficient to provide or maintain mental health. It must be accompanied by consciousness—a conscious awareness of one's intent, purpose, and truth. When energy is shaped by positive thoughts and joyful emotions, life processes are enhanced and the body expands and reflects harmony in its shape and posture. When life situations are perceived negatively, anger and fear are engendered and the body contracts and becomes awkward and disharmonious.

RATIONALE FOR USING ACTION METHODS

Action methods are used by Core Energetic therapists to correct defects in the flow of human energy. According to both Pierrakos (1987) and Reich (1948/1973), energy that streams through the body creates health, whereas energy blockages and leaks result in disease and distress. Dysfunctions in the energy field can be seen in areas of the body that are undercharged and overcharged—in an upward displacement of energy toward the head and shoulders and in rigidly held energy or fragmented energy. When energy does not flow, it is believed to affect behavior, leading to destructive life patterns and psychological symptoms and disorders. These energetic imbalances correspond to the personality types described by Reich (1945/1972) and Lowen (1958/1971): the schizoid, oral, masochistic, psychopathic, and rigid character defenses. Each character defense demonstrates particular personality issues as well as a specific body type. For example, the oral defense exhibits a lack of energy, a needy and demanding personality, and physical characteristics that include an elongated body; thin wrists, ankles, and calves; a collapsed chest; and intense eyes. In contrast, the masochistic defense is associated with held and blocked energy, a passive–aggressive personality, and physical characteristics such as a short, broad neck; a muscular build; and excess weight, particularly in the torso.

Core Energetic techniques are directed toward correcting problems in the human energy field. They are physical and emphasize movement, breathing, and self-expression. Therapeutic goals include grounding the energy so that it does not create an imbalance in the body; charging the body with energy if it is lacking; discharging energy from the body if it is blocked; containing energy in situations in which it could flood the person; eliciting repressed or out-of-awareness emotions, belief systems, and behaviors; and conveying meaning through physical action and assertive and receptive movement, including dance, journaling, art, nonverbal sounds, and role-playing.

Many interventions are used by Core Energetic therapists in addition to the breathing techniques discussed in detail in this chapter. To charge, discharge, or release repressed anger and rage, a client may be asked to hit a pile of pillows or a foam rubber block with a tennis racket. To facilitate regression to an earlier age, a client may be asked to lie down on a mattress and kick. In a group setting, one group member may stand across from the client who is hitting or kicking, role-playing the object of the negative intent. A three-pillow exercise, in which a *different* pillow represents the mask, lower self, and higher self or core, is used to elicit verbal material concerning each of these three aspects of the personality.

The roller is a Core Energetic device used to increase energy, deepen shallow breathing, ground energy flow in the legs and feet, open blockages in the pelvis, and integrate the heart and the pelvis, parts of the body that represent the forces of love and sex. This rolling pin–shaped object is about 2 feet wide and 15–18 inches in diameter. It is made of wood and a heavy cardboard material used in construction and covered with soft padding. It is laid on the floor, and the client places his or her shoulders on it and uses his or her feet to support the lower body. Exercises include rolling forward while stretching the knees toward the ground to release tight leg muscles, rolling forward while bouncing the pelvis up and down, and rolling backwards while placing the head on the floor to stretch the intercostal muscles, the diaphragm, and the solar plexus.

Other techniques involve self-massage of particular muscle groups, depending on the location of energy blockages and leaks. Clients may be directed to massage their throats to free the voice, their jaws and masseter muscles to release tears, the occipital area and eyes to reclaim memories, or their bellies to work with issues concerning control and power. All of these techniques are designed to help clients move through the four stages of Core Energetic therapy: (a) the identification and confrontation of the mask, which is hidden within tense muscles and behind ego-syntonic behavior patterns; (b) the exposure and release of the lower self in all its cruelty and destructiveness; (c) the reunion with one's authentic self; and (d) the recognition of one's universal life task. Once blockages are released from the body and energy starts to flow, clients make contact with their core and experience a revitalized life force.

DIFFERENCES BETWEEN CORE ENERGETICS AND ITS PREDECESSORS

There are differences between Core Energetics and the methodologies from which it is descended, orgonomy and bioenergetics. Both of these therapies acknowledge the roles of energy and the physiological systems in mental health, but not the role of spirituality. Orgonomy, the mode of therapy developed by Reich, requires that clients lie flat on a bed. Body techniques and breathwork are used to regress the client to early childhood. Work with physical segments (eyes, jaw, throat, upper chest, diaphragm, abdomen, and pelvis) occurs in a highly structured manner (Reich, 1945/ 1972). When Pierrakos and Lowen developed bioenergetics, they asked clients to stand up, a departure from Reich, their teacher, and taught them to ground their energy through the legs and feet, emphasizing making contact, living in the present, and taking responsibility by standing on one's own two feet (Lowen, 1976). Core Energetics moved away from bioenergetics by acknowledging spirituality as part of the therapeutic system. This difference of opinion between Pierrakos and Lowen created the original division between bioenergetics and the model of psychotherapy that came to be known as Core Energetics (J. C. Pierrakos, personal communication, May 1995). Core Energetics also differs from bioenergetics in its application of special breathing techniques designed to open the heart, its introduction of soft techniques to work with energy centers and the human energy field, its replacement of a psychoanalytic model of personality with a spiritual model, and its substitution of the roller for the bioenergetic stool. Both the roller and the stool are devices used to open muscles within the diaphragm and chest, but because the roller is built closer to the ground, it protects clients from falling and allows them to use it even when a therapist is not present. The roller therefore is an appropriate tool for between-session homework exercises.

Core Energetics practitioners are trained the same way throughout the world. However, there are a few differing areas of emphasis. Some Core Energetic therapists who remain close to their bioenergetic roots emphasize work with character defenses and techniques to open the armor and free the blockages in the body. Others stress the Reichian concept of psychosomatics, using the same techniques, often of a softer variety, to connect clients to transpersonal, spiritual, and energetic forces both within and outside of themselves.

Finally, differences exist between Core Energetics and other schools of body psychotherapy, and between Core Energetics and other spiritual schools of counseling. Examples include focusing, a method developed by Gendlin (1981), which requires clients to experience sensations in their bodies through deep concentration. This technique does not use movement to unblock energy. The Reubenfeld synergy method integrates Gestalt therapy and the Alexander method, emphasizing the identification of here-and-now feeling states and therapist manipulation of the client's body (the client lies on a massage table), but it does not acknowledge or work with energy per se (Simon, 1997). The Hakomi school (Kurtz, 1990) recognizes sensations and currents in the body but fails to stress strong physical release unless it erupts spontaneously from the client. Hakomi practitioners are trained to be extremely accepting and nonjudgmental, so as not to elicit resistance. In contrast, Core Energetic therapists welcome resistance, using confrontational techniques to bring it to consciousness to release the strong emotion repressed behind it. Holotrophic breathwork (Grof & Grof, 1990), another body technique, emphasizes breathing to resolve spiritual emergencies. However, unlike Core Energetics, it is not based on a comprehensive model of personality, nor does it use the body to diagnose underlying problems. Holotropic practitioners generally work with energy in a group format, using a form of breathing, with music in the background, that produces a state similar to hyperventilation. Finally, spiritual schools such as Jungian psychology and pastoral counseling rarely emphasize action methods or focus on the body. Instead, they use strictly verbal interactions between therapists and clients, emphasizing dreams, thoughts, metaphors, allegories, values, principles, and myths.

STACCATO BREATHING: A CORE ENERGETIC METHODOLOGY

For the ancient Greeks, breathing was related to bringing spirit into the body. They characterized a sick person as one who lacked spirit. Pierrakos also considers breathing to be the pulse of life (Pierrakos, 1997). When breathing is cut off by muscular blockages in the body so that both inhalation and exhalation are diminished, energy is found to be depleted and to flow at a minimal rate. The result is that people are less able to connect with their emotions, engage in analytic thinking, or use their creative processes.

Pierrakos (1997) observed babies in the process of nursing, noticing that, while breastfeeding, a baby sucks in air through his or her nose in several short sniffs at the same time it is sucking through its mouth. The bodies of people who were not breastfed and of those who were not properly nourished in other ways seem to have lost the ability to spontaneously engage in this pulsatory movement. To provide clients with the early nurturing and energetic experience they may have missed, Pierrakos created a form of breathing that mirrors the breathing of the nursing baby.

Staccato breathing is a Core Energetic technique designed specifically to open up several muscular blocks at once to enhance the overall flow of energy. In addition, staccato breathing helps achieve a balance between the two opposing forces in the body, the active and receptive energies.

Active energy, which flows from the heels up the back into the shoulders and the brain, is mobilized when people initiate activities. It allows them to organize, plan, and direct their efforts. Receptive energy, on the other hand, flows through the energy centers in the front of the body and represents the ability to experience spirituality, love, and many different kinds of emotions. When the active energies dominate the receptive energies, people lose their ability to experience empathy, compassion, and deep feeling. Conversely, people with dominant receptive energies have problems initiating, planning, and meeting objectives.

According to Reich (1945/1972), there are seven segments in the body that require treatment: (a) the ocular (eyes, ears, and top of the head); (b) the oral (mouth, chin, jaw, and occipital lobe); (c) the throat (neck, larynx, and tongue); (d) the chest (heart, lungs, shoulders, arms, hands, and upper back); (e) the diaphragm (solar plexus, liver, pancreas, stomach, and middle back); (f) the abdomen (the intestines and lower back); and (g) the pelvis (rectum, sexual organs, legs, and feet). Staccato breathing works with the blocks in all of these parts, encouraging a stream of energy to flow vertically through the body in the form of a figure eight. This vertical flow crosses at the diaphragm, continuing up or down the opposite side of the body from which it began. When energy is blocked, its flow moves sluggishly from side to side, as if it is trying to shake free of muscular constraints.

BASIC STACCATO BREATHING TECHNIQUE

In the following section, the basic staccato breathing technique is described. The information provided concerns the client population most able to benefit from the breathing, indicators and contraindicators for the use of this technique, the most appropriate timing for its introduction, times during the day to engage in the exercise, and specific instructions for practice. A case example is provided with a parallel commentary that explains the rationale for each aspect of the procedure.

Client Population: Indicators and Contraindicators

Staccato breathing can be used with adults of any age as an introductory technique. The breathing will vary with the physical characteristics of the individual, including type of body armor, muscular strength, gender, and age. People at many life stages, from adolescence to old age, can profit from this approach. Individuals with physical disabilities or illnesses may engage in staccato breathing as well. The exercise can be adjusted to accommodate most physical problems; it can be done in standing or sitting positions or it can be used in its original form, which is with the client lying down. Clients with lower-back injuries should proceed cautiously; it is recommended that they engage in the exercise without arching the back.

This breathing is indicated for all clients who desire to improve their mental health, raise their energy level, fully experience their emotions, and feel pleasure and contentment in their bodies. In terms of psychological diagnoses, staccato breathing benefits mood disorders such as dysthymic disorder and major depression, anxiety, and personality disorders. It is contraindicated for individuals diagnosed with psychosis, clients with medium to strong schizophrenic or schizotypal behavior patterns, and clients experiencing a bipolar episode.

Timing

Staccato breathing is taught to clients as soon as they are ready to engage in movement, energy work, and body psychotherapy. Criteria for its use include client readiness, a diagnosis of blocks in segments of the body, observed difficulties in the breathing process, and a need to open the heart and access feelings. In addition, this breathing can be assigned as homework early in the therapy. Clients may use it in the morning when they first awake while still in bed. The body tends to contract during sleep as synapses release or absorb neurotransmitters that may upset the individual's equilibrium (Pelletier, 1977). By providing freshly oxygenated air and encouraging a discharge of energy, staccato breathing can aid in blood flow and the elimination of toxins.

Instructions for Practice: Basic Staccato Breathing

There are three stages of staccato breathing: (a) expansion, the active phase; (b) contraction, the receptive phase; and (c) pausing, the relaxation phase. Reich (1945/1972) referred to similar stages—charge, discharge, and relaxation—when he described the orgasm reflex in his book, *Character Analysis*. The active movement begins the breathing. The client is asked to lie down on a couch, mat, or carpet with his or her feet flat on the floor and knees bent. The client is directed to close his or her eyes and breathe in short, strong sniffs through the nose, keeping the mouth closed, to the count of five. The therapist verbalizes, "Inhale. One. Two. Three. Four. Five." At the same time, the client's back is arched, the chest is pushed forward, and the shoulders and base of the pelvis are thrust back into the floor. The curve in the backbone creates a space between the back and the floor. While in this arched position and feeling the stretch in the spine, the client holds his or her breath for about 3 seconds before exhaling. This pause allows freshly oxygenated air to be distributed to the blood and the muscles.

During the exhalation stage, the complete expurgation of nutrient-depleted air is required. The client is told to release the breath through the mouth, continuing until all the used air is expelled, while at the same time vocalizing a sound, either "uuuhhh" or "hohohoho." Simultaneously, the physical position is reversed. The client's shoulders are lifted off the floor and rounded forward toward the heart, the lower part of the client's pelvis is tipped up about an inch, the abdomen is tightened, and the back is flattened onto the floor. The client's head may lift slightly when the shoulders curve forward and inward; however, the client's body type will determine its position. The body is now in a state of contraction.

In the third phase, the pause, the client's body relaxes. The directions are, "Now relax for a few seconds before beginning the next breath. Let your belly soften. Then start to breathe again. Take it in, one, two, three. ..." Each new breath begins in the belly. The abdomen blows up with air as the client inhales, flattens and contracts on the exhalation, and then releases for approximately 3 seconds before the next inhalation is begun. Introductory sessions of staccato breathing should be limited to between 10 and 15 minutes, and at least 10 such breaths should be taken before the client's breathing returns to normal.

Staccato breathing should not be engaged in mechanically as if it were an exercise. To bring forth the desired results, it must be experienced as a very real aspect of the client's life and connected to conscious awareness. Changes in the body and the psyche are most likely to occur if the breathing exercises are conducted daily over a period of time. When assigned as homework, the technique should be used for 10 to 15 minutes in the morning or at other times during the day. Although taught at the beginning of the therapeutic process, this technique is used throughout the therapy. Advanced techniques are described below.

CASE EXAMPLE 1: BASIC STACCATO BREATHING

Case Narrative   *Commentary*

Nora's presenting problem concerned an inability to make deep contact, especially in the form of same-sex friendships. A small woman with a slender build in her early 40s, Nora explained that although she had some acquaintances and was a wife and mother, she lacked close relationships. Diagnostically, she showed symptoms of a dysthymic disorder, including a very reduced energy level, low self-esteem, and feelings of hopelessness, all of which had been present for over 2 years. According to her family history, as a small child she received very little warmth, physical affection, or attention from either parent. Her father, manager of a department store, worked a lot, and she remembered her mother as always leaving or "going out the door."

Given Nora's presenting problem, diagnosis, and family history, the introductory staccato breathing technique was chosen to begin to break through her depression and confront her feelings of hopelessness. Staccato breathing challenges depression by encouraging deep breathing into parts of the body that usually do not receive enough oxygen. Muscular blocks are forced to release, and a vertical energy flow is created in the body. Because energy flow and the fatigue and low energy that characterize depression are mutually exclusive, Nora's depressive symptoms begin to diminish.

Analysis of Nora's body and energy flow indicated a long, narrow face with a tense and inflexible jaw; a narrow and constricted chest and diaphragm; a taut shoulder girdle that would not enable the shoulders to relax downward or move forward or backward; a straight, rigid back and neck; a well-energized and movable pelvis; and shapely, muscular legs and feet.

In our fourth meeting, which followed sessions that emphasized building rapport, conducting a thorough clinical interview, and body analysis, Nora was introduced to staccato breathing.

She was given directions that explained that the breathing involved pushing the chest forward, thrusting the shoulders and pelvis back, inhal-

Nora's narrow, tight chest and diaphragm, which were so constricted it looked as if she wore a muscular girdle, suggested little nurturance during the oral period. Her well-developed pelvis suggested that there was a connection with either her father or brother during the oedipal period. The muscles in her body also expressed a strong rigidity, portraying the desire to achieve and an ability to be successful in life. However, the blocks in the throat and jaw made it difficult for Nora to speak her truth and let her needs be known to others. Her inhalation and exhalation were diminished because of a strong contraction from the chest down into the diaphragmatic segment. This contraction protected Nora from experiencing heartbreak, separating the warm feelings in her pelvis from the rest of her body. Because of the block in the shoulder girdle, Nora's assertive energies were repressed, and she could not reach out to make contact. In addition, the solar plexus, which represents the state of the ego, indicated that Nora did not feel welcomed at birth. In response, she chose to live by taking up very little room in her family and on the planet; that is, by contracting her body into a narrow form.

The breathing was introduced at this early stage of the therapy to teach the methodology, begin the process of opening the chest and diaphragmatic segments, permit Nora to become comfortable with the technique, and allow her to experience more energy in her body.

Attention was given to teaching the correct version of both the inhalation and the exhalation. Sucking air through the nose should be demoning in short sniffs through the nose to the count of five, and exhaling through the mouth while taking the reverse physical position. She was directed to relax the abdomen for 3 seconds before breathing in again.

So I could observe her body during the breathing and note the blocks and energetic distortions, I had asked Nora to bring a pair of shorts and a halter top with her to the session. After she changed from her street clothes in an adjoining room, I demonstrated the breathing to her and took her through it step-by-step.

Once she felt comfortable with the breathing, the process was continued for approximately 10 minutes.

Nora commented several times that she was having difficulty inhaling. At one point she sat up and began to cough. Her chest could not take in the additional air. She said, "It feels too tight." I affirmed her experience, telling her that blocks in her throat and chest led to this problem. Choking and coughing continued in the next three or four sessions until the muscles relaxed. At the same time, Nora's breathing became easier, her upper chest appeared more energized, and her self-esteem began to increase.

strated and practiced in session. Inhaling in short bursts allows oxygen to go directly to the brain, thereby helping to organize the mental processes and the ego (Pierrakos, 1997). The inhalation also mobilizes several segments of the body at once, such as the pelvis, abdomen, diaphragm, and chest. In contrast, inhaling one long, deep breath can cause some of these segments to be missed.

It is important that the clinician note which parts of the body receive the breath and which parts are deprived of it. Shorts, leotards, and bathing suits, depending on the room temperature, are all appropriate clothing for the staccato breathing process.

It is also important, with fragile body types such as Nora's, to limit the amount of breathing time. A lengthy breathing period could lead to flooding (i.e., an overload of energy in a body too contracted or undernourished to process it). In Nora's case, I placed a 10-minute limit on the breathing.

Because her chest was constricted and the intercostal muscles extremely tight, Nora felt like she was suffocating. The beginning breaths were uncomfortable. There was also a certain amount of coughing, which is to be expected when there are contractions in the chest, throat, and neck.

During this period I asked her if she would be willing to work with staccato breathing at home on a daily basis. She agreed, telling me that she preferred to do so. As her therapy continued, more advanced forms of staccato breathing were introduced.

Homework is assigned in consultation with the client because the body needs continual rehearsal if the muscles are to transform. Nora's work in session and at home led to a stronger inhalation, more oxygen consumed, greater outflow of nutrient-depleted air, and an enhanced flow of energy in her body.

ADVANCED STACCATO BREATHING TECHNIQUES

This section describes a more advanced form of staccato breathing. The client population that should use advanced staccato breathing is described. In addition, indicators and contraindicators, timing for the introduction of the technique, and instructions for its use are provided. A case example with parallel commentary illustrates how this technique is used in a therapy session.

Client Population: Indicators and Contraindicators

Advanced forms of staccato breathing are used with clients who have progressed beyond the introductory stages of therapy. They are in the work phase, motivated to make changes in their behaviors, deepen their emotional experiences, and add new and better coping mechanisms to their repertoires. These individuals experience major energetic blocks in their bodies and portray other energetic problems, such as an undercharge or an overcharge in certain areas, an upper displacement of energy, energetic rigidities, energetic splits, or energetic leaks. Although the advanced breathing is not recommended for anyone experiencing a psychotic state, it is of particular benefit to those with symptoms associated with anxiety, depression, psychosomatic illnesses, and eating disorders. It also can be used successfully in group or individual therapy.

Timing

Advanced staccato breathing techniques are used in the work phase of the therapy. They may be instituted in one variation or another between the third and ninth months of therapy, and once they are initiated they can be used throughout the remainder of treatment. It is even recommended that these techniques be continued when clients complete treatment so they can maintain the therapeutic benefits and avoid regression.

Instructions for Practice: Advanced Staccato Breathing

To work with clients who need or desire more intensive therapy, the therapist introduces several techniques that are used by the client while he or she is engaged in staccato breathing. The following variations are used during the vocalized exhalation: (a) rubbing the top of the head with one hand and the throat with the other; (b) wrapping both hands around the throat and massaging it; (c) stamping the feet and hitting the mat with fists while saying "no"; (d) hitting or kicking upwards and out with extended arms or legs; (e) rubbing the knuckles into the jaws and masseter muscles; (f) raising the pelvis up and hitting it down while saying "never" or "I won't give it to you"; (g) raising the legs straight up toward the ceiling with feet pointed to the face and letting them shake and vibrate; (h) varying the pace or pitch of the breathing, from slower to faster and from louder to softer; (i) massaging the intestines with the fingers, making small circles in spots that hold tension; and (j) placing fists under the small of the back and bouncing on them. These variations occur during the exhalation phase, except for changes in speed and pace of breathing, which take place during the inhalation. Each exercise may be used alone as a specific technique to work with a particular block in the body or combined sequentially to work with several blocks in the body.

CASE EXAMPLE 2: ADVANCED STACCATO BREATHING

Case Narrative

In the work phase of the therapy, Nora continued to attend to her throat block. I asked her to wrap both hands around her throat, without squeezing the windpipe, and to inhale as before. On the exhalation, I directed her to massage the throat, helping loud sounds to escape, and, at the same time, to stamp her feet and contract her belly.

Commentary

This variation of staccato breathing in which the throat is massaged during the exhalation is used to release the throat block. It was an important exercise for Nora because of her inability to initiate communication activities or reach out with her voice to make friends. The simultaneous stamping of the feet allowed the newly discharged energy to ground rather than create an upper displacement. In addition, Nora was encouraged to tighten her belly during the exhalation to connect with the feelings held there. Most people are unaware of the belly and unconscious of the blocked energy held within it.

Continuing this exercise for several minutes, Nora allowed deep, harrowing, and dissonant sounds to emerge from her body, stopping to choke occasionally and spit phlegm into a tissue.

After repeating this inhalation/exhalation/throat-release combination approximately 12 times, I suggested she relax, place her hands at her sides, and breathe normally. Her body eased into the sofa.

A lot of energy had been released with the breathing, but its flow stopped at the knees, where it seemed to block again.

Therefore, on the next exhalation, I asked Nora to stamp her feet, hit the mat with her fists, and say "no" with her lower jaw extended. When she released her breath, she began to pound, kick, and scream at the top of her lungs, moving wildly for a minute or two. She repeated this combination several times.

When she stopped the movement, I suggested she discharge more energy by raising her legs and pointing them toward the ceiling with her feet directed toward her face. This position created a stretch in her hamstring muscles, and her legs began to shake

Tensions in the throat and neck exist to decrease sensation in the body and control anxiety. They result in a muscular obstruction that thwarts people from speaking their truth. By massaging the masseter and sterno-cleidomastoid muscles and releasing foreign and unpleasant sounds, contractions in the vocal apparatus are eliminated.

It is equally important to allow the body to relax during different stages of the breathing, providing an opportunity for energy redistribution and for sensations and feelings to be identified and experienced.

With training, clinicians can learn to see energy release and to chart its flow. The information gained can help determine the next intervention. Because the staccato breathing, a charging technique, increased Nora's energy level, it became necessary to discharge some of this energy so it did not move to another place in the body and create new blocks.

Nora was asked to stamp her feet and hit with her fists to discharge the excess energy. (Stamping and hitting also may be used to charge the body.) Saying "no" was initiated to work with Nora's resistance. She had to say "no" to having friends before she could reach out and bring close relationships into her life. By fully experiencing her resistance, Nora could move beyond it and create the opposite state in her life.

The hamstring stretching exercise continued to discharge the energy, releasing blocks in the legs and allowing it to flow through her body. During discharge, the vibrations moved from her legs into her trunk and upper body.

and vibrate. Although the vibrations were "a little scary," she said that they felt great.

The exercise also created a grounding experience for Nora. Standing up, she observed that her energy had distributed itself throughout her body. As we summarized what was accomplished in the session, Nora commented, "Something inside me was definitely freed up in here today."

About 2 weeks later, another advanced staccato breathing technique was integrated into Nora's therapy. This involved working with the shoulders and arms. I requested that during the next series of exhalations she raise her arms and hands toward the ceiling, fingers stretching upwards, asking for help. I directed her to make several verbal requests, such as "Please help me. I want your friendship. I want to be close." Nora had a strong reaction to this reaching aspect of the exercise. Her fingers would not stretch up; instead they folded over, drooping down. She kept repeating, "It's hopeless, no one is there." Then she began to sob deeply.

I did not interrupt the sobbing, but when it decreased, I asked her to continue the staccato breathing. On the exhalation, I requested that she strike out in front of her with her arms and fists, saying "I hate you" as loudly and fiercely as possible while moving her legs at the same time.

The aggressive punching helped her to regain a sense of power. Once she attained it, I suggested she continue the breathing and again try reaching with her arms. Encouraging her, I said, "Reach. Really reach. Ask for help. Claim your right to friends."

Work such as this also enhances grounding, permitting clients to experience energy in the lower body, pelvis, legs, and feet.

Reaching with her shoulders and arms helped Nora experience her infantile pain: the image of her mother's back going out the door. Her blocked shoulders and listless arm muscles reflected repressed feelings of hopelessness and anger.

By striking out, Nora was able to bring her hidden resentment toward her mother to consciousness.

Reaching with her arms aggressively while asserting for what she needed (i.e., help, contact, and friends) encouraged muscular repatterning of early belief systems and schemata.

She was able to maintain this position for a while, stretching through her shoulders and her arms, asking for help. Her face changed and brightened. She whispered, "Help me. I deserve love."

Following this exercise, I suggested she give love to herself. I asked Nora to let her breathing return to normal and to place her hands on her heart. She laid for a while, crying softly. The work ended with a beautiful smile on Nora's face.

I ended the exercise with Nora's hands on her heart so that she could experience her chest without armor. By reaching for love from the universe, she received a sense of empowerment in place of the old expectation of rejection she had carried with her from early childhood.

RESISTANCE

Because of its psychoanalytic origins, Core Energetic therapists generally treat resistance as a product of unconscious forces that attempt to thwart change (Reich, 1945/1972). However, there is also a resistance to action techniques that stems from client doubts and concerns about the methodology. Because many people view psychotherapy as sitting and talking to another person, an image that has been supported by the media as well as by academic institutions, resistance to action therapies should be expected and accepted. For the traditional client, action methods may seem weird, touchy–feely, and not to be taken seriously.

People who come for therapy often are inhibited, self-conscious, perfectionistic, and low in self-esteem. Using methods that make them feel uncomfortable or ashamed, such as various forms of movement, may hinder the therapy. Therefore, clients may request that certain procedures or techniques be stopped. In general, resistance to Core Energetic sessions should be handled in specific ways. First, clients need to be supported; their resistance should be heard and understood. Second, clients should be given an opportunity to participate in the selection of techniques to be used. Third, therapy may begin with verbal interventions until the clients request a more active approach. For particularly unstable clients, impulsive clients, and clients with a strong schizoid defense, verbal therapy provides a safer way in which to begin the work.

Additionally, resistance to action methods can be transformed through psychoeducational processes. When clients understand how the body affects the mind and vice versa, they usually decide to participate. It is important that clients be educated about the expected outcome and how it will be achieved. Core Energetic therapists' offices often contain boards on which to draw models, writing utensils for note taking, and other equipment, such as tape recorders for those who wish to record sessions.

Because Core Energetic therapists are required to look at a client's body to analyze energetic patterns and muscular blocks, clients must be informed about this procedure. Although a body analysis does not take place before the client is completely comfortable with the idea, and bathing suits or workout clothes are worn during the session, people with negative body images may experience discomfort. Therefore, it is essential that the therapist establish a safe environment before this diagnostic session. Education provides safety as well as understanding and participation.

One last form of resistance is encountered from some people who are familiar with the therapy—a resistance to the kinesthetic experience of energy flowing within the body. Although the energetic flow feels good, enhances pleasure, and creates sexual and loving feelings, many people fear such pleasure as a result of earlier experiences with the loss of it (Pierrakos, 1987). Therefore, a conditioned response to limit pleasure occurs, creating by association a resistance to these exercises. This resistance is dealt with through homework assignments for clients and supervision for therapists.

REPEATED AND SUCCESSIVE USES

Because it is not an easy task to release a physical block that has formed over a number of years or to revamp an energy system that has been overcharged or undercharged, techniques must be used repeatedly to achieve success. Clients like the familiarity of certain techniques, and each time a technique is repeated it leads to slightly different results. For example, striking a pillow with a racket in successive sessions releases muscular blocks at increasing depths and allows clients to attain a greater understanding of the multiple layers that make up their repressed negativity. Because many techniques have several versions that serve the same purpose, others may be substituted if one becomes boring. In addition, homework, a repetitive tool that brings about overlearning, is a necessary part of the therapeutic structure. Clients are expected to continue the work at home on a daily basis, because a weekly or biweekly therapy session can only initiate change; implementation and actualization of change processes require daily exercise and reinforcement.

Successive use of action techniques is also important, because both the body and the personality change in relationship to the energetic work. For instance, as the therapy continues, the body shifts from one defensive structure to another, reflecting earlier, unresolved wounds. Clients may begin working with undercharged oral areas of the body, reflecting their neediness. However, once the body becomes charged in that area, overcharged, masochistic areas of the body may come to the attention of therapist and client, representing a passive–aggressive tendency or a need to withhold. Therefore, the therapeutic technique might shift from one of reaching out with the arms and saying "I need you" to one of stamping with the feet and saying "Get away." Clients work in layers, generally moving from less stressful to more stressful areas of concern. The body mirrors these same strata in the musculoskeletal system.

EMPIRICAL SUPPORT

Pierrakos (1974) and Brennan (1987) conducted exploratory research in support of the Core Energetic theoretical stance, but they did not provide evidence concerning the method's efficacy. In contrast, some of Reich's disciples conducted research supporting orgone therapy's efficacy (Mann, 1989), but these earlier studies have been criticized because of design problems. Therefore, evidence of the effectiveness of the Core Energetic approach is still lacking. Studies that are most supportive come from the area of health psychology and involve research with individuals with cardiovascular problems and cancer or in exercise programs.

Investigations of the role of anger and hostility in cardiovascular disease (Lai & Linden, 1992; Wolman, 1988) and cancer (Fawzy et al., 1990; Simonton, Creighton, & Simonton, 1978) shed light on the effectiveness of the verbal expression or mental imaging of anger. Research concerning the use of Core Energetic methods to release anger needs to be conducted, especially regarding their effect on blood pressure, immune response, stress level, and degree of depression or anxiety. Research exists (Gauvin, Rejeski, & Norris, 1996; Slaven & Lee, 1997) that shows the effects of physical exercise on emotional states and indicates that vigorous physical activity is related to significant improvement in affect and feeling states. Similar research needs to be conducted in a Core Energetic therapy setting to test the generalizability of these results.

Much more empirical research on Core Energetic methods is needed to determine (a) whether Core Energetic interventions are more effective than verbal therapy alone; (b) what the effects are of Core Energetic techniques when combined with another methodology (e.g., cognitive–behavioral therapy); (c) whether a Core Energetic body analysis can help clinicians make more efficient diagnoses and treatment plan designs; (d) which Core Energetic techniques are most helpful to people with specific diagnoses; and (e) which techniques best enhance problem solving, coping skills, and the attainment of pleasure in life.

THERAPIST CHARACTERISTICS, EDUCATION, AND TRAINING

The Core Energetics training program is a 4-year professional program that generally follows an advanced degree. Graduates include physicians, psychologists, social workers, counselors, and pastoral counselors. The curriculum stresses psychology, energy dynamics, character analysis, bioenergetic and Core Energetic techniques, diagnosis, psychosomatics, psychopathology, spiritual studies, anatomy, and group leadership. During the training, students are required to have individual therapy with Core Energetic therapists, group process work, and both group and individual supervision sessions. In addition, it is necessary for trainees to work with their own processes, transforming their masks, releasing their negativity, and opening their hearts toward themselves and others (Institute for Core Energetics, 1996). They are encouraged to experience love and pleasure in their lives and to search for their unique truths.

In the first year of training, students learn concepts of energy and consciousness, methods of diagnosis, and how to identify the different character defense systems. They also learn about themselves: their life tasks, core qualities, and character structure. The second year of training focuses on techniques for working with the body, psychosomatic theory as detailed by Reich (1972/1945) and therapeutic interventions developed by Pierrakos (1987). The third year integrates spirituality with methods designed specifically to work with the human energy field (the aura), the energy centers (the chakras), and the character defense structures. Trainees need to see and sense subtle energies to be effective practitioners. The final year of training involves practice sessions and reviews of transference, countertransference, resistance, ethics, and sexuality. A postgraduate year, for those who plan to teach, emphasizes a deepening of the work and many aspects of practice, including individual, group, couples, family, and sex therapies.

CONCLUSION

Core Energetics, an action therapy that integrates body, mind, spirit, and emotion, emphasizes that energy flow in the body is necessary for the attainment of love, pleasure, and mental and physical health. The model teaches that love is basic to the life force. When the core, or authentic self, is no longer overshadowed by the destructive characteristics of the mask or lower self, love is free to nourish people and help them transform their lives. The correction of energetic blocks, leaks, displacements, rigidities, and fragmentations facilitates the diminishment of the mask and the release of repressed lower-self emotions. The dysfunctional belief systems and out-of-awareness negative affect that are elicited are transformed, and the body is revitalized. Flowing energy plus consciousness facilitate the attainment of emotional truth, creative cognitions, activities combining receptive and assertive forces, spiritual experiences, and mental health in general. Through the many techniques and interventions offered by Core Energetic therapists, clients achieve healthier patterns of living and better coping mechanisms.

REFERENCES

Brennan, B. A. (1987). *Hands of light: A guide to healing through the human energy field*. New York: Bantam Books.

Fawzy, I. F., Cousins, N., Elashoff, R., Fahey, J. L., Fawzy, N. W., Kemeny, M. E., & Morton, D. (1990). A structured psychiatric intervention for cancer patients: Changes over time in immunological measures. *Archives in General Psychiatry, 47,* 729–735.

Gauvin, L., Rejeski, W. J., & Norris, J. L. (1996). A naturalistic study of the impact of acute physical activity of feeling states and affect in women. *Health Psychology, 15,* 391–397.

Gendlin, E. (1981). *Focusing* (2nd ed.). New York: Bantam Books.

Grof, G., & Grof, S. (1990). *The stormy search for the self*. Los Angeles: Jeremy P. Tarcher.

Institute for Core Energetics. (1996). *Core Energetics evolutionary process: A four year training program for helping professionals*. New York: Author.

Kurtz, R. (1990). *Body-centered psychotherapy: The Hakomi method*. Mendocino, CA: LifeRhythm.

Lai, R. Y., & Linden, W. (1992). Gender, anger expression style, and opportunity for anger release determine cardiovascular reaction to a recovery from anger provocation. *Psychosomatic Medicine, 54,* 297–310.

Lowen, A. (1971). *The language of the body*. New York: Collier Books. (Original work published 1958)

Lowen, A. (1976). *Bioenergetics*. New York: Penguin Books.

Mann, E. W. (1989). *Vital energy and health: Dr. Wilhelm Reich's revolutionary discoveries and supporting evidence*. Toronto: Houslow Press.

Pelletier, K. R. (1977). *Mind as healer, mind as slayer*. New York: Dell.

Pierrakos, J. C. (1974). *The case of the broken heart*. The Institute for The New Age Publishing. (Available from the Institute for Core Energetics, 115 East 23rd Street, 12th Floor, New York, NY 10010)

Pierrakos, J. C. (1986, October). *The history of Core Energetics*. Paper presented at a meeting of Core Energetic therapists, New York.

Pierrakos, J. C. (1987). *Core Energetics: Developing the capacity to love and heal*. Mendocino, CA: LifeRhythm.

Pierrakos, J. C. (1997, August). *Breathing: The pulse of life*. Paper presented at the

International Conference of the Association for Core Energetics, Phoenicia, NY.

Reich, W. (1972). *Character analysis* (3rd ed., V. R. Carfagno, Trans.). New York: Farrar, Straus & Giroux. (Original work published 1945)

Reich, W. (1973). *The cancer biopathy* (A. White, M. Higgins, & M. R. Chester, Trans.). New York: Farrar, Straus & Giroux. (Original work published 1948)

Simon, R. (1997, September/October). Listening hands: An interview with Ilana Reufenfeld. *Family Therapy Networker, 20*(5), 62–73.

Simonton, O. C., Creighton, J., & Simonton, S. (1978). *Getting well again: A step-by-step, self-help guide to overcoming cancer for patients and their families*. Los Angeles: Jeremy P. Tarcher.

Slaven, L., & Lee, C. (1997). Mood and symptom reporting among middle-aged women: The relationship between menopausal status, hormone replacement therapy, and exercise participation. *Health Psychology, 16*, 203–208.

Wolman, B. (1988). *Psychosomatic disorders*. New York: Plenum.

ADDITIONAL RESOURCES

Publications

Core Energetic Newsletter. New York: The Institute of Core Energetics.

Journal of Energy and Consciousness. New York: The Institute of Core Energetics.

Pierrakos, J. C. (1997). *Eros, love and sexuality: The forces that unify man and woman*. Mendocino, CA: LifeRhythm.

Training Programs

The Institute of Core Energetics
115 East 23rd Street, 12th Floor
New York, NY 10010
(212) 982-9637/(212) 505-6767 (telephones)
(212) 673-5939 (fax)
E-mail: jagroom11@aol.com
Web site: www.core-energetics.org

10

PHOENIX RISING YOGA THERAPY

MICHAEL LEE

For thousands of years the practices of yoga have offered systematic ways to bring body, mind, and spirit into harmony. Phoenix Rising Yoga Therapy (PRYT) uses selected traditional yoga practices, along with contemporary approaches to focusing awareness, to bridge and integrate these same aspects. PRYT is a nondirective, client-centered process for facilitating the client's awareness of what is happening in his or her body and life, for integrating this information, and for using it to initiate desirable changes. All Phoenix Rising practices and methods are compatible with certain yogic principles or beliefs that are discussed below, but they stem from the core belief that "most of our fundamental attitudes in life have their physical counterparts in the body" (Iyengar & Menuhin, 1995).

One of the earliest documents outlining the practice of yoga is the Yoga Sutras of Patanjali (Feuerstein, 1990), which is believed to have been first recorded some 4,000 to 6,000 years ago. (The exact date of recording is unknown.) These "yoga sutras," or short aphorisms, present directions for understanding life more fully and offer techniques, including the use of the body and breath and meditation, for attaining deeper wisdom.

Over the years, the tradition of yoga has been developed and passed on by many teachers, each with his or her own particular emphasis. When yoga was first introduced to North America in the early 20th century, it came through several different teachers with different emphases. This trend multiplied further midcentury as various teachers from India arrived in the United States in response to the shift in consciousness that was occurring, popularized in part by the Beatles' sojourns with Maharishi Mahesh Yogi. Some of the teachers of this time chose a purely physical approach (hatha yoga) and downplayed the spiritual and transformational aspects of the practice. Other yogis, like Paramahansa Yogananda at the Self Realization Fellowship in Encinitas, California, did the opposite, openly teaching practices that encompassed all the spiritual aspects of the ancient tradition (Walters, 1991).

Although the therapeutic benefits of yoga have been apparent for a long time, it has only been in the last 30 years that therapeutic practices based directly on yoga have become more widely practiced and gained more widespread acceptance (Kleinman, 1996). There are forms of deep therapeutic work involving breath, body, and mind, such as those taught by Stanislov Grof and others (Grof, 1993), that originate from yogic techniques. There are forms of structural yoga therapy for improving the physical posture of the body and alleviating chronic pain, such as those taught by Larry Payne (1986). Yoga-based meditation techniques are used in mainstream stress-reduction programs, heart disease recovery programs such as that of Dean Ornish (1990), and the mindfulness meditation practices based on the work of Jon Kabat Zinn (Kabat Zinn & Santorelli, 1994) taught in hospitals in Massachusetts and elsewhere. The deeper psychotherapeutic benefits of yoga-based practices are also now finding widespread acceptance through such modalities as PRYT, which was developed in 1986, although the relevance of these practices was clearly envisioned 10 years earlier (Rama, Ballantine, & Ajaya, 1976).

PRYT developed from the realization that certain yoga practices, delivered and taught in a particular form, could quickly and easily support greater mental clarity, increased emotional awareness, and heightened capacity for living life more in touch with inner self-knowledge (Lee, 1997). In developing the modality, certain traditional yoga-based practices were adapted to enable the therapist to work one-on-one with a client, guiding the client through various body, breath, and meditative yoga experiences while at the same time using dialogue and other contemporary humanistic psychology techniques to facilitate access to deeper levels of awareness. These modern techniques were, however, considered completely compatible with the yogic tradition with which they were matched. The principles and core beliefs coming from the yogic tradition, and on which PRYT is based, include the following:

- All people have within them the capacity for their own healing.
- There is inner knowledge and wisdom that is available that

lies beyond what can be accessed with the conscious mind alone.

- Healing and growth are supported by expanding awareness on all levels—physical, emotional, mental, and spiritual.
- Whatever insights this new awareness offers, their acceptance without judgment further supports the healing process, especially if integrated into people's day-to-day lives.
- The physical body is a useful tool for accessing awareness on all levels of being. This is achieved through the process of *attunement*—the act of paying attention in detail to one's total experience (Lee, 1985).

THE PHOENIX RISING APPROACH

The PRYT approach consists of a repertoire of assisted yoga postures, dialogue techniques, and a guided integration process to support clients in releasing physical tension, which often results in some kind of emotional, mental, or spiritual shift. The basic technique is to support the client in holding a yoga posture at "the edge"—a place of neither too much nor too little stretching (Lee, 1995). Then, with coaching to focus awareness on his or her immediate experience, the client is invited to dialogue with the therapist about what he or she is experiencing on all levels—body sensations, thoughts, and feelings. The supportive, caring, and yet unobtrusive presence of the therapist is an essential part of the process. It is important that PRYT practitioners not try to "fix" clients or take them away from their experience, which can sometimes be tempting, especially for professionals trained in traditional psychotherapy. Instead, practitioners are to engage clients in a physical experience and then simply trust the wisdom of the client's body and the client's capacity to be fully present without offering any planned outcome-oriented intervention. The importance of this "loving presence" aspect of the PRYT approach has been researched and documented (Kokinakis, 1995).

Another key element in the PRYT process is the integration of the moment-to-moment yoga experience with the client's life experience. Questions like "What significant things happened here?" and "How does what happened here connect to your life experience?" help to make this bridge. Such questions form the basis of the Phoenix Rising integration process (Lee, 1997).

PRYT has served many different populations, and elements of the modality can be used in a variety of contexts. Many PRYT clients are attracted to the work as a vehicle for enhancing their personal growth and quality of life. Most are short-term clients who receive an average of between 6 and 10 sessions initially, but many often return for further work when they feel the need. After a series of sessions clients often will report finding greater clarity around significant life issues; greater freedom of movement; less tension in their bodies; more finely tuned awareness of their physical, emotional, and mental states; and better connection with their inner spirit for guidance.

Somewhat surprisingly, the above-mentioned benefits do not depend on the client's physical condition. Both those clients who are in good physical condition and those who are not in touch with their bodies or who are suffering from some physical disability or illness can receive this work and find benefit. Physical differences do, however, require different approaches from the practitioner. For those clients who are flexible and have good body awareness, it is possible to move very easily into more complex assisted yoga postures, to remain longer at the edge, and to engage in dialogue sooner. Clients who are less flexible and less aware of their bodies generally need to be coached carefully and patiently as to how to receive the work, with particular emphasis on working with their breath, working at their edge, and focusing their attention on the moment-to-moment experience. Once this has happened, however, those in this category often have deep and profound experiences with the work very quickly. In many instances, some of these initial experiences are the most memorable and revealing (Lee, 1997).

Although the above descriptions fit the most likely PRYT clients, some practitioners use the work with other populations, including those in recovery from substance abuse. The deep levels of awareness that come from the yoga-based body experiences, together with the deeper states of relaxation produced, can create somewhat of a paradox for such clients. They tap into a more honest and yet potentially painful knowledge of the self, but at the same time create the feeling that all is well, regardless. Generally, addictions therapists who use PRYT prefer to introduce it only after clients have been in recovery for some time and can work with the deeper levels of awareness that are likely to surface.

PRYT techniques are also practiced by some family therapists as a means of creating deeper awareness of family issues and the belief systems held by family members. Insight gained through the wisdom of the body can provide the foundation for healing in family relationships (Markowitz, 1996). For clients who have had traumatic experiences in childhood that continue to manifest in various ways in their adult lives and require deeper integration, therapists use PRYT as a way of helping support the healing of both emotional and physical wounds from a client's past. Although some use a strict Phoenix Rising approach, others use PRYT sessions as an adjunct to more traditional forms of therapy. Other Phoenix Rising practitioners use the work with clients dealing with emotional and physical issues arising during the rehabilitation period following an injury or surgery. A nondirective, body–mind approach like PRYT appears to be very effective in such cases (DiBella, 1996).

Other areas in which PRYT has been and is being used as either the primary or an adjunct modality include chronic pain management; pre- and postnatal support; smoking cessation; weight loss; stress reduction; juvenile hyperactivity reduction; and adjustment of handicapped adolescents and special needs populations in school settings. The PRYT experience is generally delivered in a one-on-one setting between a trained practitioner and the client. Two of the methods used in PRYT sessions are described below: *body scanning* and *therapist-assisted yoga postures*. Both are accompanied by dialogue and integration of body experience with life experience.

BODY SCANNING

Body scanning in PRYT is an adaptation of the yogic technique of using different parts of the body as foci for awareness to aid in relaxation. Whereas most traditional yoga practitioners use the method with the client lying on his or her back, PRYT clients are usually guided through the experience while in a standing position facing the practitioner. PRYT practitioners generally lead clients through a body scan in one of the first three sessions. It is a valuable introductory method because it invites clients to practice attunement to body experience and begin making connections between that physical experience and their lives. The body scan is led in a way that is relatively nonthreatening and, because the client is relatively passive (compared to later, when more advanced methods are used), it is easy for the client to focus. Also, as part of PRYT, this technique is used to support clients in deepening their body awareness and to prepare them to use the body more easily in later work. It is also an appropriate method for clients with physical limitations who might not be able to work with more complex methods. At the same time, it often is possible for the client to receive meaningful and helpful insights and awareness from this beginning method, as the following case illustrates.

CASE EXAMPLE 1: THE BODY SCAN

Sylvia, who was in her late 30s, was a successful real estate broker/ investor. She experienced numerous physical and emotional symptoms of stress: headaches; neck and back pain; fatigue; angry outbursts with family and close friends followed by remorse; fear of "losing her touch"; and fear of failure and of losing her ability to function effectively.

A close friend in whom she had confided recommended that she take yoga classes and get bodywork in the form of PRYT. The friend had received several PRYT sessions and said they had helped her "lighten up." In her initial interview and screening, Sylvia displayed typical signs of stress-related muscular contraction around her neck and shoulders and spoke rapidly without full breaths between sentences. It was agreed that she would receive an initial series of six PRYT sessions followed by an evaluation of the effectiveness of the work in meeting her needs.

Case Narrative	*Commentary*
In her second session, Sylvia was guided through a body scan.	
While standing with her eyes closed, Sylvia was asked to focus on different parts of her body and to hold her focus on each part long enough to fully experience all the feelings and sensations as well as to be aware of her thoughts and monitor her inner experience as she shifted her focus from one part to another. Toward the end, she was also asked to focus on each side of her body in turn.	Although it was only her second session, Sylvia entered the experience easily and was able to stay with it to allow for a longer and more comprehensive version of the body scan technique to be used, taking around 20 minutes. Although this is not difficult for most clients, some find it difficult to remain standing with their eyes closed.
She was then asked to thank her body and to open her eyes, sit, and talk about what she experienced.	Some clients also find it easy to enter into the experience and follow along with the therapist's guidance, as Sylvia did. Visual cues such as facial expression, will indicate to the therapist if this is occurring.
Sylvia was amazed at what she discovered. She described her experience in great detail, noting in particular that as she focused on her legs she recalled herself as a small child running through an open meadow on the farm in Ohio where she grew up. She also noticed near the end that she had a very different experience of the left side of her body compared to the right. Her left side felt soft and childlike. Her right side felt rigid and hard. And, as she focused her attention there, she could also feel her jaw and neck muscles tighten.	As often happens in the body scan experience, Sylvia's body has transported her to another time in her life. In this case, her childhood memories were significant as they reflected a state of being that had been somewhat ignored in her life recently. She also became aware from the different experiences of her left and right sides of a corresponding split in her experience of her life.

When guided through an integration of her experience the following dialogue with Sylvia took place.

Th [Therapist]: So, tell me, Sylvia, if there was anything you noticed during your body scan experience that has some connection with your life.

Sylvia: Well, I'm aware of how much I miss that feeling of being that carefree little girl. I want that feeling back but I'm so damned obsessed with work right now that there is no time for it.

Th: So you want to reconnect with the part of you that can express herself like the girl running through the meadow? And you don't seem to have created enough time for her right now?

Sylvia: Right on. All work and no play. That's my life.

Th: Was there anything else that you noticed that connects to your life?

Sylvia: Yes, and it's around the same theme. Like my right and left sides. My right side felt rigid and hard just like I am at work. My left side felt soft and childlike. And the two seemed to be in conflict—just like in my life. And that's what I need to resolve.

Th: You want to resolve this conflict between work and play in your life?

Sylvia: Yes.

Th: So close your eyes and let's find out if your body can help you with that. [The therapist guides Sylvia through an exercise in visualizing resolution of the conflict in her body. She then asks her to talk about how it occurred.]

The integration of the body scan is minimally guided, in that the client selects from his or her experience what he or she deems important. The client also is asked to decide what is significant about the experience and how it shows up in her life. Further, the client is empowered to determine what course of action to take as a result.

Sylvia is typical of many PRYT clients. She is aware and quick to make the connections between her body experience and her life. This is not always the case at this stage but it is a learned process with most PRYT clients arriving at the capacity to do this relatively easily after about six sessions. In Sylvia's case the therapist moves right along with her as she realizes Sylvia's capacity to move quickly from body experience to life experience, and then to integration and application.

There are several different ways that PRYT practitioners can guide this part of the integration process. In this case, as Sylvia has learned to connect so well to her body, the therapist used a body-oriented approach. Sylvia also appeared open

Sylvia: Well, it was somewhat of a struggle. Both sides want to hold on to their territory but reached an agreement to let each other share the space. I noticed when they did that, that the tension around my neck and jaw seemed to relax.

Th: So it took some effort but they could share the space. I wonder what that would look like in your life?

Syliva: For one thing, it would mean they would have to share my time.

The therapist continues brief conversation with Sylvia about how she might do that. She then asks Sylvia if there is anything she might do to begin the process within the next week.

Sylvia: Yes. . . . I'm going to go for it, right away. I'm going to take this weekend off and go visit my family and friends in Ohio. I might even go out and find that meadow and run and play like I remember doing as a child.

Th: And it's feasible for you to do that?

Sylvia: Sure.

Th: Great. Then I'll see you next week and look forward to hearing about it. One suggestion, though, that might be helpful with all of this: As you go about making your plans for the weekend, traveling, meeting family and friends, running in the meadow, or whatever you do, just be aware as much as possible as to what is happening in your body as you do it. I'd like to hear about that, too.

and accepting of her new awareness. Were this not the case the therapist would guide an experience to support the client in the loving acceptance of her new awareness before moving to address possible resolution.

When the client makes a new choice around some aspect of their life, the therapist will guide him or her in finding some kind of 'homework' to support the new choice within the next week and to also connect the new choice in some way with their body experience. The homework is also always reality checked as well.

A MORE ADVANCED TECHNIQUE: ASSISTED YOGA POSTURES

With the more advanced technique of assisted yoga postures, the PRYT practitioner guides and supports the client into an assisted yoga posture while providing dialogue opportunities. Dialogue helps clients verbalize their physical experience and integrate it with their life experience. Another important element in this method is the loving presence aspect of the work, as previously mentioned (Kokinakis, 1995).

Before clients can be introduced to this method, however, they need to have become familiar and comfortable with the basic physical aspects of the work and to be able to focus their awareness inward to the sensations in their bodies. To reach this point, the therapist will structure lead-up sessions using simple stretches to familiarize the client with the edge and as opportunities to coach the client in focusing his or her awareness (Lee, 1995). Not all Phoenix Rising clients necessarily reach this stage, but with coaching by the therapist, most will reach this point by their fifth session. Clients who have been practicing yoga or some other body-oriented discipline accompanied by inner awareness tools generally will be able to move to this method by their second session.

Depending on the assisted yoga postures used, this method may be contraindicated for clients with injuries or recent surgeries. The method is also contraindicated for clients who have not reached the state of readiness described above. The potential for physical injury with this method is negligible with a trained therapist and a client with some level of body awareness and the capacity to focus on the moment-to-moment physical experience. For clients diagnosed with or showing symptoms of a mental disorder, a history of severe abuse, or on prescribed medication, this method may be beneficial, provided the PRYT practitioner obtains the consent and collaboration of the client's primary health care provider. These techniques are powerful, and PRYT practitioners should be aware of their possible effects on clients. This advanced method is strongly indicated for clients wishing to deepen their awareness of the self and make life changes based on that awareness (Lee & Reynolds, 1992).

CASE EXAMPLE 2: ASSISTED YOGA POSTURES

Case Narrative	Commentary
Ted, a man in his early 40s, has college education including a graduate degree in literature. He has had two long-term relationships but is currently not in a committed relation-	Ted looks older than his age. His face is wrinkled from frowning, which he does frequently as he talks. His shoulders are both rounded toward the front of his body and drawn

ship. He has been practicing yoga on and off for a few years and has dabbled in several of the new-age personal growth modalities. In his initial session, Ted talked about needing to make some changes in his life, including having more fun.

Ted received instructions on how to position himself physically to enter the posture. It involved him sitting or kneeling. His hands were joined together behind his back and his bent forward on a soft pad on the floor in front of his knees while raising both arms up behind his body. The therapist supported Ted's arms in position, giving traction and support to maintain the edge. As Ted approached his edge, the following dialogue took place.

Th: Ted, as we approach your edge, I want you to let me know.

Ted: Yes. We're coming to it now.

Th: OK, take a few long deep breaths and let your inner focus go right to the sensations.

[Client breathed. Therapist supported posture at the edge.]

Th: So what's happening now, Ted?

Ted: I can really feel the stretch between my shoulder blades. It's a hot prickly sensation but when I take a deep breath it feels OK.

[Long pause in dialogue. Ted makes sounds as he exhales and begins to move his jaw up and down.]

upward. In the initial body scan done in his first session, much of his awareness focused on the tightness in his shoulders and neck. It appears that this might be an area of his body to focus on when beginning work with assisted postures. Although he is very tight in his musculature, Ted has done sufficient work with his body in yoga and other practices that he is able to focus his awareness and determine where his edge is.

This assisted posture is a variation of the classic yoga posture known as *yoga mudra*. It was chosen because it specifically opens up the shoulders and upper back, releasing muscular tension and associated emotional tension held there.

At this point the posture is engaged. The dialogue began sparingly, allowing Ted time to focus on his body and reach a deeper state of presence. The therapist listens for breathing as a sign that he was fully engaged in the experience.

The jaw movement indicated that physical release of tension could have been occurring.

[Sounds changed to long "aaahhh's" on the exhale]

Th: And now, what's happening for you, Ted?

Ted: I want to yell!

Th: You want to yell?

Ted: Yes I want to yell. Its like there is this sensation there in my back that will be relieved if I can just yell.

Th: . . . if you can just yell?

Ted: Yes I want to yell 'Get off my back'

Th: [mirroring the intensity of feeling in Ted's words]. Get off my back?

Ted [in a very loud voice]: Yes. . . . Get off my back you damn son of a bitch. Get off my back.

Ted [in a quieter voice]: God it feels good to say that.

Th: It feels good to say that?

Ted: Oh yeah, I've wanted to tell him that so many times. In fact I wanted to tell both of them.

Th: Both of them?

Ted: Yes, both my godammed father and his godammed father—my [expletive] grandfather . . . the old [expletive].

Th: So you wanted to tell both of them to get off your back for a long time?

Ted: Oh yeah . . . [quieter barely audible sounds, maybe sobbing]

[Long pause in dialogue—client continues to make sounds. Therapist continues to support client in posture. Sounds subside. Therapist guides client out of posture and they proceed to the Integration phase of the session.]

The client has moved from the physical to the emotional state. The physical release in his shoulders is most likely accompanied by a release of whatever created the tension there emotionally.

The therapist stays present for the client by offering physical support in holding the assisted yoga posture while offering verbal support by mirroring. The therapist does not probe or analyze. The loving presence and the physical support enable the client to feel safe to express himself as much or as little as he wants.

There is of course a story behind what is occurring for Ted. This is discussed in the integration phase following the assisted posture. Here Ted talks further about his relationship with both his father and grandfather and of their high expectations of him. He feel like a failure a lot of the time because, unlike them, he has never achieved anything worthwhile with his life. He has carried the burden of knowing this for many years. The burden has been carried in his shoulders, tension building there through restraining the urge to yell at them both, to tell them off, to get off his back, to let him live his own life, and to meet his own expectations. At this point in time, however, the therapist does not have this information, and although there is the temptation to ask the kinds of questions that will elicit it, she instead stays with the standard PRYT process. This involves resisting the temptation to seek explanations or rationale for behavior and to stay focused in the present at both the physical and emotional levels.

The therapist will allow and be present for the client's emotional release however it occurs, and will only intervene to stop it if it becomes dangerous to herself or her client. Likewise, she will continue to support the client in the assisted yoga posture for a time, as long as the client does not go beyond the edge or become physically distressed in a way that could hurt him. Like all PRYT practitioners she watches for any signs of this as she continues the dialogue.

Ted reported feeling much lighter after the experience. His shoulders felt free of tension, he stood taller, and he felt more power in his belly and less afraid to follow his own direction in life. Ted returned for several more sessions and developed a greater sense of empowerment, including working with the fears that he had held onto that had kept him vulnerable to the criticism of his elders.

In cases like Ted's, the PRYT practitioner should be aware of the potential dangers in the sudden release of long-held anger. It may be appropriate to bring the client out of the posture early, before a complete release has occurred, and to proceed more slowly over several sessions. A referral to a practitioner more specialized in dealing with anger, and with whom the PRYT practitioner can work adjunctively, might also be indicated. It is difficult to make such a judgment in advance and may need to be made by the PRYT practitioner in light of what transpires for the client in the first use of this technique.

RESISTANCE

Most clients who come to PRYT are open to the use of action methods such as the ones described above. As the very name *yoga therapy* implies use of action methods, client resistance to their use is rare. Even so, therapists practicing this work must be careful to explain the methods being used and to invite the client's participation. Therapists who practice more traditional forms of therapy as well as PRYT should be selective in choosing which clients might be suited to these action methods. Clients who have been working for many years using only verbal techniques may be threatened by body-oriented methods. In such cases, the therapist may choose not to use PRYT or may proceed slowly in the introduction phase to help clients become more comfortable with this way of working. Similarly, PRYT is a nondirective approach, without analysis and interpretation by the therapist for the client. Clients who have worked with more directive approaches may require education and an adjustment period to work with a method that requires more from them in determining their own body–mind connections.

SUCCESSIVE USES

For clients like Ted, successive uses of action methods like the ones described further enhance their self-awareness and support a deepening of their commitment to make desired life changes. Homework also supports this process. In the integration phase of the work clients often will come up with their own homework. Ted in the example above chose to visit his father and talk with him about how he had been trying so hard to please him and that he was now letting go of that. Although he hoped to create a fuller relationship with his father, he was also open to the possibility of rejection. If rejected, he would use that experience as an opportunity to maintain his resolve to make his own choices and not surrender his power. In many cases, clients also are supported by beginning a daily yoga practice for self-empowerment as a part of their homework. They use many of the same Phoenix Rising techniques of focusing awareness at the edge, breathing, and relaxing into the experience, moment to moment. After several Phoenix Rising sessions, they are also able to do their own inner dialogue and integration, as well as consciously apply their day-to-day experience on the yoga mat to their day-to-day life experiences. This was particularly useful in Ted's case. A subsequent session was devoted to teaching him six standing yoga poses that he could practice on his own. The postures were to be accompanied by affirmation, imagery, and inner work to support the process of empowerment.

EMPIRICAL SUPPORT

Fishkind (1991) worked with a group of clients diagnosed with cerebral palsy, each of whom received a weekly PRYT session over the course of the study. On the basis of pre- and posttreatment measures, Fishkind concluded that the clients had become more empowered and self-responsible as well as more physically able.

The most significant piece of research on PRYT to date is the study cited earlier by Kokinakis (1995), which addressed the implications for teaching professional standards with regard to the aspect of PRYT known as loving presence. In her conclusions, Kokinakis noted the similarity between the loving presence as practiced in PRYT and the notion of "unconditional positive regard" in the client-centered therapy of Carl Rogers (1957), as well as evidence supporting the importance of the relationship between therapist and client for facilitating life changes. Most other research into PRYT has been in the form of collected case material supporting the broad hypotheses that clients receiving PRYT do experience beneficial changes in their lifestyles, behavior, attitudes, relationships, and many facets of their spiritual and material lives. Many clients attribute these changes directly to awareness that they have received during their PRYT work and on which they have taken action. Methodologically rigorous research is needed to test these outcomes as well as to investigate what physiological, emotional, and mental changes result from the sustained holding of a yoga posture accompanied by certain breathing and focusing techniques as practiced by PRYT practitioners.

There has been a significant increase in the popularity of yoga generally, and PRYT specifically, in the last 5 years. This is due, in part, to changes occurring in our society. As individuals become more technologically dependent and live more complex lives that require significant and frequent adjustments of focus and modes of being, they are more in need of a body–mind–spirit technology that can support them in making those transitions with minimal stress. The action methods of PRYT can contribute in making such transitions.

THERAPIST CHARACTERISTICS

Since 1987, there have been approximately 800 practitioners certified to practice PRYT. Psychotherapists are one of the largest occupational groups drawn to study PRYT. They often are drawn to the work through their interest in the body–mind connection and the relative ease with which PRYT seems to facilitate and integrate it. Many are also interested in the psychospiritual dimension of PRYT and its processes for empowering the individual through both body and mind to find his or her own path in life. Many PRYT practitioners also have a background in yoga, often as teachers. They have seen the possibilities that exist in yoga to enhance life generally, but often they are particularly interested in learning more about the body–mind connection that they have seen their students experience in their classes and want to learn how to work with it in a more focused, one-on-one approach, as offered through PRYT. Medical practitioners, chiropractors, bodyworkers, and counselors are some of the other professionals who have studied and practice PRYT.

Most successful PRYT practitioners tend to be those who were drawn to the work as a result of their own direct experience of it. They are often more in touch with their bodies than the general population; have developed a finely tuned awareness of the self, others, and their surroundings; and could be regarded as adventurers on the journey of life, appreciating their own and others' personal learning through life experiences.

TRAINING

The training program for PRYT practitioners currently consists of three levels and is offered in several locations in the United States and in selected foreign locations by certified teachers working with the parent organization, Phoenix Rising Yoga Therapy, Inc., which is located in Housatonic, Massachusetts. The first two levels (4 days and 6 days, respectively) usually are combined as a 10-day residential program that uses both experiential and didactic teaching modes. Students are introduced to the basic principles of PRYT and given extensive and intensive guided practice and coaching sessions. The third level of the training program is now a 6-month part-time program that refines, expands, and enhances the work done in the earlier levels. Each student is assigned a mentor/coach and receives coaching on a required number of practice sessions with volunteer clients. During this time, students also attend a number of advanced workshops on topics such as advanced dialogue techniques, advanced bodywork techniques, the client–therapist relationship, professional ethics, and the anatomy of yoga. There is also an assigned reading requirement as well as an experiential yoga/personal-growth self-study during this part of the program. In addition to the requisite skill development, one of the emphases of this part of the training is on enhancing students' clarity as to their own motivations and increasing their understanding of themselves in the practitioner role. Students also take electives or required additional courses to supplement their background in yoga and other experiences and education before entering the program. For example, a psychotherapist with little knowledge of yoga would be asked to include several additional yoga programs in his or her course of study, whereas a yoga teacher without a strong background in the areas of personal growth or counseling would be required to receive additional training in these areas. There currently is no national certification of yoga therapists specializing in somatic therapy in the United States or elsewhere. Phoenix Rising Yoga Therapy, Inc., has therefore established its own certification and continuing education requirements. Before graduating, students are required to meet various demonstrated skill requirements, including the satisfactory completion of an observed evaluation session. For practicing PRYT practitioners, there is an active practitioners support association that provides referrals, a monthly newsletter, and an Internet site. Additionally, this organization seeks and supports ongoing research opportunities for its members.

CONCLUSION

After little more than a decade of practice, it appears that PRYT is offering viable approaches and techniques that go beyond talk therapy in supporting clients to deeper levels of awareness and the implementation of change in their lives. There is still much to be learned about these techniques, but there is also much that has been learned already. Case material as contained in the studies discussed in this chapter suggest that clients do find these approaches revealing, effective, helpful, and fast. On the surface, the approaches might appear simple and yet are capable of creating profound awareness. Despite the apparent simplicity, it is also known that therapists who use them need to be multiskilled. As well as directing and supporting their clients' body experiences, they also must guide their emotional and mental process and provide a framework for integration. These PRYT techniques also demand a degree of faith on the part of the therapist that clients will be able to use their bodies as a source for their own healing. Such faith in the client is not new to therapy in general, as evidenced by the work of Rogers (1957). Perhaps what is relatively new is the extention of this faith to the domain of the body within the therapeutic context. It is ironic that these new techniques derive in part from the ancient practice of yoga and represent not only the integration of mind and body but also the integration of ancient and modern wisdom surrounding the nature of human development.

REFERENCES

DiBella, P. (1996, September/October). Can your body advise you toward recovery? *The Healing News, 1*(5), 7.

Feuerstein, G. (1990). *The yoga-sutra of Patanjali: A new translation and commentary.* Inner Traditions.

Fishkind, R. (1991). *The effects of hatha yoga therapy on adolescents with cerebral palsy.* Unpublished master's thesis, Lesley College, Cambridge, MA.

Grof, S. (1993). *The holotropic mind: Three levels of human consciousness and how they shape our lives.* San Francisco: Harper.

Iyengar, B. K. S., & Menuhin, Y. (1995). *Light on pranayama and the yogic art of breathing.* London: Crossroad.

Kabat Zinn, J., & Santorelli, S. (1993). *Mindfulness-based stress reduction professional training resource manual.* Boston: University of Massachusetts Medical Center.

Kleinman, S. (1996). Yoga therapy: A panel discussion. *The Journal of the International Association of Yoga Therapists, 7,* 1–5.

Kokinakis, C. L. (1995). *Teaching professional standards: Training yoga therapists in loving presence.* Unpublished doctoral dissertation, Michigan State University, East Lansing.

Lee, M. (1985). *The therapeutic effects of yoga.* Unpublished master's thesis, Norwich University, Montpelier, VT.

Lee, M. (1995, March/April). The edge. *Yoga Journal, 121,* 104–106.

Lee, M. (1997). *Phoenix Rising Yoga Therapy: A bridge from body to soul.* Deerfield Beach, FL: Health Communications.

Lee, M., & Reynolds, N. (1992). *Phoenix Rising Yoga Therapy training manual.* Housatonic, MA: Phoenix Rising Yoga Therapy, Inc.

Markowitz, L. (1996). Minding the body, embodying the mind. *Family Therapy Networker, 20*(5), 21–33.

Ornish, D. (1990). *Dr. Dean Ornish's program for reversing heart disease.* New York: Random House.

Payne, L. (1986). *Healthy back exercises for high stress professionals.* Los Angeles: Samata International.

Rama, S., Ballantine, R., & Ajaya, S. (1976). *Yoga and psychotherapy: The evolution of consciousness.* Honesdale, PA: Himalayan International Institute.

Rogers, C. (1957). The necessary and sufficient conditions of therapeutic personality change. *Journal of Consulting Psychology, 21*(2), 95–103.

Walters, D. (1991). *Essence of self-realization: The wisdom of Paramahansa Yogananda.* Grass Valley, CA: Crystal Clarity Publications.

ADDITIONAL RESOURCES

Folan, L. (1998). The inner smile [CD]. Relaxation Company.

Norian, T. (1997). Yoga at the edge [Cassette]. Todd Norian.

Norian, T. (1998). Yoga for rebalancing [CD]. Todd Norian.

IV

EXPRESSIVE ARTS
THERAPIES

11

ART MAKING IN FAMILY THERAPY

DEBRA LINESCH

Throughout the history of psychotherapy, clinicians of many disciplines have used art making in the service of self-expression. However, the defined field of art therapy has existed only since the 1950s. The practice of art therapy is based on the premise that art is the primary communication method of psychotherapy. The practice embraces the idea that the graphic arts provide opportunities for individuals to express themselves in ways that are creative, nonlinear, and less rigidified by defense mechanisms and that reveal many levels of potential meanings. Although there are as many approaches to facilitating art therapy as there are approaches to therapy in general, all art therapists share a central commitment to art process.

Art therapy is most simply described as the practice of psychotherapy using the visual arts as the expressive modality between client and therapist. This simplification, however, risks the possibly limited understanding of the process as that of simply an alternative modality. Art therapy is much more; when psychotherapy fully engages art making, the process becomes greater than simply an alternative to verbal interaction. It takes on all the inherent healing properties of the arts. By harnessing creativity and imagery, it typically can deepen the client's experience of the self and often accesses previously unacknowledged resources.

Art therapy is currently used in all types of settings in which mental

225

health services are provided. It is often found in psychiatric hospitals and day-treatment facilities in which art therapists practice as part of treatment teams that use art therapy techniques to support overall psychiatric treatment goals. It is also found in specialized agencies that provide services for a variety of populations, including substance abuse clients, victims of domestic violence, and the elderly. Art therapy is also used in outpatient clinics, child guidance centers, and family counseling centers where the process is more likely to be a primary therapy method rather than adjunctive as in the earlier examples. The art therapy techniques described in this chapter are illustrative of art therapy practiced in an outpatient setting.

Art therapy can incorporate all the visual arts, although simple materials and techniques are typically used. Because the process of doing the art task is much more significant than the created product, the teaching of art techniques is not emphasized, and easy, nonthreatening media generally are used. Materials range from those easiest to manipulate, such as colored pencils and collage materials, to those most psychologically stimulating and able to provoke primitive kinds of experiences, such as wet clay and finger paint. Although the techniques outlined in this chapter describe fairly simple art projects, the enormous breadth of the spectrum of available media illustrates the need for comprehensive training. The therapist who understands and wants to make available the tremendous potential for growth inherent in art processes needs to be skilled at assessing and managing the client's comfort with the unfamiliar experiences of art making.

Because the dominant psychotherapeutic framework at the time of art therapy's emergence was psychoanalytic, its roots (and, indeed, many of its tenets) have a psychodynamic orientation. However, the practice of using the visual arts as the predominant communication method of psychotherapy transcends the Freudian language with which it was first described (Kramer, 1971; Naumberg, 1966). Art making is, by definition, an activity, an experience that uses and integrates elements of the body, the intellect, and the emotions. All art therapy processes involve action. Although art therapy theory often emphasizes insight (Naumberg, 1966), interpretation (Kramer, 1971), self-awareness (Betensky, 1973), and language, the client's fundamental experience is of engaging in a physical task. The question of whether or not to use action methods within art therapy misses the point; all of art therapy is action. Only the degree to which the art therapist facilitates or embraces action determines whether art therapy becomes more or less of an action method.

ACTION METHODS IN ART THERAPY

The actual role that the art plays in the process of art therapy has been debated throughout the development of the field, and it is only recently that art therapists have begun to understand that diversity in the approaches in the field strengthens rather than weakens it. Historically, the debate was polarized between art therapists who believed that the art process was inherently curative and that the psychodynamic phenomena of catharsis and sublimation were responsible for healing (Kramer, 1971) and art therapists who insisted that the art was only valuable to the degree that verbal processing and language about the imagery facilitated insight (Naumberg, 1966; Rubin, 1987). This debate, which has continued to the present, seems to beg the issue; the art is intrinsically more multidimensional than either side of this dichotomous thinking presents. Both theoretical approaches, and others as well, inform a comprehensive understanding of the art process that actually comes close to the orientation of action methods. The art task that is the pivotal phenomenon of the art therapy session involves the client's physical interaction with art media, a process intended to shift the client's experience. This shift may involve feelings, awareness, thoughts, and verbalizations, but it arises fundamentally from the art activity.

Even the early articulators of art therapy, despite being locked into Freudian interpretations of the art therapy process, understood that it was the action of the art making that facilitated the benefits of which they spoke. Kramer (1987) may have used complicated language to describe sublimation—"to designate the processes whereby primitive urges emanating from the id are transformed by the ego into complex acts that do not serve direct instinctual gratification" (p. 26)—but, it is clear that she believed that it was in the physical action of the art process that these phenomena occurred. Rubin (1987) also put forth the notion that the art process facilitated a secondary, and perhaps more important, experience, that of insight, saying, "I am convinced that art can greatly enhance the analytic experience of insight ('seeing in'). This is probably true because art is concrete and visual, in addition to its value in 'uncovering' unconscious imagery" (p. 21). However, it is also apparent that it was the activity of art making itself that created the opportunities for the psychotherapeutic benefits of which she spoke. It is interesting that these two philosophies, so often discussed as antagonistic because of their differing attitudes regarding the role of insight, are actually very similar: The art is pivotal, the art is experiential, and the art creates change.

One of the most important nonpsychoanalytic art therapy theorists, Mala Betensky, who first moved the debate away from the art-as-therapy/ art-in-therapy polarization, described the art therapy process in phenomenological terms, and in so doing indirectly supported the connection between art therapy and the practice of action methods in psychotherapy. Betensky claimed, "First clients in art therapy produce an art projection that is a direct experience. Then they experience its appearance in their eyes and in their immediate consciousness, and this is a second direct experience" (Betensky, 1987, p. 150). It is in Betensky's emphasis on the experience that she seems to move more directly into a description of the actual art therapy process and not its benefits or results.

In the years since early debates defined the field, many art therapists have written about the art therapy process from different theoretical orientations (e.g., McNiff [1988] and humanism, Moon [1990] and existentialism, Nucho [1987] and cybernetics, Landgarten [1987] and family systems, and Riley [1994] and social constructionism). Each theoretical dimension adds depth to the practitioner's understanding of the process but distracts from the centrality of the art itself. My own theoretical and professional identity is based on an openness to diverse conceptualizations of the work but rooted most deeply in a commitment to the art making itself. It is obvious that theoretical musing has enhanced the field of art therapy, establishing its clinical validity and inspiring its clinicians. However, as illustrated in this chapter, it is the experience with imagery that is directly beneficial to art therapy clients.

In the following sections, three examples of art processes used as action methods with families are described. Art making as a tool with families facilitates the pictorial or graphic communication of all family members. It supports each member's attempt to find an alternative (i.e., nonverbal) form of self-expression while simultaneously allowing for the emergence of a graphical depiction of the family system itself. The resulting depictions, often richly symbolic and laden with multiple levels of meaning, offer the family the opportunity to shift patterns of speaking to each other, of listening to each other, and of interacting with each other. The three art tasks discussed were all used with one family during their participation in a multifamily art therapy group. Progression through the three tasks can be observed, demonstrating the ways in which art tasks can be more or less complicated as the client (or, in this case, the family) becomes more open to the opportunities presented.

BEGINNING ACTION METHOD 1: THE FAMILY DRAWING

The family drawing comes from an extensive tradition of family art therapy (Kwiatkowska, 1978; Landgarten, 1987; Linesch, 1993; Riley, 1994) and provides the family with the opportunity to visually represent the dynamics or patterns in which it functions. By having each member of the family pick a separate color and use that color throughout the drawing, the art therapist is able to facilitate a two-dimensional picture or map of the family's experience participating in an activity together. This technique works extremely well with families with children or adolescents, leveling the playing field so that the nonverbal or less verbal (i.e., child or adolescent) can communicate on an equal footing with the very verbal (i.e., adult).

The family drawing is an excellent assessment tool and is ideally suited for first sessions as a means to familiarize the client or family with the art process as a psychotherapeutic tool. It also is an excellent way to immediately involve all members of the family simultaneously.

CASE EXAMPLE 1: THE FAMILY DRAWING

Simple art supplies are needed for this task: large drawing paper and a variety of colored markers. The family is instructed to select markers, being careful that each member has her or his own color, and then create a drawing. No instructions about talking or decision making or taking turns are given. This gives the therapist the opportunity to observe the family's process. A time limit is provided; usually 10 to 15 minutes is more than sufficient, and the therapist can sit back and allow the activity to facilitate the family's experience. When the family indicates that the drawing is complete, the therapist may or may not lead the discussion by asking questions about leadership, roles, and alliances reflected by concrete observations in the artwork rather than vague abstractions about the family's described perceptions and experiences.

Case Narrative

The J family consists of a 36-year-old single mother and her two sons, Jimmy (12) and Joey (10). The boys' father abandoned the family when the boys were young and has had only sporadic contact with them since. Neither boy is functioning well academically, and their mother describes them as "out of control" at home. Joey, the identified client, was referred for treatment by school personnel.

At the second group meeting, when only the mother and Joey represented the J family, all the families were asked to work together to create family drawings (Figure 11-1). Joey chose a green marker and drew a house on the right side of the page while his mother chose a blue

Commentary

The agency from which the family sought treatment recommended participation in a multiple-family art therapy group. The family began attending weekly and connected quickly with the other families, all of whom were headed by single mothers experiencing similar feelings of frustration and being overwhelmed. Directed art tasks were given in each session to support treatment goals.

Both Mrs. J and Joey apparently found the art process helpful in two ways, experiencing pleasure in the collaborative and expressive activity and experiencing relief at the opportunity to safely express their concerns nonverbally and symbolically. Not only did their drawing depict Mrs. J's marker and drew the family on the left side of the page and three clouds above her son's image of a house. They worked quietly and intensely on the picture, and the resulting image graphically portrayed the family dynamics.

The families were invited to speak about their pictures, and the J family did so somewhat tentatively.

When Mrs. J spoke about her picture of her own state of frustration with her boys' "bickering," the other mothers in the group nodded and sighed empathetically.

Joey pointed out how he had depicted the "interior" of his home, specifically how he and his brother climbed the stairs to get to their mother's bedroom.

fundamental state of feeling overwhelmed as a parent, it simultaneously included Joey's primitive attempt to articulate his "interior" conflicts, with particular focus on the availability and accessibility of his mother (whose bedroom in the drawings was sealed and a leap away from the two ascending staircases (possibly representing Jimmy and Joey's rivalry for their mother's attention).

Mrs. J particularly enjoyed the responses of the other mothers in the group, feeling gratified by her role as the one who could depict the way they all felt.

It is interesting to note that the J family actually lived in a one-level apartment.

The drawing process facilitated the depiction of the family's emotional conflict and provided the art therapist and other group members with an opportunity to acknowledge and comment on unverbalized feelings present in the imagery.

As illustrated, the family drawing is a powerful tool that can immediately present a graphic depiction of family dynamics. This technique is well suited to the assessment stages of therapy, but it can easily probe deeper as family members indicate their willingness to explore meaning and embrace interpretive complexities.

BEGINNING ACTION METHOD 2: THE COMMUNICATION COLLAGE

The general use of collage material in the practice of art psychotherapy is supported most articulately by Landgarten (1993). She claimed, "The collage mode is a meaningful tool for the discovery of problem areas. Clients conflicts, defense mechanisms, and styles of functioning are revealed in a short time" (p. 2). Because the client does not have to draw or in any way initiate the image, the experience of making a collage is not bounded by the apprehension and intimidation many individuals feel about the art

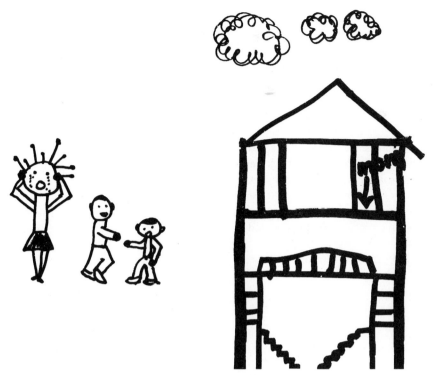

Figure 11-1.

process itself. Anyone can select and glue magazine pictures and, in doing so, gain greater access to self-expressive and self-explorative opportunities.

Many clinicians use collage processes during the assessment phase of therapy because they are quick to execute and nonthreatening but able to expose both interpersonal and intrapersonal material. However, the use of collage throughout the course of treatment can be sensitively handled if the therapist pays attention to the ebb and flow of defense mechanisms and guides clients appropriately to manage more or less threatening explorations by shifting and suggesting media options.

To use collage making in therapy, simple materials are required: a collection of precut images (of various sizes, styles, content, colors, and cultures), scissors, glue sticks, and large sheets of drawing paper. Although the process can be directive or nondirective, very specific use of collage making in organized tasks seems to be consistent with it as an action methods model. The specific directed way of using the collage process in the next case example involved instructing family members in the following three steps:

1. Pick out pictures of people who are communicating.
2. Glue them on the paper in relation to the pictures picked out by other family members.

3. Add words underneath the images to give voice to what you believe each person is communicating.

CASE EXAMPLE 2: THE COMMUNICATION COLLAGE

Case Narrative

Commentary

The J family returned for the fourth group meeting, once again with only Mrs. J and Joey present. For the first art task of the evening, each member of the group was asked to select a collage picture of someone communicating. They were then instructed to glue the picture on a sheet of paper with their family members' selections and to use the markers to write what that person was communicating.

It seemed that Mrs. J remained unwilling to bring both her boys to the art therapy group, choosing instead to work with one at a time. The directive to have the family members make communication collages was based on the assessment that all the families in the group were stuck in redundant and ineffective patterns of communicating with each other. It was hoped that the art task would provide alternative opportunities that might facilitate shifts in interactions.

The J family created Figure 11-2, a collage depicting two young boys and a maternal figure. Mrs. J's collage selection [on the left side of the page] was an image of a waiflike, pleading youth under which she wrote the caption, "I am so hungry." Joey's collage selection [on the right side of the page] was an image of a young boy being shown something by a caretaking woman. As articulated by Joey, the maternal figure was saying, "What would you like?" Together, the two decided to name the piece, "I'll help you!", and Joey wrote the title at the bottom of the page.

The J family's collage demonstrates some of the fundamental difficulties experienced by this family; the overwhelmed, resource-depleted mother ambivalently parenting the role-confused and unindividuated child. Mrs. J's collage selection poignantly depicted her own sense of deprivation, whereas Joey's picture suggested his compensatory efforts and his difficulties in experiencing his own identity and sense of self within this family system. The collage process and, in particular, the activity of connecting their selected imagery served to facilitate deeper levels of interaction and communication between them than that in which they typically engaged.

The two were pleased with their production and asked if they could use the collage pictures to make more interactive stories. Joey particularly enjoyed having his mother write down the words he made up for the characters he selected.

The task provided the family with a quiet and conflict-free experience in which they were freed from patterned attention-getting behaviors. Although the art product suggested deep systemic dysfunction, the art process allowed the mother and son to experience each other differently.

I am so hungry!

What would you like?

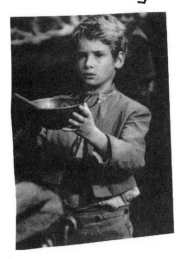

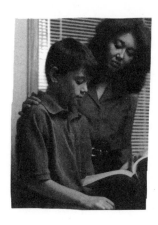

I'll Help You

Figure 11-2.

Unlike the first art task discussed, this project contained a specific intervention (i.e., to expand the dyad's communicative repertoire). This task is a useful technique that supports the augmentation of interfamilial behaviors. Additionally (like all art making), it offers the clients, the therapist, and, in this case, the other group participants the opportunity to grapple with the meanings embedded in the imagery. With the J family, even at this early point in treatment, the evident pleasure and relief in the communicative collaboration of the project suggested that insight-probing explorations of meaning would best be left for later. The therapist can feel assured that further art making will facilitate the emergence of unexplored dynamics.

AN ADVANCED ACTION METHOD: THE INTERACTIVE FAMILY AND GROUP PROJECT

This art task, the interactive family and group project, is a slight modification of a traditional art therapy approach that asks family members to draw themselves as animals, involves several steps, and is based on the goal of including group dynamics as a strategy to support family treatment goals. Its richness and multidimensionality lie in the layering of processes from one step to another as the family moves through the sequential activities, deepening their expressed sense of self and using the resources of other group members to expand and augment their repertoires of adaptive techniques.

The task demonstrates the powerful potential of the art process in both family and group therapy and its particular potency when these two modalities are integrated. As with all art psychotherapy techniques, very simple supplies are needed: markers, scissors, glue sticks, and large sheets of drawing paper. Careful instructions need to be given for this task, however, and it is best broken down into three simple steps with the directions for each being given only after the preceding step is completed:

1. Each family member is asked to draw himself or herself as an animal.
2. Each family is asked to organize its members' animal representations into a whole and to embellish the image.
3. Each family is asked to share their work with a different family and to exchange ideas about additions or changes that could be made.

CASE EXAMPLE 3: THE INTERACTIVE FAMILY AND GROUP PROJECT

Case Narrative

The S family (mother, age 40, and Samuel, age 8) joined the multifamily art therapy group in which the J family had been participating 3 months after it had started. On the S family's first night, when only Mrs. J and Joey represented the J family, group members were asked to draw themselves as animals. Figure 11-3 is the cat drawn by Mrs. S to represent herself, and Figure 11-4 is the unidentified creature drawn by Samuel to represent himself.

Although Mrs. S was reluctant to discuss her cat drawing, Samuel enjoyed the group's excited response to his creature drawing and delighted in sharing the growling noises its ferocious voice could project.

Commentary

Attending their first group session was difficult for the S family, and they appeared shy and somewhat awkward with the art directives with which the other families had become familiar and comfortable.

Mrs. S was embarrassed by her cat drawing, recognizing its childlikeness, but on a deeper level seeming also to be aware of its expression of fragility and isolation. It was perhaps too early for these difficult feelings to emerge in the art process, and Mrs. S

The second step in the art task was to have family members cut out their self-representational animal drawings, glue them on one piece of paper for the whole family, and use markers to add an environment in which the animals could live. Figure 11-5 depicts how Mrs. S and Samuel quickly cut out their animals, glued them on the provided paper, and minimally embellished their picture. Samuel used a thick blue marker to create what he described as a "cage" for his creature, and Mrs. S added faint green "grass" for her cat.

For the third step in this art activity, each family was asked to share its picture with another family and exchange ideas and suggestions about additions and changes that could be made to the imagery. The S family connected with the J family and somewhat hesitantly spoke about their cat/creature imagery. Mrs. J and Joey appeared eager to help the S family embellish their picture, and although Mrs. S and Samuel seemed disinterested in making changes, Mrs. J and Joey asked permission to add to the drawing themselves. Figure 11-6 shows the result of this collaborative effort. Mrs. J added a collar, leash, and rider to Samuel's creature, and Joey sheltered Mrs. S's cat in a solid structure he labeled *home*.

had difficulty engaging with the group and indeed even with her son, who seemed surprised by the group's positive response to his imagery and their subsequent encouragement for his continued and expanded self-expression.

Mrs. S's shy and withdrawn behavior catalyzed sympathetic and supportive responses from the other mothers, who murmured support for and interest in her cat image. It was this empathic response from her peers that enabled Mrs. S to add the green grass (however feeble and minimal) to the drawing. Mrs. S's cat appeared vulnerable, overwhelmed, and out of its element relative to the strong and somewhat contained ferociousness of her son's creature. With his cage of bars, Samuel seemed to have separated himself from his mother and temporarily contained his aggression.

The J family gravitated to the S family in apparent recognition of similar dynamics. Mrs. J clearly understood the ways in which Mrs. S's sense of being overwhelmed echoed her own. For Mrs. J and Joey, the opportunity to add resources (metaphorically and symbolically) to the S family's systemically representative drawing (resourceless as it was) was extraordinarily empowering. The cross-familial and cross-generational support (i.e., Mrs. J taming Samuel's barely controlled creature and Joey sheltering Mrs. S's forlorn, homeless cat), took advantage of an opportunity that verbal therapy alone could not have provided. It was the activity—or action—of art making that facilitated this curative process of pooling limited resources.

Both families appeared very satisfied with the results of this art task and requested the opportunity to do more joint tasks in the future.

Both families experienced many things in this project: pleasure in working together, a shift in their patterned or redundant behaviors, and the opportunity to experience increased understandings of family.

This art task illustrates the way in which art making in therapy is not formulaic, but rather is directed by the therapist's own creative response to the needs of the client, family, or group. When art making is understood as the language of therapy, the art tasks become the here-and-now responses of the therapist to the here-and-now experiences and needs of the client, family, or group.

RESISTANCE

When resistance is defined as a divergent alignment of purpose between therapist and client, the art therapy process can be viewed as offering very special kinds of opportunities to respond to it. By incorporating creative processes to support the client's experiences and to realign the purpose of the therapist more closely to the client's experience, the art therapist is uniquely equipped to bypass those obstacles to treatment progress often categorized as resistance. Because art making is experiential and action oriented, it is possible and indeed exciting for the therapist to discover, along with the client, the processes and materials that are ego-syntonic with the person's current experience:

- If the client's unwillingness to make art is experienced by the therapist as resistance, then the therapist needs to shift the art-making activity to reflect (either directly or symbolically) the reluctance the client is feeling about self-expression.
- If the client's unwillingness to discuss feelings is experienced by the therapist as resistance, then the therapist needs to shift the art-making activity to support (either directly or symbolically) the client's exploration of the emergence of feelings within the art itself.

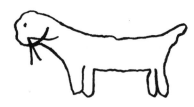

Figure 11-3.

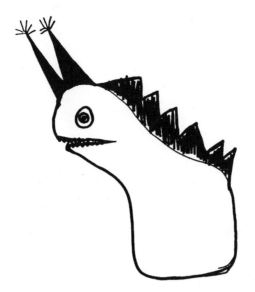

Figure 11-4.

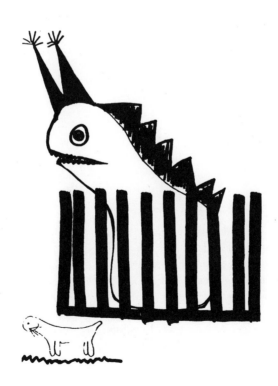

Figure 11-5.

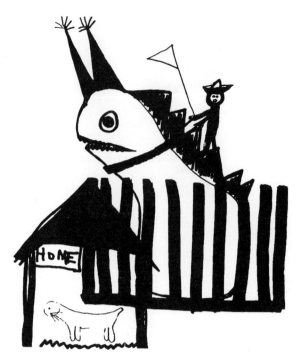

Figure 11-6.

- If the client's apparent lack of movement toward the achievement of treatment goals is experienced by the therapist as resistance, then the therapist needs to shift the art-making activity to reflect (either directly or symbolically) the ways in which the client currently is engaged in treatment.

These guidelines illustrate the ways in which the art therapist becomes the guide of the client's experience, alertly offering, encouraging, and supporting the client's artistic efforts as experiential self-representations with materials, direction, and understanding. A brief vignette from art therapy treatment with a 15-year-old boy diagnosed with conduct disorder richly depicts this process:

> Sean had decided that the art therapist, like his school counselor, his probation officer, and his parents, was of no use to him, and he entered his first art therapy session cursing and insisting that he hated art and "would not be caught dead making art." Rather than interpreting his resistance as an obstacle to treatment, the art therapist remained alert to Sean's terror and need to stay in control and engaged the boy by asking him to first assume that the white piece of drawing paper on the table was a representation of the art therapy session and to then use any material to show where he would place a representation of himself in relation to that now symbolically meaningful piece of paper.

> When Sean angrily picked up a piece of chalk and made an aggressive X on the wall, as far away from the paper as possible within the therapy room, he began to be engaged in treatment.

When chalk marks on the wall are understood as legitimate an art form as oil pastels on paper, and when clients are allowed to authentically represent their experiences of disengagement, disorientation, and distrust, resistance does not occur.

VALUE OF SUCCESSIVE USES

As demonstrated in this chapter's case examples, art-making processes are ideally used as successive and continuous processes that support and reflect the shifting experiences of clients as they make use of art making and their own imagery. Because the supplies used in most art therapy activities are simple and easy to manipulate, it is often feasible to encourage clients to continue art making at home between sessions. Such homework endeavors serve many functions: They allow the client to feel a continuous connection to the therapeutic process and to the art therapist; they allow the client to continue the exploration begun in a therapy session (e.g., the J family, discussed earlier, asked permission to continue with their communication collages at home); and they provide the art therapist an opportunity to view the client's experiences as recorded in the art product outside of the therapy room.

EMPIRICAL SUPPORT

The current controversies around the validity of traditional scientific investigations into psychotherapeutic processes are nowhere more intensely manifested than within the debates and dialogues between art therapists. It is interesting that just as the field of art therapy tends to polarize its clinical approaches between art-as-therapy and art-in-therapy, it has polarized its scholarly debates in a parallel manner; that is, nontraditional research that incorporates the art versus traditional research that validates the art. Just as the answer to the original dichotomous question is "neither and both," the answer to the research debate is encouragement toward diversity and inclusion. The field of art therapy desperately needs scholarship of all kinds: empirical research that tests the assessment, diagnostic, and treatment implications that abound in its published case materials as well as more exploratory and phenomenological research that attempts to understand the depths of the art psychotherapy process. Sean McNiff poetically reminded us that the arts have always been validated by practitioners' own experiences when he encouraged all art therapists interested in research to adopt artistic standards of inquiry. He said, "Rather than attempt to prove the significance of what we do according to standards incapable of articulating complexity and depth, I suggest a sustained focus on practice. Research in the creative arts therapies is inseparable from doing the work and its demonstration to others" (McNiff, 1993, p. 9).

THERAPIST CHARACTERISTICS, EDUCATION, AND TRAINING

As in any therapeutic process, the presence and use of the self by the therapist is crucial to the therapeutic experience of the client. Unique to all creative art therapies, however, is the singular importance of the therapist's belief in the healing potential within the creative process, and unique to art therapy is the therapist's primary focus on the use of visual arts for self-expression. The best way that this value or belief system can be cultivated and demonstrated is by the art therapist's own involvement in his or her creativity and his or her incorporation of art processes for personal growth. Without firsthand experience (not necessarily talent but depth exploration) of the dynamics of making art, the therapist cannot fully access the rich dimensions inherent within the processes. It is hard to imagine a therapist inexperienced with his or her own artistic explorations being able to encourage an angry adolescent like Sean to find a way to become engaged. Without a deep-seated personal belief in the power of imagery, the inexperienced therapist would consequently be less likely to appreciate the profound significance of Sean's hastily executed X.

Personal commitment to the healing potential within the visual arts is not enough; the art therapist must be trained in the assessment and treatment principles of clinical practice for the transformative powers of the art processes to be most available. Art therapy training programs that focus (as most do) on working with individual clients typically require 2 years of full-time didactic and practicum training. Family art therapy training programs require additional coursework in family systems theory and family therapy techniques. The work discussed in this chapter requires a comprehensive understanding of family therapy and a commitment to understanding both the artwork and the family as part of a system.

The practice of art therapy is more than the combination of art and therapy. Rather, it is a synergistic integration that produces an entirely new entity and catalyzes the existence of a discrete professional identity. Those who practice art therapy are art therapists, practitioners substantively different from other psychotherapists who use art in their practice. In recognition of this differentiation, training programs have been established throughout the country, typically providing master's-level degrees, but also awarding bachelor's degrees, doctorates, and certificates. Since 1969, the American Art Therapy Association (AATA) has established standards for education, registration, and certification processes. The most comprehensive way to pursue registration is through a master's degree in art therapy (currently offered in 32 AATA-approved and 30 other training programs) and subsequent postgraduate supervised hours in the practice of art therapy. Certification follows registration but requires passage of a comprehensive examination.

CONCLUSION

As described in this chapter, art therapy is an effective and powerful action method that can facilitate expanded self-expression, increased awareness, and experimentation with changes in behavior. Although art therapy techniques can be and often are used by clinicians with a very rudimentary understanding of the visual arts and their power in psychotherapy, the field itself has both more breadth and more depth than these techniques illustrate. The symbolic process and creativity are of course the complex processes that underscore the power of the visual arts in psychotherapy and demand comprehensive respect. To understand the techniques of art therapy as an action method is a first step; to increasingly acknowledge the multiple levels on which this process occurs is the task faced by everyone interested in both the arts and psychotherapy.

REFERENCES

Betensky, M. (1973). *Self-discovery through self-expression: Use of art in psychotherapy with children and adolescents.* Springfield, IL: Charles C Thomas.

Betensky, M. (1987). Phenomenology of therapeutic art expression and art therapy. In J. Rubin (Ed.), *Approaches to art therapy: Theory and technique* (pp. 26–43). New York: Brunner/Mazel.

Kramer, E. (1971). *Art as therapy with children.* New York: Schocken Books.

Kramer, E. (1987). Sublimation and art therapy. In J. Rubin (Ed.), *Approaches to art therapy: Theory and technique.* New York: Brunner/Mazel.

Kwiatkowska, H. (1978). *Family therapy and evaluation through art.* Springfield, IL: Charles C Thomas.

Landgarten, H. (1987). *Family art psychotherapy.* New York: Brunner/Mazel.

Landgarten, H. (1993). *Magazine photo collage: A multicultural assessment and treatment technique.* New York: Brunner/Mazel.

Linesch, D. (1993). *Art therapy with families in crisis.* New York: Brunner/Mazel.

McNiff, S. (1988). *Fundamentals of art therapy.* Springfield, IL: Charles C Thomas.

McNiff, S. (1993). The authority of experience. *The Arts in Psychotherapy, 20*(1), 3–9.

Moon, B. (1990). *Existential art therapy.* Springfield, IL: Charles C Thomas.

Naumberg, M. (1966). *Dynamically oriented art therapy: Its principles and practices.* New York: Grune & Stratton.

Nucho, A. (1987). *The psychocybernetic model of art therapy.* Springfield, IL: Charles C Thomas.

Riley, S. (1994). *Integrative approaches to family art therapy.* Chicago: Magnolia Street Publishers.

Rubin, J. (1987). *Approaches to art therapy: Theory and technique.* New York: Brunner/Mazel.

ADDITIONAL RESOURCES

Books

Junge, M., & Asawa, P. (1994). *A history of art therapy in the United States.* Mundelein, IL: American Art Therapy Association.

Kramer, E. (1958). *Art therapy in a children's community.* Springfield, IL: Charles C Thomas.

Landgarten, H. (1981). *Clinical art therapy: A comprehensive guide.* New York: Brunner/Mazel.

Landgarten, H., & Lubbers, D. (Eds.). (1991). *Adult art psychotherapy: Issues and applications.* New York: Brunner/Mazel.

Linesch, D. (1988). *Adolescent art therapy.* New York: Brunner/Mazel.

Malchiodi, C. (1990). *Breaking the silence: Art therapy with children from violent homes.* New York: Brunner/Mazel.

Naumberg, M. (1953). *Psychoneurotic art: Its function in psychotherapy.* New York: Grune & Stratton.

Robbins, A. (1989). *The psychoaesthetic experience.* New York: Human Sciences Press.

Rubin, J. (1978). *Child art therapy.* New York: Van Nostrand Reinhold.

Rubin, J. (1984). *The art of art therapy.* New York: Brunner/Mazel.

Wadeson, H. (1980). *Art psychotherapy.* New York: Wiley.

Journals

The American Journal of Art Therapy. Northfield, VT: Vermont College of Norwich University.

Art Therapy. Mundelein, IL: American Art Therapy Association.

The Arts in Psychotherapy. New York: Pergamon Press.

Professional Association

American Art Therapy Association
1202 Allanson Road
Mundelein, Illinois 60060
(847) 949-6064 (telephone)
(847) 566-4580 (fax)
E-mail: arttherapy@ntr.net
Web site: http://www.arttherapy.org

Represents over 4,000 art therapists in the United States and abroad. Its purposes are as follows:

- the progressive development of the therapeutic use of art;
- the advancement of standards of practice, ethical standards, education, and research;
- the provision of professional communication and exchange with colleagues;
- the provision of legislative efforts to promote and improve the status of professional practice; and
- the promotion of the field of art therapy through the dissemination of public information.

12

A PSYCHOANALYTICALLY INFORMED APPLICATION OF DANCE/MOVEMENT THERAPY

IRMA DOSAMANTES-BEAUDRY

The emergence of dance/movement therapy (DMT) as a clinical discipline and practice in the United States during the 1950s represented a modern rediscovery and reconstruction of those integrative and transformative properties of dance acknowledged long ago by tribal communities (Bartenieff, 1972). This phenomenon was in large measure facilitated by the humanistic psychology movement of the 1950s and 1960s (Dosamantes-Alperson, 1974). This movement, which was critical of mainstream society's obsession with control and extreme reliance on verbal communication and rational thought, emphasized empathic phenomenological observation and bodily felt experiencing and expression in its clinical practices. The inclusion of intersubjective relatedness, bodily experiencing, and expression into the broader psychotherapeutic community created a climate more open to all arts- and body-movement–based psychotherapies.

First-generation DMT pioneers (e.g., Marian Chace, Liljan Espenak, and Blanche Evan on the East Coast and Alma Hawkins, Trudi Schoop, and Mary Whitehouse on the West Coast) were strong and creative modern dancers who intuitively understood the value of embodied experience in altering human consciousness (Dosamantes-Beaudry, 1997a). They recognized that the creative and healing elements of modern dance—bodily awareness, individual expressiveness, spontaneity, and creativity—could be made accessible to ordinary people who were not trained as dance performers, as well as to those who were institutionalized with emotional disorders (Levy, 1988).

During the period between 1940 and 1970, each of these pioneers developed distinctive versions of DMT that in part reflected their cultural traditions, personalities, dance training, views of the creative process, understanding of health and emotional disturbance, and kinds of clients with whom they chose to work and who sought them out.

The creation of the American Dance Therapy Association (ADTA) in 1966 led to the professionalization of the field and to a psychotherapeutic definition of DMT that emphasized the integration of soma and psyche. This association officially defined DMT as "the psychotherapeutic use of movement as a process which furthers the emotional and physical integration of the individual" (Bunney, 1980, pp. 24–25).

During the 1970s, as dance therapists became increasingly familiar with the clinical methods and theoretical concepts of the humanistic psychotherapies of that era, hybrid DMT approaches combining methods derived from both DMT and humanistic psychotherapies (e.g., Gestalt and experiential DMT approaches) began to surface (Levy, 1988). During the next decade and extending into the 1990s, psychoanalytic and analytic concepts (e.g., personal and collective unconsciousness, transference and countertransference, active imagination and object-relations perspective of human development) greatly influenced the work of many second-generation dance therapists (Dosamantes-Beaudry, 1997a). The hybridized versions of DMT that resulted from the inclusion of these concepts forged a more psychodynamic and intersubjective view of the DMT process. These psychodynamic approaches placed greater emphasis on unconscious processes taking place within intersubjective and interpersonal fields created between the dance therapist and the client.

For example, within a psychoanalytically informed type of DMT (hereafter referred to as PSY-DMT), clients bear major responsibility for initiating and directing the content of their sessions. The therapist generally abstains from recommending the content that a client should explore. In this form of treatment, the therapist's focus is on the unfolding psychodynamic process, including the quality and types of transference and countertransference relationships being developed between the client and the therapist, the client's internalization of needed psychological functions, and the forging of new identifications with others (Dosamantes-Alperson, 1985–1986).

PSY-DMT offers clients a new chance for a creative "play space," a space in which they can play freely with their sensations, object-related movements, images, feelings, and thoughts in the presence of another who does not intrude, but instead quietly mirrors their reality as an empathic observer and communicator. This space is analogous to the child's transitional space, for it is neither inside nor outside of the person, but both simultaneously (Winnicott, 1965). The client's perception of the therapist alternates between that of a character half-created by the client's imaged action fantasies and an outside person who is an interested yet impartial observer, listener, and interpreter. At some point in treatment, clients begin to select for identification particular therapist functions that they cannot perform for themselves (e.g., the capacity to contain unpleasant affects). They accomplish this through the creation of imaginary action fantasies that involve them with the therapist in some way that replicates the needed psychological function. For example, they may imagine themselves sitting on the therapist's lap while being held securely and gently rocked by her or him (Dosamantes-Alperson, 1985–1986).

Historically, as the number of "marriages" between dance/movement-based and psychotherapy-based theories and practices increased, they gave rise to a wide array of DMT clinical approaches and pressed the field to delineate its boundaries and unique features as a psychotherapeutic practice distinct from both existing verbal psychotherapies and various kinds of body therapies. In a report submitted to the Commission on Psychiatric Therapies, the ADTA delineated the following premises on which DMT was founded as a clinical discipline (Dosamantes-Alperson, 1981, pp. 4–5):

- Emotional well-being is reflected in the integration of soma and psyche. Emotional disorder is manifested in the dissociation of mind from body.
- Body movement is a medium through which an individual may experience, express and communicate elements of experience not readily communicable through verbal means (this experience is usually less conscious in nature).
- When individuals move spontaneously, their movement reflect and reveals something about their emotional state of the moment as well as the manner in which they ward off the expression of particular affects and experiences.
- When individuals move in relation to one or more persons their movement reflects something about the emotional nature of their ongoing relationship.
- It is possible for an individual to explore intrapsychic and interpersonal emotional concerns or problems within the safe

bounds of a therapeutic relationship established with a trained dance therapist.

In the same report, dance therapists were distinguished from body therapists by virtue of their paying greater systematic attention to the evolving psychodynamics triggered by the movement experience and to the processing of the emotional meaning of the experience (Dosamantes-Alperson, 1981).

SCOPE OF DANCE/MOVEMENT THERAPY PRACTICES

Dance therapists work within a wide variety of clinical settings—in hospitals, outpatient clinics, correctional facilities, day-care centers, homeless shelters, alternative medicine clinics, holistic healing centers, pain clinics, wellness centers, counseling centers, and schools. Some teach in universities or colleges and engage in research. Many are in private practice (Duggan et al., 1979). Client populations served by dance therapists include the severely emotionally disturbed, the mentally retarded, the physically disabled, nonhospitalized individuals with varying degrees of self-pathology, individuals with psychosomatic and immunological disorders, victims of domestic abuse, and individuals engaged in health-maintenance and illness-prevention programs.

Both the type of DMT training received and the particular psychotherapeutic school subscribed to by an individual practitioner influence the clinical positions adopted by him or her regarding the kinds of clinical populations she or he feels might benefit from a particular DMT approach; the choice of brief or long-term treatment; the choice of working with individuals, groups, or families; the relative weight given to nonverbal and verbal modes of experience and expression during treatment; and whether or not to attend to the transferential reactions of client and therapist. The clinical decision concerning the benefit of any DMT approach for a particular individual depends in part on the individual's preference for or need for a predominantly nonverbal form of treatment focusing on bodily experience and expression. For individuals who have access only to nonverbal modes of expression and communication (e.g., mute or autistic individuals), DMT may well be the treatment of choice. In instances in which somatic and psychosomatic symptoms prevail, or where body-image problems are the predominant features, DMT can be of singular value, as the relationship between soma and psyche is a primary focus and concern of this form of treatment. DMT is also well suited for individuals with varying degrees of self-pathology for whom the origins of their emotional difficulties can be traced back to preverbal stages of emotional development (Dosamantes, 1992a).

A PSYCHOANALYTICALLY INFORMED APPLICATION OF DANCE/MOVEMENT THERAPY

Adults with self-pathology have been characterized by the absence of reliable, emotionally attuned caregivers who were responsive to their affective inner lives and emotional needs while they were growing up (Stolorow & Lachman, 1980). These individuals tend to rely on others excessively for their sense of cohesiveness and self-esteem. By adopting relevant clinical concepts from object-relations, self, and intersubjective psychologies, in DMT work with these clients, I am able to observe their enactment of traumatic or narcissistically wounding experiences that date back to early significant relationships. The emotional meaning contained in these enactments is conveyed by clients through somatic symptomatology and symbolic movement metaphors (Dosamantes, 1992a; Dosamantes-Alperson, 1987; Dosamantes-Beaudry, 1997b).

As a dance therapist also trained as a clinical psychologist and psychoanalyst, I conduct a private practice with these kinds of adult clients. Some of them choose to work within PSY-DMT rather than the more traditional psychoanalytic framework, which relies more heavily on words, makes use of the couch, and requires a greater number of sessions per week. In working with PSY-DMT, I see clients for hour-long sessions, preferably at least twice weekly. The room in which we meet is a large, private room that is empty of all furniture except for two large, comfortable futon chairs. The client and I use these chairs when he or she is not moving and is instead engaged in a verbal dialogue with me.

In this work, I adopt the free-associative method and nonintrusive stance of psychoanalysis. This means that clients are free to move or not and in whatever way they choose. When a client leaves the safety of her or his comfortable chair, she or he enters the large, empty movement space, which for many symbolizes entering the unknown. As they begin to move spontaneously and to follow receptively their own inner impulses to move, clients frequently close their eyes. This puts them in touch with their internal world of sensations and images. As they continue moving, they begin to enact experiences that appear to them in the form of imaged memories or fantasies. When they stop moving, they return to their chair and share their movement experiences verbally with me.

I consider my role to be that of a "container" for all client productions. I act as a transitional object until a client can provide for himself or herself those emotional functions I originally served for him or her. I act as a kinesthetically and affectively attuned empathic observer, silently tracking clients as they move while simultaneously tracking my own bodily and imagistic reactions to them. I do this to gauge clients' emotional states as well as to sense the type of object relation they may be constellating with introjected others as they move (Dosamantes, 1992a; Dosamantes-

Beaudry, 1997b). These relationships also tend to mirror the kind of transference relationship that is being established with me. Throughout the treatment process, particularly during the later phases, I act as an interpreter of the emotional meanings contained in client enactments and in the intersubjective relationship transacted between a client and myself.

An excerpt from a first PSY-DMT session with an adult client illustrates the method I use and describes the process that unfolded between us. It shows how directly unconscious meanings are revealed when a client's internal world is approached initially through a receptive, bodily felt movement process.

CASE EXAMPLE 1: SPONTANEOUS MOVEMENT— A FIRST SESSION

Case Narrative	*Commentary*
Lorna, 38 years old, a White, heavyset, intellectually brilliant woman, sought DMT treatment because she found that whenever she attempted to dance spontaneously, she was moved to tears but could not explain why. She had some vague notion that a part of her was "untouched," and she wanted to find out more about this part of herself.	I noted Lorna's familiarity with movement and sensed her ambivalence (a mixture of curiosity and fear) of "spontaneous" movement that stirred up painful emotions that were dissociated from cognitions (reflective of a body–mind split). As I listened, I had an image of Lorna as a lonely infant with a large head and an undifferentiated body (a clue to me of her emotional developmental level).
When she stopped talking, I suggested that she move to a place in the room where she might be comfortable moving, sense an ongoing pulse in her body, and allow this pulse to be moved outward without passing judgment on it; that is, simply let herself follow it wherever it took her.	I sensed her need to end verbal contact with me. By shifting her focus from the verbal to the kinesthetic or enactive mode, she could do so while simultaneously beginning to risk moving in a self-directed, spontaneous way while in my presence. As a quiet observer, I would be able to perceive her movement dynamics and bodily defenses.
She responded by selecting a place that was some distance from me, and she assumed a sitting position facing away from me. She closed her eyes and began to move slowly and tenta-	

250   IRMA DOSAMANTES-BEAUDRY

tively. The movement I observed appeared to originate in her upper torso. She led with her chest held forward and moved her upper torso in a circular, pivotal fashion. In contrast to her active top half, her lower torso remained perfectly still and appeared rooted to the floor. She indicated that she was finished moving by opening up her eyes. Her first verbal association to her movement was that she felt she moved in the studio in the same way she moved in the outside world. I asked her to expand on what she meant.

As she sought to explain further, she took a deep breath, expanded her chest, and placed both hands on her hips in a confrontative or challenging posture. She explained that the attitude she has assumed represented the way she related to the world outside. She called it "my attitude to the world at large." She went on to describe the "feeling tone" of this

I perceived the body split Lorna was exhibiting and thought that perhaps the stillness I observed in her lower torso might be related to some sexual inhibition or trauma. However, because Lorna might have had very different emotional meaning associations to this bodily experience, I needed to wait for her to confirm or disconfirm this perception.

During the initial phases of therapy, I am most interested in the emotional meaning clients attach to their bodily felt experiencing. I abstain from sharing my observations with them, because this would divert the focus away from them and onto me (i.e., my perceptions and my projections) and, in effect, would replicate for them the kinds of pathological relational patterns that had been established with them earlier by their caregivers. In later phases, when clients have become more familiar with the therapeutic process, have established a collaborative therapeutic working relationship with me, and are emotionally ready, I may offer verbal interpretations to enhance or integrate their understanding of the experiential process.

posture "as though I'm angry and as if I'm saying, 'I'll show you'." She then stated that she felt "nothing below her waist." Almost as an afterthought, she wondered whether this sense of no feeling might have something to do with her "current lack of sexual excitement." Following these more immediate associations, she recalled a childhood memory that had been triggered while she was moving. The memory was that of her father comparing her unfavorably to her younger, prettier sister and berating her by calling her "big" and "clumsy."

As she spoke, she stuck out her tongue several times. However, she seemed quite unaware of this action.

This unconscious gesture seemed to me to be perfectly congruent with the feelings of resentment she was expressing toward her father.

She concluded her verbal narrative of her childhood memory with a prophetic comment about her existential condition: "It must have been then (referring to her childhood) that I must have decided to excel in the world through my intellect rather than my physical looks."

I was pleasantly surprised by the easy flow and volume of Lorna's verbal associations. Not all patients are as self-revealing during their first session. I also became aware of how bright and perceptive she was (ego strengths that would serve her well during subsequent sessions).

First sessions tend to be very rich clinically, often revealing several core self-identity issues and conflicted significant object relationships. These concerns are subsequently revisited many times throughout the course of treatment, until their full emotional meaning for the client in the present has been worked through.

The length of PSY-DMT treatment varies depending on the extent and depth of psychological change sought by the client and his or her tolerance for increasing levels of anxiety. Treatment can last from several months to several years. In this form of psychotherapy, movement and verbalization always are used as modes of communication. However, during the initial phases of treatment, clients tend to move more and talk less, whereas during the later phases (the working-through and terminal phases), the reverse appears to be the case (i.e., clients talk more and move less). Initially, the therapist functions as an observer, listener, and container for the client's experience and productions, whereas later, she or he also offers a greater number of verbal interpretations. During the later phases of treatment, clients also exhibit an increased ability to symbolize their own experience into words and to regulate their affective states (Dosamantes, 1990).

CASE EXAMPLE 2: DREAM ENACTMENT—A LATER SESSION

The following case example is of a client who had been in treatment for several months. It demonstrates how a conflict she initially encountered in a disturbing dream was worked through using an embodied movement process.

Case Narrative

Commentary

Helen, 30 years old, a White, slender, attractive, brunette woman began her session by verbally recounting a dream from the previous evening. She dreamt that a large ship was stranded at sea and had lost its bearings. It first went in one direction, then another. "Totally lost, the ship was laden down with heavy cargo, and so it could not move very fast through the water." She woke up suddenly and was very upset by the dream although she did not know why.

I asked her which aspect of the dream she wanted to explore through movement.

She responded that she would like to move like the lost ship. She stepped into the movement space, closed her eyes, and began to move as the ship

By shifting to a kinesthetic-movement mode, Helen could explore further her kinetic identification with the ship "that could not move very fast through the water."

she had envisioned in her dream. She surged and lunged in one direction after another.

She suddenly stopped moving, opened her eyes, and said, "I am totally lost. Where am I going? I have no center."

I asked Helen if she had felt that way before. She blurted out that her movement reminded her of her father, whom she described as "forgetful, irresponsible, and untrustworthy, so unlike mother." She described her mother as "firm, very responsible, and at times very angry; she seemed so burdened."

She decided to move again, but this time as "the burdened ship." She stood up, closed her eyes, and began to move. Gradually, I observed her collapse under the weight of the cargo that she appeared to be carrying until ultimately she wound up lying belly-down, flat on the floor. She spurted, "My burden is so heavy." She went on to describe her mother as "not only a burdened person but also a burdensome person" who was "very resentful." She then noted that she recently had found herself "assuming too many responsibilities and, like her mother, she found herself becoming "increasingly irritated and angry."

I stated, "I wonder if whether, as with your mother, you might not be in greater need of support from me."

She responded that she "felt understood" by me and proceeded to recount how her parents "had divorced because they could not possibly live together any more." She then announced that she would like to move

As she continued darting in various directions and frantically increasing the speed of her movement, I could sense her becoming increasingly anxious.

Helen's embodied movement identification with the lost ship of her dream put her in touch with her fear of losing a core sense of herself.

This question was intended to help Helen locate the past self–other relational context of her movement metaphor of the lost ship.

This question was intended to serve as a bridge, to relate Helen's past experience to her present experience.

again. She resumed moving like the directionless ship.

When she finally stopped moving, she explained that she "had enjoyed the spontaneity of moving freely" and that in the past, she had associated "being bad, out of control, and not being serious with being spontaneous."

As Helen moved in different directions and at varying speeds, I observed the emotional tenor of her movement begin to shift from discomfort to exhilaration. Her movements began to assume a more carefree quality. I also observed that, after each change of direction, she returned to a clearly defined location on the floor.

Within the context of an emotionally understanding therapeutic environment, Helen was able to reclaim and reintegrate into her sense of self those disavowed qualities she previously had associated with her father —her "bad" self, which included loss of control and spontaneity.

Two critical characteristics of the working-through stage of PSY-DMT are illustrated in this example: (a) the retrieval of disavowed self-identifications pertaining to earlier ruptured significant relationships and (b) their symbolization, transformation, and reintegration by the client into a more benign form.

RESISTANCE

As a psychoanalytically oriented dance therapist, I define *resistance* as any block or interference to the flow of the therapeutic process. Resistance can manifest itself in a variety of ways.

Clients who are unfamiliar with the use of movement as an instrument of consciousness, for example, may—at the beginning of treatment—express fear of engaging in a spontaneous movement process. These feelings appear to be related to fear of self-disclosure and correlative feelings of doubt and shame. Clients who lack a cohesive sense of self seem to be particularly susceptible to experiencing intense feelings of vulnerability. This is the case even when they possess an extensive movement vocabulary and use movement frequently as a performance skill, as many professional dancers do.

By focusing on the client's bodily felt experience, the dance therapist can access the client's fears, retrieve avoided feelings, and permit the content associated with these feelings to surface and be clarified, as illustrated by the following example:

> Diana, a young professional ballet dancer, originally came to see me because she was distressed over critics' comments that although her performances were technically brilliant, they lacked emotional depth.
>
> Initially, she spent several DMT sessions executing her familiar virtuoso ballet repertoire. However, by the end of the third session, I sensed that both she and I had become bored with her performances, so I asked her what she experienced while moving in the room. She replied that she felt "detached," "like a puppet," and "sleepy."
>
> She showed me how sleepy she felt by lying flat on her back for a long time. When she "awoke," she suddenly and quite spontaneously curled herself up into a fetuslike position. Then, while maintaining that position, she managed to roll herself over into the furthest corner of the room.
>
> When she stopped moving, she began to sob uncontrollably and cried out that she felt "like a baby who needed to be protected." Then, she added that she found the movement she had just done to be "very difficult" because she was "afraid of losing control" and "could not anticipate what [she] might dredge up that [she] would dread."

As this case illustrates, a client's avoidances or resistances serve a useful defensive function for her or him. Therefore, they must be sensitively broached by the therapist and understood by him or her within the context of the client's emotional life history, capacity for emotional containment, prior movement experience, and capacity for initiating self-directed spontaneous movement; the nature of the evolving client–therapist transference relationship; and the point within the treatment process at which they are enacted.

Throughout the treatment process, resistance continues to surface, and the therapist—in collaboration with the client—must untangle the emotional and symbolic meaning they hold for the client. Resistance can be recognized, for example, when either the client or the therapist, or both, begins to feel stymied or stuck, the verbal or nonverbal content expressed by either becomes repetitious, the prevailing affective tone of the therapeutic process becomes one of deadness or boredom, or the therapist experiences a strong sense that nothing is happening.

EMPIRICAL SUPPORT

Ritter and Low (1996) conducted a review of all studies published between 1974 and 1993 to evaluate the efficacy of DMT with children, nondisturbed adults, adult psychiatric clients, disabled individuals, the elderly, and clients with neurological deficits. Their search yielded a total of 95 studies.

In reviewing these studies, Ritter and Low (1996) found serious methodological problems with many of them (e.g., lack of appropriate control groups and inadequate sampling and assessment measures). They applied meta-statistical techniques to 23 studies that they felt met the criteria for adequate research design. They culled from the reports of these studies some of the positive effects attributable to DMT. Some of the more cogent findings they cited included (a) modest positive effects relative to movement and spatial awareness among developmentally disabled children; (b) positive changes in body attitude, self-acceptance, and movement integration and lowered anxiety and depression among noninstitutionalized adults; (c) although confounded by heterogeneous diagnoses, increased group cohesion among psychiatric clients in residential settings; (d) improved body-image changes among adult arthritic clients; (e) increased range of motion and feelings of camaraderie among women with breast cancer seen in groups; and (f) increased capacity for independence, level of comfort with personal space, and degree of relaxation in individuals affected by traumatic brain injuries.

In their review, Ritter and Low (1996) did not differentiate between studies in terms of the type of DMT approach used. Three empirical studies that evaluated several short- and long-term effects and processes generated by psychodynamic DMT groups are described in greater detail below as their findings bear more directly on the approach presented in this chapter.

The first, an outcome study, sought to evaluate the effectiveness of DMT with noninstitutionalized adults (Dosamantes-Alperson & Merrill, 1980). It compared two dance therapy groups with two control groups on several psychological and expressive movement measures. DMT was found to promote significantly greater change in participants' feeling reactivity, spontaneity, self-acceptance, capacity for intimate contact, and body–self acceptance. Preliminary findings also indicated a shift toward lighter and more confident, extraverted, explorative, and integrative movement qualities for participants in the DMT groups compared with the control groups.

The second, a process study, traced several psychodynamic and expressive movement changes taking place in two long-term DMT groups each lasting 2 years (Dosamantes, 1990). Behaviorally, participants in these groups showed greater initiation of movement, increased eye contact with others, increased capacity for defining personal space relative to others, and increased capacity for attunement to others' movements following their exposure to DMT.

This study also revealed that although the object choice of participants' prevailing fantasy and the affective themes explored by participants varied during the 2-year period of the study, members' trust in the group and their self-esteem increased over the course of treatment. When participants rated the various functions served by the therapist during the 2 years, it was found that during the first year the therapist was more frequently perceived by participants as a provider of emotional containment and movement structure, while during the second year, the therapist was most frequently perceived as a provider of verbal interpretations. This finding is of clinical interest, because it appears that the perceived functions served by the therapist at different points in the groups' treatment followed the same developmental sequence generally adopted by a primary caregiver during the first 2 years of an infant's life. Additionally, the direction of expressive movement changes observed among participants during the course of treatment indicated a shift toward increased flow, expansiveness, and focus and more integrated, engrossed, spontaneous, and varied movement patterns.

Another process study, conducted on the same participants as the 2-year-long psychodynamic DMT group study cited above, examined the kinds of spatial patterns generated by group participants during four stages of the groups' treatment process (Dosamantes, 1992b). It provided evidence for the appearance of specific spatial patterns corresponding to different stages in the life of a group. Further, the study found that distinctive emotional states and psychodynamic spatial patterns appeared to prevail for each stage. The results of this study provide support for a view originally posited by Schilder (1950) that people continually and unconsciously physically shape and mold themselves in response to their social–emotional environment. When individuals feel open and receptive they tend to move toward others and to reduce or dissolve their body boundaries, whereas when they feel threatened, they retreat from others and shore up their body boundaries.

Two basic questions that are likely to receive greater attention from DMT researchers in the future include the following: (a) What kinds of research methodologies might be most appropriate for the study of creative body-movement–based psychotherapies such as DMT approaches? and (b) How are clinical methods developed by DMT practitioners in the United States applicable with clients from other cultures who possess different worldviews?

THERAPIST CHARACTERISTICS AND TRAINING

Graduate training programs in DMT generally require that applicants have a background in dance and psychology. At present, the training required to become a dance therapist entails the completion of a DMT master's degree or alternate training that complies with the graduate training guidelines established by the ADTA. This training consists of 2 years of academic coursework and includes a 700-hour clinical internship supervised by a qualified DMT supervisor. Following the completion of training, graduates may pursue credentialing from the ADTA.

There are several graduate programs located throughout the United States that offer DMT training. The training received by graduate students in these programs teaches them to observe, ethically intervene, and conduct research in DMT using methods appropriate to a creative body-movement–based practice that take into consideration clients' emotional developmental level and needs.

The possession of kinesthetic sensitivity and the capacity to accurately perceive somatic experience and movement dynamics, to become emotionally attuned to others, and to engage in improvisational body movement expression are all prerequisite characteristics for becoming an effective dance/movement therapist (Dosamantes-Alperson, 1981). Additional psychological characteristics that are likely to ensure a DMT practitioner's effectiveness include the capacity for self-insight, empathy, self-integration, the ability to contain intense emotions, and the ability to conceptualize the treatment process (Van Wagoner, Gelso, Hayes, & Diemer, 1991). These physical and psychological characteristics may be acquired through educational, studio, and clinical training, as well as through the therapist's own psychotherapeutic treatment.

For dance/movement therapists interested in conducting a PSY-DMT practice, additional training in psychoanalytic psychotherapy or psychoanalysis is essential. Although the ADTA does not require such specialized training for the generic practice of DMT, such training helps to ensure that clinicians receive in-depth clinical supervision working with difficult patients and undergo their own treatment—two features that will help them to work more effectively.

CONCLUSION

The clinical discipline of DMT can be viewed as a modern rediscovery and reconstruction of several integrative and transformative aspects of dance acknowledged by tribal communities long ago. In its modern incarnation, however, it has been transformed into a creative, body-movement–based psychotherapy that makes its central foci the integration of psyche and soma and the exploration of individuals' intersubjective and interpersonal worlds. Because the overwhelming majority of practitioners have been and continue to be women, DMT—as both a clinical discipline and a set of practices—also reflects and represents a distinctive kind of embodied female consciousness within the broader psychotherapeutic community.

PSY-DMT, a psychoanalytically informed type of DMT, focuses on clients' self-directed spontaneous movement, enactments, movement metaphors, imaged-action fantasies, and verbal insights derived from bodily felt experiencing. In this approach, the therapist serves a variety of functions: as a container for all client productions; as a transitional object for functions the client lacks at the outset of treatment; as an affectively attuned, empathic observer of the client's nonverbal and verbal expressions; and as an interpreter of the emotional meanings enacted and transacted within the evolving intersubjective relationship created between client and therapist throughout the treatment process. By working through the phases of the PSY-DMT process, adult clients with varying degrees of self-pathology begin to exhibit an increased capacity for symbolizing their bodily felt experience, regulating their affective states, and creating more benign identifications with others.

REFERENCES

Bartenieff, I. (1972). Dance therapy: A new profession or a rediscovery of an ancient role of dance? *Scope*, 7, 6–18.

Bunney, J. (1980). Dance therapy: An overview. In R. Gibson (Ed.), *The use of the creative arts in therapy* (pp. 24–26). Washington, DC: American Psychiatric Association.

Dosamantes, E. (1990). Movement and psychodynamic pattern changes in long-term dance/movement therapy groups. *American Journal of Dance Therapy, 12,* 27–44.

Dosamantes, I. (1992a). The intersubjective relationship between therapist and patient: A key to understanding denied and denigrated aspects of the patient's self. *The Arts in Psychotherapy Journal, 19,* 359–365.

Dosamantes, I. (1992b). Spatial patterns associated with the separation–individuation process in adult long-term psychodynamic movement therapy groups. *The Arts in Psychotherapy Journal, 19,* 3–11.

Dosamantes-Alperson, E. (1974). The creation of meaning through body movement. In A. I. Rabin (Ed.), *Clinical psychology: Issues of the seventies*. East Lansing, MI: Michigan State University Press.

Dosamantes-Alperson, E. (1981). *Dance therapy: Psychiatric manual*. Columbia, MD: American Dance Therapy Association, Commission on Psychiatric Therapies.

Dosamantes-Alperson, E. (1985–1986). A current perspective of imagery in psychoanalysis. *Imagination, Cognition and Personality,* 5(3), 199–209.

Dosamantes-Alperson, E. (1987). Transference and countertransference issues in movement psychotherapy. *The Arts in Psychotherapy Journal, 14,* 209–214.

Dosamantes-Alperson, E., & Merrill, N. (1980). Growth effects of experiential movement psychotherapy. *Psychotherapy: Theory, Research and Practice, 17,* 63–68.

Dosamantes-Beaudry, I. (1997a). Reconfiguring identity. *The Arts in Psychotherapy Journal, 24,* 51–57.

Dosamantes-Beaudry, I. (1997b). Somatic experience in psychoanalysis. *Psychoanalytic Psychology, 14*(4), 517–530.

Duggan, D., Bell, A., Orleans, F., Wexler, L., Bennett, R., & Greenberg, M. (1979). *Dance therapy.* Columbia, MD: American Dance Therapy Association.

Levy, F. J. (1988). *Dance/movement therapy: A healing art.* Reston, VA: American Alliance for Health, Physical Education, Recreation and Dance.

Ritter, M., & Low, K. G. (1996). Effects of dance/movement therapy: A meta-analysis. *The Arts in Psychotherapy Journal, 23,* 249–260.

Schilder, P. (1950). *The image and appearance of the human body.* New York: International Universities Press.

Stolorow, R. D., & Lachman, F. (1980). *Psychoanalysis of developmental arrests: Theory and treatment.* Madison, CT: International Universities Press.

Van Wagoner, S. L., Gelso, C. J., Hayes, J. A., & Diemer, R. A. (1991). Countertransference and the reputedly excellent therapist. *Psychotherapy: Theory, Research, Practice, and Training, 28,* 411–421.

Winnicott, D. (1965). *The maturational processes and the facilitating environment.* New York: International Universities Press.

ADDITIONAL RESOURCES

Journals

American Journal of Dance Therapy. New York: Human Sciences Press. National professional journal that publishes DMT articles.

The Arts in Psychotherapy Journal. New York: Elsevier Science. International, interdisciplinary professional journal that publishes articles featuring the creative arts therapies (art, dance, drama, music, and poetry).

Professional Association

American Dance Therapy Association
2000 Century Plaza, Suite 108
Columbia, Maryland 21044-3263

National professional DMT organization that disseminates information about the field. Also offers current list of training programs.

Training Programs

Professor Irma Dosamantes-Beaudry
UCLA
Graduate DMT Program

World Arts and Cultures Department
Box 951608
Los Angeles, CA 90095-1608

Graduate specialization, Dance As Healing and Therapy, featuring interdisciplinary cross-cultural perspective

A current list of additional training programs may be obtained by contacting the ADTA office.
(410) 997-4040 (telephone)
(410) 997-4048 (fax)
E-mail: info@ADTA.org
Web site: http://www.ADTA.org

13

MUSIC AS SYMBOLIC EXPRESSION: ANALYTICAL MUSIC THERAPY

BENEDIKTE B. SCHEIBY

Music therapy is a broad field with definitions and practices that vary according to whether one is considering a psychotherapeutic, rehabilitative, or medical treatment model. Although the concepts and methods used by analytically informed music therapists usually are modeled after the particular psychological theory with which the therapist identifies, other music therapists are more concerned with creating theory from the musical practice and do not rely on existing psychological rationales. Other factors determining practice are the specific population that the music therapy is directed toward and the cultural context. A general definition used in the United States is as follows: "Music therapy is the use of music in the accomplishment of therapeutic aims: the restoration, maintenance and improvement of mental and physical health" (National Association for Music Therapy, 1980, p. 1). I propose a more specific working definition:

> Music therapy is the systematic use of improvised or composed music as intervention in order to effect therapeutic change. Musical experiences and the musical relationship between client and music therapist are the main dynamic factors in the therapeutic process.

The following are the methods most commonly used in music psychotherapy: musical improvisation, music imaging, musical psychodrama, learning and performing music, songwriting, and song discussion. The most frequently used theories are psychodynamic, existential–humanistic, Gestalt, transpersonal, and cognitive–behavioral approaches.

DIFFERENCES BETWEEN MAJOR PROPONENTS IN THE USES OF ACTION METHODS WITHIN MUSIC THERAPY

Music therapists work from all of the existing psychotherapeutic orientations, including the various psychoanalytic perspectives, as well as the cognitive–behavioral, humanistic, and transpersonal belief systems. Those working in a behavioral vein use music "as a contingent reinforcement or stimulus cue to increase or modify adaptive behaviors and extinguish maladaptive behaviors" (Bruscia, 1989, p. 85). Music often is presented or withheld as an independent variable to influence dependent behaviors, especially in the special education setting. Music therapists working within a humanistic perspective often consider music a means of bypassing pathology or disability to access the individual's healthy, undamaged core. In addition, the potential of music to create a safe, nonthreatening therapeutic environment is emphasized, and theorists such as Carl Rogers and Abraham Maslow are frequently referenced. Humanistic music therapists also are concerned with the role of the music therapist in the community at large rather than in the purely institutional use of music therapy (Broucek, 1987). Those music therapists who work from a transpersonal perspective emphasize the power of music to effect changes in states of consciousness, create transcendent experiences, and generally stimulate processes of self-actualization. This is done through active music making and receptive music experiences such as embodied in the technique of guided imagery and music (Bonny & Savary, 1990). The work of theorists such as Roberto Assagioli, Abraham Maslow, and Ken Wilber often serves as the foundation for transpersonal music therapy approaches.

In this brief review, I emphasize the various psychoanalytic orientations within music therapy. Differences among clinicians result more from theoretical orientation and model of interpretation of the music than in their use of action methods. The different music therapy methods based on psychoanalytic thought make use of similar action methods, but the underlying theoretical frameworks and interpretation models vary.

At one end of the spectrum is the strictly Freudian-oriented music therapist who never actively plays together with the client but is an instrument for verbal interpretation and reflection of the client's musical expressions. This therapist can be a facilitator of the process up to the actual improvisation by identifying the issue, suggesting the appropriate action method, and leading the verbal processing and integration after the improvisation. The Freudian-oriented music therapist will make use of action methods, but only the client actually acts.

The Jungian-inspired analytical music therapist will sometimes actively participate in the improvisations and sometimes not, depending on the focus and intention of the improvisation. This type of therapist might focus more on musical gestalts and ways of expression that can be related to as musical archetypes, such as projections of the animus/anima or identification of the musical shadow or persona, while at the same time focusing on facilitating a musical individuation process. (See Austin, 1993, for an example of this type of work.)

The analytical music therapist who uses an object-relations approach will actively participate in the improvisations and during the action techniques focus on the client's developmental stage through the qualities of the client's music that reflect problems of symbiosis, separation, and rapprochement. This music therapist might focus on identifying in the music the client's developmental stage and use action methods in music that facilitate movement to the age-relevant stage. The music often will be understood and used as a transitional object. (See Dvorkin, 1991, for a clinical case study using an object-relations approach in music therapy.)

In Gestalt therapy–inspired work, the analytical music therapist most often will actively participate in the improvisations. The focus during the action techniques will be on the intrapersonal and interpersonal contact with the here and now, awareness, and energy during the improvisations. This includes work on musical relatedness to "the other" (that is, the other person[s] who are involved in the improvisational communication), instrument use, musical expressivity, and body language during the action technique. (See Stephens, 1983, for further information on this type of work.)

Some of the major theoretical orientations in music therapy are distinguished by whether the music is used *as* therapy or *in* therapy. In the former, music-as-therapy, music is used as the primary change agent and field for interaction; verbalization is not considered necessary for important and lasting changes to occur. In the latter, music-in-therapy, musical experiences are seen as one component of an approach that includes elements of traditional psychotherapies. Individual practitioners often draw from both perspectives, depending on what is clinically indicated. In both orientations, the experiential techniques of music therapy engage the client in issues through active involvement in various forms of musical activity rather than in purely verbal explorations. Through the musical action the client is engaged at a physical level, where body and mind act together, facilitating an integrated result closer to outer reality. There are relationship aspects as well; when accompanied by the music therapist's music, many clients express relief that they are not alone in the musical action process.

The level of intervention in music psychotherapy can be considered as falling into one of two primary categories: supportive music psychotherapy or insight music psychotherapy. In insight music psychotherapy, the primary goal is to facilitate insight into the client's conscious and unconscious lives to stimulate desired changes. The primary intent is to eliminate psychological disturbances and reconstruct the development of personality. Goals are either reconstructive (i.e., to discover unconscious determinants of the client's conflicts and make in-depth changes in the client's personality structure) or reeducative (i.e., to effect behavior change, environmental readjustment, goal modification, or self-actualization).

In supportive music psychotherapy, the primary goal is to facilitate emotional and physical growth based on support, maintenance, and building up of the ego. The music therapist helps the client to function better in daily life with no intent to alter the client's personality structure. Both types of work can be used in individual, couples, family, or group therapy settings. The following typical applications can be used in institutions or offered in private practice: short- and long-term programs in psychiatry and substance abuse; short- and long-term neurological rehabilitation; crisis intervention for clients experiencing trauma, acute illness, or loss; and work with incarcerated clients, nursing home residents, hospice patients, and personal encounter-workshop participants. Supportive music psychotherapy may also be used with functional clients who want to improve their life quality, enhance personal growth, and increase self-actualization.

ANALYTICAL MUSIC THERAPY

The focus of this chapter is a form of music psychotherapy that is used both as a supportive and an insight form: analytical music therapy (AMT). I was trained by AMT's founder, Mary Priestley, who developed it in Great Britain in the 1970s. According to Priestley (1994), AMT is "the analytically-informed symbolic use of improvised music by the music therapist and client. It is used as a creative tool with which to explore the client's inner life so as to provide the way forward for growth and greater self-knowledge" (p. 3).

AMT is considered one of the major approaches in the field of music therapy; its tenets and practices are taught in major graduate programs in music therapy. The term *analytical* refers, on one hand, to Priestley's inspiration from psychoanalysts such as Freud, Jung, Klein, and Adler, and on the other, to the client's verbal processing of musical improvisation to better integrate emotions, bodily awareness, and cognitive insights.

Since 1980, I have used AMT with individuals from the following populations: psychiatric inpatients; neurological rehabilitation clients; geriatric clients; victims of sexual, physical, or emotional abuse; and clients with eating disorders, substance abuse problems, and mental retardation. Clients who are not able to understand or use language do not profit as much as those who can verbalize their experiences in the improvisations, but they still can benefit from the approach and achieve therapeutic change.

The overall aim of AMT is to remove obstacles that prevent the client from realizing his or her full potential and from achieving specific personal goals through the active use and experience of music. The music therapist does not have specific goals for the client at the outset of the therapy process. In the foreground are the specific goals that the client expresses or develops through the emerging therapy process; it is then up to the music therapist and client to define objectives together that make reaching these goals possible. For clients who are nonverbal or who are very cognitively or physically impaired, the music therapist alone develops the goals and objectives for the client's musical actions and responses.

No prior musical skill or training is required of the client. The improvisations are performed vocally and on instruments that do not require any special skill or knowledge to play. These can include a variety of percussion instruments such as Chinese gongs, chromatic xylophones, metallophones, cymbals, different types and sizes of drums, maracas, shakers, rain sticks, claves, wood blocks, bells, and tambourines. Symphonic instruments that are more difficult to play are also available, such as piano, guitar, violin, cello, accordion, recorder, saxophone, and harp. For patients who are very limited physically, body suits are available that produce musical sounds that are triggered by client movement. In general, clients choose the instruments that they want to play and are encouraged in self-expression rather than in meeting any performance standards. The AMT format is either individual, dyadic, or group sessions. The ideal size for groups is four to eight members, including the music therapist. Individual and dyadic sessions generally last for 1 hour, whereas group sessions last 60 to 90 minutes.

The primary agents of therapeutic change in AMT are (a) the expressive qualities and structural components of music; (b) the musical relationship between the music therapist and the client; and (c) the action modality (i.e., the fact that the client is acting by singing, playing, or moving in the process of producing music).

Music rivals verbal language in its complexity and is well suited to conveying the subtleties and ambiguities of emotional expression. For readers not familiar with improvised music I list below aspects of the music that the music therapist uses with clinical intent: intensity, emotional content, melodic contour, rhythmic contour (i.e., Is the client able to keep a steady beat?), tonal/atonal language, sense of time, pauses, articulation, sudden changes or monotony, energy flow, patterns of tension and relaxation, wholeness and fragmentation, sense of form versus chaos, experimentation, spontaneity, spirituality, mood, antiphonal (dialogic) quality, timbre, polarities, choice of instrumental or vocal sound, developmental level (oral, anal, phallic, or genital music), repetition, flexibility, receptiveness, phrasing ability, sense of beginnings and endings, boundaries, symbiotic qualities, regressive qualities, musical scales, preferred idioms and styles, pitch, initiative, choice of instruments, and use of instruments. The music therapist also considers which images and feelings the client is getting in touch with by the improvisational action. The philosophy behind using music in this way is that the improvisational action reflects psychological, physical, spiritual, and cultural aspects of both the client's intrapersonal and interpersonal lives. Both process and content of the sessions are described in musical terms and in terms of psychoanalytic concepts, such as musical transference, musical countertransference, resistance, etc.

An important part of the method involves documenting the sessions through audio- or videotaping (with the client's consent). The client can listen to the playback of the session to explore its significance with the therapist's guidance. Compositions or songs can be worked on in the session; the recording also can be used to stimulate the creation of artwork or support expression through movement. After the session, the tape is reviewed by the therapist so that important events and expressions not observed during the session can be noted. The tapes are also used for supervision purposes.

TECHNIQUES

There are different categories of techniques that involve the client taking action in AMT. The most common ones are as follows: programmed or spontaneous regression, entering into somatic communication, free association, splitting, reality rehearsal, dreamwork, role-playing, ritual acts, guided imagery, myths, and holding. The following describes some of the action techniques used in the later case examples.

Programmed or Spontaneous Regression

The client is instructed to return, or perhaps returns spontaneously, in the music to a certain age in his or her life when unresolved conflicts, traumas, or other problematic events took place. He or she then has an opportunity to relive and resolve these problems in a safe, creative context. The music therapist helps to establish the "stage" musically and dramatically and provides musical support for emotional expression in the improvisation. Audiotaping can be used to reflect on the experience.

Entering Into Somatic Communication

When clients are dealing with psychosomatic symptoms, music can help uncover what the underlying emotion or emotions could be or reveal possible reasons for the physical manifestations. The client may improvise being the symptom (headache, stomachache, tic, etc.) while the music therapist reinforces, mirrors, or expresses musically the bypassed emotion or emotions. The client is encouraged to follow and express his or her free associations as they appear during the improvisation. Afterwards, the taped recording of the improvisation can be played back for verbal exploration.

Free Association

In this technique, the client improvises alone without title, focus, or specific intention and follows free associations, images, emotions, and physical actions as they emerge. The client is encouraged to vocalize while playing to keep the therapist aware of what is going on. The therapist can reinforce or mirror the client in his or her accompaniment, or he or she can simply be an active listener. This technique is often used when the client is not able to communicate verbally or to focus on a particular issue. It also can be used when the client is verbally defensive.

CLARIFICATION OF PLACE AND IMPORTANCE OF MUSICAL ACTION AND VERBAL ASPECTS OF ANALYTICAL MUSIC THERAPY

There are no rules about the order of musical or verbal aspects in music therapy. Some clients start talking, and through verbalization an issue is identified, whereupon a choice of relevant musical action is then decided. Aspects of the musical action often will be processed verbally after the end of the improvisation, but this does not always occur, because the music itself often has done the actual work. One musical action method can also lead to another one without verbal processing between them. Some clients start playing or singing right away, and it is not necessary to identify an issue verbally. Some clients improvise musically throughout the entire session, and, at times, verbalization is not necessary. Some clients may verbalize constantly, and the music therapist might accompany the client's words musically to try to help the client take musical action. Some clients neither verbalize nor play music or sing in the beginning of treatment (e.g., autistic children), and the music therapist may musically mirror the client's bodily expressions and movements or try to find a way to reach out musically or vocally. My position is that the diagnosis, goals, context, and individual characteristics determine which choices are made regarding musical action and verbalization.

SUPPORTIVE MUSIC PSYCHOTHERAPY

CASE EXAMPLE 1: SUPPORTIVE MUSIC PSYCHOTHERAPEUTIC APPROACH[1]

The music therapy group in this case example consists of four clients ranging in age from 42 to 92. They are all in a long-term care facility, have mild to severe dementia and depression, and have experienced a variety of neurological traumas.

W, an 83-year-old African-American man with severe glaucoma, is almost totally blind and has had a stroke that left him with impaired speech and little mobility in his legs. He has been singing in a church choir for 30 years and has some knowledge of music theory. J is a 42-year-old African-American man with severe brain damage caused by an accident that left him in a coma for 6 months. He has little mobility in his left leg but some in his right and has severe memory loss and cannot remember things from one moment to another. He was interested in listening to rock music before the accident. G is a 44-year-old African-American woman with severe tremors stemming from a stroke. She is without mobility in her legs and right arm and has a little mobility in her left hand. Her speech is severely impaired, and it takes a long time for her to form a word or sentence. She likes to sing and listen to music. M is a 92-year-old White female with severe senile dementia, paranoia, and behavioral problems. She sometimes talks excessively, at times hits and bites, has severe mood swings, and has reduced mobility in her legs. She likes to sing and listen to music.

This group has been receiving hour-long music therapy sessions three times weekly for 4 weeks. The main goals of the therapy are as follows: relieving depression, slowing the progress of dementia, and improving memory and life quality. At this point, M has been helped with her feelings of loneliness and sadness by two interventions that got her in touch with the fact that this is a group of her friends. The group had offered their support by singing "You've Got a Friend," replacing the original lyrics with their own words addressed to M. After the end of the song, I asked how the rest of the group members were feeling. Their answers seemed very short and superficial, and no one wanted to take further initiative. To help them take action and get more in touch with their emotions and memories

---

[1]This case example is part of a larger research project funded through the New York State Department of Health, Long-Term Care Dementia Program, 1997–1999, and Beth Abraham Health Services.

at this point, I used the action technique of free association by suggesting an improvisation theme: "What we see and feel right now."

J picks the jimbe (a big Senegalese drum) that he holds between his legs. This is a change from former sessions in which he was indifferent about choices of instruments. W is indifferent, so I offer him a bass drum for his left hand and the cymbal for his right hand. G asks for the Tibetan gong bowl, whereas M accepts a hand drum I offer her.

Case Narrative	*Commentary*
M starts rambling in an angry mood, shouting, "Get up!"	M gets in touch with the anger that is underlying her depression.
J has already started a rhythm on his jimbe, and the rest of the group is following. I support the rhythm on a floor tom-tom drum and with my voice.	J takes the initiative and moves out of his isolated position. The group shows cohesiveness by playing together in the same rhythm.
I encourage M to get her anger out in the music. She beats the hand drum energetically, shouting unintelligibly. The drumming reminds me of elders drumming in an African village as a part of their daily ritual.	
During the collective drumming, W starts talking about his memories of sitting in Central Park near a certain subway station when he was younger, listening to people drumming every Sunday.	W starts to reminisce and inspires the rest of the group to do the same.
M starts rambling again very loudly, and W says in an angry voice, "I do not understand one word of what she is saying."	W expresses anger for the first time. He usually is very polite, quiet, and introverted, with his head bent downwards. Now he looks straight at M.
I realize that the gong bowl is too difficult for G to play and give her a small shaker. I ask G which park she used to go to. She struggles with finding the words and finally says, "We used to go out to the park on the Fourth of July." The other group members try to help her with the words. I ask her where she used to live, and she answers right away,	G rarely says longer sentences, and the group often "forgets" about her existence. Now she gets the support of the group, and a "flirting" relationship initiated by J begins in this session.

"The Bronx." J says, "She lived in the Bronx. I used to live in Far Rockaway. I used to go to Flushing Meadow Park." M now mentions her park, Fordham Park, and suddenly gets very angry and begins talking very loudly and quickly.

Nobody understands what she is saying, and J says, "Slow down, M." M becomes increasingly out of control and tries to hit with her hand drum. I give her a tambourine instead and start improvising a gospel tune at the piano.

J takes over the leadership of the group for a while.

I sing, "We are all going to the park to get together and have some fun." M gets very engaged in the music; everybody seems to have found a common rhythm and to enjoy it.

I intervene and initiate a guided imagery to help the group stay focused on the subject.

After the end of the improvisation, M says, "We are all jokers." After this exchange of laughter and humorous sentences from each group member, we move on to another improvisation inspired by a remark from W: "We are all at the end of the subway."

The music seems to elicit humor from the group members, an important resource for persons who are depressed and have a poor quality of life.

As a result of this session, the following positive outcomes emerged: (a) M and W got in touch with their repressed anger, the alleviation of which provided some relief for their depression; (b) M, J, G, and W were all able to use and exercise aspects of those memory functions that remained intact; (c) G improved her ability to speak; (d) all got in touch with their sense of humor and became less isolated than in former sessions; and (e) interpersonal communication skills improved for W, J, and G. The whole group was working on the issue of being out of control, a major issue for this population. In this session, they achieved the feeling of being in control of their own lives and got a sense of what they could do to obtain this sense of control. This was accomplished by playing instruments and using the music to facilitate interaction with each other, exchanging emotions (e.g., anger, humor, caring, and affection), and taking initiative and leadership roles.

This action technique can be used with any group of clients who are depressed, isolated, physically impaired, or having intra- or interpersonal communication problems. It can be used with adults as well as children in any beginning music therapeutic treatment. This intervention is contraindicated for clients who are psychotic or hallucinating. Other action techniques could have been used, such as (a) every group member picking out a song that is significant for him or her concerning the issue of being lonely and the whole group singing those songs and then processing them verbally, or (b) each group member reaching out musically or vocally to another person in the group and experiencing the emotional and physical effects of doing so.

INSIGHT MUSIC PSYCHOTHERAPY

For clients who have experienced physical, emotional, or sexual abuse, individual AMT can offer a safe place for them to relive emotions attached to the trauma, rebuild self-esteem, and regain the feeling of being in control. Undesired or repressed material that spontaneously comes to the surface by improvising together often is perceived as not as threatening as when it is expressed verbally, primarily because the client has the option of taking action regarding the difficult material and is not relegated to a passive stance. The idea of music therapy in this work is to relive aspects of the trauma through the action form of the music, doing so in a safe context in the presence of a witness, who also may act with the client. Some clients who have been victims of abuse are not able to articulate or consciously symbolize what went on during the abuse. Therefore, the music can serve as an expressive tool in the reparation process to contain and maintain the material in musical form until the client is ready to verbalize its nature. As clients quite often have somatic reactions and sensations that originate in their traumatic experiences, these can be explored through the action methods mentioned previously.

A variety of action methods have been found to be extremely helpful in this work:

- *Entering into somatic communication.* See Case Example 2.
- *Role-playing.* In working with victims of trauma, a very important part of treatment is to let the client reenact, reexperience, and address the emotions behind some of the relational positions—the sadistic abuser; the helpless, impotently enraged victim; the unseeing, uninvolved parent; the unseen, neglected child; the seducer; the seduced; the idealized, omnipotent rescuer; and the entitled child—that the client might have internalized during or after the trauma and that always come up in the improvisations, unconsciously or consciously. Improvised music is an excellent tool for this purpose.

- *Programmed or spontaneous regression.* The client is instructed to return, or perhaps returns spontaneously in the music to a certain age in his or her life where unresolved conflicts, traumas, or other problematic events took place, and then has an opportunity to relive and resolve these problems in a safe, creative context. The music therapist helps to establish the "stage" musically and dramatically, and provides the musical support for the emotional expression in the improvisation. The audiotape can be used to reflect on the experience.
- *Free association.* This process can be used when the client is not able to communicate at a verbal level. Repressed material often will come to the surface during the improvisation. Encouraging clients to vocalize during music making often opens up their ability to speak the previously unspeakable.
- *Splitting.* This process can be very helpful when the work is about resolving the different splits and polarities that the client experiences as a result of the trauma. The music therapist can facilitate improvisations that reinforce bridges and integrative possibilities. For example, if a client is working on issues regarding his or her mother, the therapist can offer to play the mother musically while the client plays himself or herself. The client also can choose to play the important individual with whom current issues are focused on while the therapist plays the client.
- *Dreamwork.* If the client can remember dreams, a musical dramatization of them in different variations can help the client verbalize and understand difficult material.

CASE EXAMPLE 2: AN ADVANCED METHOD—ENTERING INTO SOMATIC COMMUNICATION

Kate, a 38-year-old woman with a history of sexual and emotional abuse, is also a recovering alcoholic. Her mother died when Kate was 14 years old; her father, an alcoholic who suffered from depression, is still alive. She has two sisters and one foster brother. Kate had been sexually and emotionally abused by her foster brother, a female teacher, and several men with whom she had been involved. She has been married unhappily for 4 years and intermittently works part time. Kate uses music and art at an amateur level at home as healing media. In the initial client assessment, she expressed the primary goals of becoming more assertive, more skilled in improvising on the piano, and more emotionally stable and of working on issues around her sexual identity. The following case example represents about 30 minutes of a music therapy session that took place within the first 2 months of a 3-year course of therapy.

Case Narrative	Commentary
Kate brings up verbally an overwhelming number of issues in a brief time. In chronological order, they are as follows: (1) feeling in control and being assertive versus caving in and being ashamed; (2) not wanting to be touched by anybody; (3) a dream that stirred up questions about her sexual identity and caused her to wonder if she were gay; (4) a physical pain in her vagina; (5) considering confronting her foster brother, who had sexually abused her; (6) confronting denial from a parent; (7) anger; and (8) the pain in her vagina again.	An overwhelming amount of material is brought up in a short time, which is characteristic of victims of trauma. They often feel like they are being flooded with feelings and have difficulties in focusing. Listening to Kate, I feel myself flooded by potential material for musical improvisation (traumatic countertransference). To stop the flooding and to concentrate on the physical pain, which is very concrete, and to help Kate to a place where she can take action and deal with the issues that are causing her pain. . . .
Therapist: How about making an improvisation titled "The Pain in My Vagina"? I will support you in the music in whatever comes up. See if you can allow yourself to share that pain with me in the music. You can choose whatever instrument you feel like playing.	I make use of the action technique "entering somatic communication." Another choice could have been free association, with the improvisation theme: "My feelings right now."
Kate: I think I would like to play the cello.	Kate's experiences illustrate common phenomena for these clients: (a) somatic pain related to the trauma; (b) feeling flooded by feelings, ideas, and associations; (c) feeling out of control; (d) being manipulative in relationships; (e) acting out the role of the abuser in intimate relationships; (f) seductive behavior; (g) lability; and (h) having the ability to verbalize but not acting.
Therapist: I will be responsible for the time keeping, and I will leave some time for talking after the improvisation so that we may talk about it.	
Kate: OK.	
Therapist: It is OK to stop in the improvisation if you don't feel like going on or if you feel like changing instruments or something like that.	
[Kate starts plucking the strings on the cello.]	
Kate [laughing]: I have never really done this.	

Therapist: So it is a real challenge.

[I start playing the accordion along with Kate.]

The sounds that Kate makes are explorative as she experiments with the various tones that the cello can produce.

Her body language holding the cello, her laughter, and the cello sounds are similar to a young, shy child holding and examining a new toy and its sounds.

As I listen to her music, I introduce a dissonant cluster to reflect the pain aspect of the improvisation's title. Kate immediately plays dissonant sounds with the bow on the cello strings, hitting them very hard. I add tremolos in the interval of a minor second, and Kate starts playing tremolos on the strings.

At the same time, she makes guttural sounds like a person who is beginning to vomit and then begins to cough uncontrollably. Her movements and body language indicate that Kate is undergoing a regression. I dampen my dissonances into a pianissimo (soft) dynamic. The cough-

I chose the accordion for a variety of reasons: (a) Because Kate chose to play the cello, I wanted to use an instrument that clearly contrasted in form and sound to hers to create an experience of autonomy for her. (b) I wanted to be able to move around in the room and to turn my back to Kate in case it became too threatening for her to look at me face to face. (c) With the accordion I could play melody, rhythm, and harmony at the same time in all possible dynamics, which might be needed in the situation. (d) The accordion is held close to the body, as is the cello, reflecting Kate's relationship to her instrument.

The action technique stimulated a spontaneous regression that I choose to support.

It sounds like a drama is starting to unfold. It seems to reflect aspects of abuse in the form of the dissonances, the hitting on the strings, the tremolos, and the fast tempo, reflecting musical transference, which is defined as follows: "Transferential music is discovered by hearing sound patterns that reflect the client's reexperiences and reenactings of unfinished gestalts from previous relationships or distortions of experiences of the present" (Scheiby, 1997, p. 187).

When Kate starts coughing very hard and suddenly changes her musical expression to appealing glissandi, my internal images evoked by the music are of somebody getting raped and somebody trying to seduce. The evoked images and connected feelings can be identified as musical

ing stops suddenly, and Kate changes her musical expression into very appealing ascending and descending vocal glissandi (slides).

countertransference: "Countertransferential music can have the following characteristics: It can be music that does not seem to belong in the musical context at that moment; music that does not seem to be appropriate from the therapist's perspective; musical expressions from the therapist that surprise him/herself; a sense of not knowing where the music comes from" (Scheiby, 1997, p. 187).

The music seems to reflect a reenactment of the relational positions of the seducer and the seduced.

I accompany Kate's vocal glissandi with music that reflects the anxiety, anger, confusion, and drama that emanate from Kate's music and that are also released through my countertransference. I am feeling as if my music has become a part of Kate's music, so it is hard to distinguish who is playing what. Musically, this is expressed by my tremolo clusters with fluctuating tonality and unstable rhythms in a forte dynamic. The music seems to reflect the relational position of the helpless, impotently enraged victim.

Kate reinforces her vocal glissandi with cello glissandi. Then she takes over the therapist's tremoli, shaking the bow on the strings of the cello. The music ends in a loud confrontation between the cello and the accordion, after which the music slowly dies out.

I am not sure if the improvisation has ended or if there is more to come. This ending seems very inorganic.

Kate starts making guttural sounds again as if she needs to vomit. At the same time, she hits the cello strings very violently with the bow. I play dissonant tones firmly on the accordion. Kate suddenly changes the mood back again to inviting vocal

My musical contribution reflected my countertransference, as I have images of being in a physical fight, with the cello and the accordion engaged in a loud, noisy conflict. I mirror Kate vocally with my own voice and offer musical support on the accordion.

glissandi. This expression turns gradually into heavy loud coughing that sounds like that before vomiting. Kate stops coughing and ends the improvisation.

The musically induced association at that point is the image of a person getting an object forced down the throat. I sense the musical presence of a fourth position, that of a sadistic abuser. I end the improvisation by holding supportive accords in a soft dynamic.

There was a long pause. I then suggested that we play a song to the child inside Kate who has been exposed to that pain. "Sing a song to that child or make some music that this child needs," I said, using the splitting technique to access and address the needs of Kate's child part. This intervention provided a safe, musical structure and holding or a "musical mother." Kate improvised a song vocally and accompanied herself at the piano. The song was addressed to the abused child in her. I accompanied with my voice and the accordion. Kate looked very content and smiled. When I asked her afterwards how it was to play and sing the two different improvisations, she said, "It was good. It was. . . . I feel self-conscious, like I am being judged. And I feel like, when I was playing the cello, in some ways I didn't have that in the feelings, because I didn't play it before. And then I worried about, when I started hitting it, whether I would hurt it, you know, or hurt the bow. And I sort of liked doing it, sort of, and some of it was like P [a female teacher who had also sexually abused Kate for several years in her teens]. But it was like—she used to always perform for me—like I was supposed to be her audience and everything [P was a cello teacher]. So it was nice for me to play instead of her." I responded, "Like you were the soloist?" Kate then replied, "Yeah. So that was great—and with this I just felt like playing the fifths (on the piano), because they are very safe, and then I just felt. . . . I don't know—I just like the way they sound and . . . it is hard to sing because I feel so emotional, but that was great—that felt safe and to hear my own voice sing. I felt in control."

As Kate's physical symptoms slowly disappeared, she divorced her husband, moved to her own apartment, began to look into more gratifying job possibilities, and resumed piano and organ lessons with the goal of becoming an organist. Listening to and playing music became a major interest, a tool to explore her spiritual life and resources, and a source of joy and creativity. This example of an action technique can be used in any individual music therapy session in which the client is an adult victim of abuse. The typical sequence resulting from this intervention is well illustrated: The cause of the physical symptoms is revealed, the client begins to feel safe and in control, the client works through some of the relational positions that were activated through the abuse, and the client takes action instead of being passive. In the longer run, the physical symptoms disappear and the client becomes stabilized and takes charge of his or her life. The music therapist must have established a trusting relationship with the client, and the client has to be ready to face and possibly relive the trauma in a safe environment.

RESISTANCE

There are two forms of resistance common in this type of therapy. The first is resistance toward playing instruments or vocalizing. Playing music together often is perceived as being extremely intimate and revealing, so a frequent reaction in the beginning of the therapeutic relationship is rejection, often voiced in the following ways: "I am not musical," "I never played an instrument," "My voice sounds terrible," or "I am afraid of my emotions." In some instances, to overcome the resistance, the therapist can start improvising or singing for the client or to the client. Another approach is to ask the client to bring in recorded music that has special meaning and value. The therapist and client can listen to the music and start the musical relationship that way. Slowly, the client may become motivated to move into action.

The second form is resistance observed within the client's musical expression. Resistance manifested in the musical action can be expressed in many ways: (a) The client expresses his or her emotions freely in the improvisation, but when he or she is verbalizing about the music, he or she blocks intellectually and cannot connect feelings expressed in the music with thoughts. (b) There is repetitiveness in the music (repetition of motifs, rhythms, melodies, tones, harmonies, dynamic, or lyrics). (c) The client is very inactive in the musical process. (d) There is a lack of affect in the music. (e) There is a contradiction between the musical affect and the affect that the client is talking about. (f) The client has a tendency to stop playing or singing abruptly and prematurely. (g) The client repeatedly refuses to begin the improvisation. (h) The client repeatedly refuses to choose certain instruments. (i) The tempo in the client's music is colored by extremes; either the client is racing through the improvisation or playing extremely slowly. (j) The client refuses to participate in the process of developing an action technique that could be helpful. (k) The client refuses to create a title for the improvisation.

When the therapist becomes aware of resistance, he or she should initially respect it and encourage its expression because it is present for a good reason. The timing for challenging client resistance cannot be generalized; it depends on each individual treatment process and client response. If the time has arrived to confront the resistance, there are different ways that this can be done. First, it can be very helpful to listen to an audio recording of the improvisation in the session. Bits and pieces can be pointed out; sometimes the client can be encouraged to move physically to his or her music to lessen the possibility of dissociation. Another approach is to ask the client to take the music just played one step further. The therapist can also suggest that the client repeat the musical experience in the hope that a deepening of awareness will occur. The therapist can also suggest ways to alter the tempo, rhythm, dynamic, form, harmonics, melody, and articulation. If the client has been playing alone, the therapist can offer to play together with the client and intervene musically where insights or changes need to happen. (For further reading on this subject, see Austin & Dvorkin, 1993.)

THERAPEUTIC VALUE OF SUCCESSIVE USES

Clients who repeatedly experience how it feels to take action, to be in touch with emotions connected to action, and to sing or speak out loud words that usually would get stuck in the throat survive and feel better just by becoming physically and vocally active. The benefits of a lengthier course of music therapy are numerous. Clients show improvement in various aspects of the personality, including enhanced playfulness, flexibility, spontaneity, and emotional expressivity. They also demonstrate enhanced capacities for enduring positive change, frequently seen in a willingness to move between reflection and action and between past and present and a willingness to take risks and experiment with and explore alternate behaviors and solutions to problems. A lessening of overly rigid inner controls is often demonstrated by an increased ability to regenerate the sense of a natural flow in processes. AMT is also useful in helping clients differentiate between self and other (through listening to another person's musical response), be more able to live completely in the moment (making the sound that fits to the action), and experience an interpersonal relationship through musical interaction with the therapist.

Sometimes homework is recommended to further facilitate the treatment process. The audiotaped music produced in a session often can be used by the client outside the session to serve a variety of functions: increase relaxation (reduce sleeping problems and stress); reduce pain; send a nonverbal message to a partner, family member, or friend; encourage and support the client in transferring to reality what was experienced in the session; or serve as accompaniment for art, poetry, or movement expression. Homework also can consist of practicing playing a certain instrument, singing certain songs, or composing or listening to specific music relating to issues being addressed in therapy.

EMPIRICAL SUPPORT

Outcomes studies on the efficacy of various music therapy approaches have been undertaken by university faculty and published in referred journals such as the *Journal of Music Therapy*, *Music Therapy Perspectives*, *Music Therapy*, *Musiktherapeutische Umschau*, and *The Arts in Psychotherapy* (see also Langenberg, Frommer, & Tress, 1993, 1995; Nygaard-Pedersen & Scheiby, 1988). Although the situation is changing in the United States as music therapy moves to increasing emphasis on graduate education and advanced credentials, clinical specializations such as AMT have not been part of academic training so much as a topic for institute training in nonacademic programs. As a result, this particular approach has not been researched extensively in either North America or Great Britain, two areas where the clinical approach has been applied. In Germany, however, there has been ongoing qualitative research (Langenberg, 1988; Langenberg, Frommer, & Langenbach, 1996; Langenberg, Frommer, & Tress, 1992, 1993, 1995) on one of the theoretical foundations of AMT: the resonator function—that is, the "personal instrument of relating and understanding by which the therapist resonates to the latent content of the music, which allows it to become conscious and serve as an inspiration for clinical interventions" (Langenberg et al., 1993, p. 61). In the research, a clinical excerpt was played for and analyzed by a panel of psychologists and psychiatrists who were given instructions to report the content of images and feelings evoked by the music as well as the qualities of the music itself. The therapist and client performed their own listening subsequent to the session, and their accounts were also recorded. All of the accounts were analyzed for the presence of common themes and clinical motifs. The motifs resulting from the qualitative analysis were then compared to the case material to determine if the salient aspects of treatment could be discerned by a panel who had access to the music from the sessions but none of the case material. The overall focus was to evaluate both the degree to which improvised music can express important clinical material and the capacity of the therapist to discern the nature of this material.

In general, the research showed that there were commonalities in the reactions of the research panel and that these commonalities clearly related to the clinical issues being addressed through the music. The researchers claim that they "have found a valid instrument for the research of processes in music therapy" (Langenberg et al., 1993, p. 83). They believe that their methodological design shows how to perform comparative analyses of different treatment theories and is a way of detecting the personal influences of specific therapists on the clinical processes.

TRAINING AND QUALIFICATION REQUIREMENTS

To be able to work successfully with AMT as an action method and treatment modality, a therapist needs a master's degree in music therapy plus specific postgraduate training in AMT, including individual and group music therapy self-experience, AMT clinical supervision, and a theoretical understanding of the basics of the method. It is recommended that the clinically active music therapist receive weekly supervision by a trained AMT supervisor.

There are close to 80 music therapy programs in American universities offering BA, MA, and doctoral training. Information on these programs is available from the AMTA. At the present, AMT can be studied in graduate music therapy programs in Denmark (Aalborg University) and in Germany (Hamburg). None of the American programs presently offer this specialized training.

A large inventory of entry-level and advanced competencies serve as the basis for the approval of university music therapy degree programs (Bruscia, 1986; Bruscia, Hesser, & Boxill, 1981). Certain of these skills (as well as other personality attributes) have relatively more importance in AMT practice: improvisational skills on a variety of musical instruments; comfort with one's voice used as an instrument; the ability to spontaneously compose music and songs; intermediate-level competency on one major instrument; and the ability to be a good listener and observer of musical and verbal expressions. It is necessary that the music therapist possess the psychological and therapeutic expertise to integrate therapeutic objectives into musical interaction. It also helps that the therapist be a bit of an actor and have an extensive musical repertoire.

Typical AMT supervision, either individual or group, focuses on processing issues of countertransference, transference, resistance, projective identification, and parallel process as they occur in the musical actions of the client and the music therapist. Such processing is done mostly through music. Often, the supervisee brings in audiotaped examples from clinical sessions; the supervision session itself is usually audiotaped. (For readings on music therapy supervision see Scheiby & Montello, 1994; for readings on music therapy education see Nygaard-Pedersen & Scheiby, 1988, and Scheiby, 1991.)

CONCLUSION

As demonstrated in the case examples, AMT can provide a variety of nonverbal expressive techniques, which facilitates intrapersonal and interpersonal communication, clarification, and integration between emotional and cognitive content generated in sessions. The music moves behind the defenses and elicits a dialog between the conscious and the unconscious. It also serves as a vehicle that can bring the client to unexpected places and insights, which aid in the process of healing. Repressed emotions are expressed through sound, and the inner music of the client starts playing by itself. Conscious use of the concepts of musical transference, musical countertransference, and musical resistance emphasizes the analytical part of the approach. AMT can be applied to a broad variety of populations and is specifically indicated whenever clients are having difficulties in verbalizing.

REFERENCES

Austin, D. S. (1993). Projection of parts of the self onto music and musical instruments. In G. M. Rolla (Ed.), *Your inner music*. Wilmette, IL: Chiron.

Austin, D. S., & Dvorkin, J. M. (1993). Resistance in individual music therapy. *The Arts in Psychotherapy, 20,* 423–429.

Bonny, H. L., & Savary, L. M. (1990). *Music and your mind: Listening with a new consciousness*. Barrytown, NY: Station Hill Press.

Broucek, M. (1987). Beyond healing to "whole-ing": A voice for the deinstitutionalization of music therapy. *Music Therapy, 6*(2), 50–58.

Bruscia, K. E. (1986). Advanced competencies in music therapy. *Music Therapy, 6A,* 57–67.

Bruscia, K. E. (1989). *Defining music therapy*. Spring City, PA: Spring House Books.

Bruscia, K. E., Hesser, B., & Boxill, E. (1981). Essential competencies for the practice of music therapy. *Music Therapy, 1*(1), 43–49.

Dvorkin, J. M. (1991). Individual music therapy for an adolescent with borderline personality disorder. An object relations approach. In K. E. Bruscia (Ed.), *Case studies in music therapy*. Phoenixville, PA: Barcelona.

Langenberg, M. (1988). *Vom Handeln zum Behandeln: Darstellung besonderer Merkmale der musiktherapeutischen Behandlungssituation im Zusammenhang mit der freien Improvisation* (From action to treatment: Description of specific characteristics of the music therapeutic treatment situation in the context of free improvisation). Stuttgart, Germany: Fischer.

Langenberg, M., Frommer, J., & Langenbach, M. (1996). Fusion and separation: Experiencing opposites in music, music therapy, and music therapy research. In M. Langenberg, K. Aigen, & J. Frommer (Eds.), *Qualitative music therapy research: Beginning dialogues*. Phoenixville, PA: Barcelona.

Langenberg, M., Frommer, J., & Tress, W. (1992). Qualitative Methodik zur Beschreibung und Interpretation musiktherapeutischer Behandlungswerke (A qualitative method to describe and interpret music therapy works of treatment). *Musiktherapeutische Umschau, 4,* 258–278.

Langenberg, M., Frommer, J., & Tress, W. (1993). A qualitative research approach to analytical music therapy. *Music Therapy, 12*(1), 59–84.

Langenberg, M., Frommer, J., & Tress, W. (1995). From isolation to bonding: A music therapy case study of a patient with chronic migraines. *The Arts in Psychotherapy, 22,* 87–101.

National Association for Music Therapy. (1980). *A career in music therapy* [Brochure]. Washington, DC: Author.

Nygaard-Pedersen, I., & Scheiby, B. B. (1988). Intermusiktherapie innerhalb der Ausbildung (Intertherapy integrated in education). *Musiktherapeutische Umschau, 9,* 140–162.

Priestley, M. (1994). *Essays on analytical music therapy.* Phoenixville, PA: Barcelona.

Scheiby, B. B. (1991). Mia's fourteenth—The symphony of fate: Psychodynamic improvisation therapy with a music therapy student in training. In K. E. Bruscia (Ed.), *Case studies in music therapy.* Phoenixville, PA: Barcelona.

Scheiby, B. B. (1997). Listen to the music of the unconscious: Using countertransference as a compass in analytical music therapy. In A. Robbins (Ed.), *Therapeutic presence.* Bristol, PA: Jessica Kingsley.

Scheiby, B. B., & Montello, L. (1994). Introduction to psychodynamic peer supervision in music therapy. In Connections: Integrating our work and play. *Proceedings of the Annual Conference of the American Association for Music Therapy.*

Stephens, G. (1983). The use of improvisation in developing relatedness in the adult client. *Music Therapy, 3*(1), 29–42.

ADDITIONAL RESOURCES

Books

Bruscia, K. E. (1987). *Improvisational models of music therapy.* Springfield, IL: Charles C Thomas. Includes a detailed description and analysis of AMT.

Bruscia, K. E. (Ed.). (1991). *Case studies in music therapy.* Phoenixville, PA: Barcelona. Gives thorough definitions and descriptions of major music therapy approaches, clarifies key concepts in the discipline of music therapy, describes the variety of the field, and explains how different populations are worked with in different methods.

Bruscia, K. E. (Ed.). (1998). *The dynamics of music psychotherapy.* Gilsum, NH: Barcelona.

Priestley, M. (1975). *Music therapy in action.* London: Constable.

Scheiby, B. B. (1995). Death and rebirth experiences in music and music therapy. In Carolyn B. Kenny (Ed.), *Listening, playing, creating: Essays on the power of sound.* Albany: State University of New York Press.

Wheeler, B. L. (1995). *Music therapy research. Quantitative and qualitative perspectives.* Philadelphia, PA: Barcelona.

Journals

The Arts in Psychotherapy. New York: Elsevier Science.

British Journal of Music Therapy. Middlesex, England: Adept Press. The journal of the British Association for Music Therapy.

Journal of Music Therapy. Silver Spring MD: American Music Therapy Association. Previously published by the National Association for Music Therapy.

Music Therapy (the journal of the American Association for Music Therapy). Ceased publication with volume 14 in 1996.

Music Therapy Perspectives. Silver Spring, MD: American Music Therapy Association. Previously published by the National Association for Music Therapy.

Professional Associations and Organizations

American Music Therapy Association
8455 Colesville Road, Suite 1000
Silver Spring, MD 20910
(301) 589-3300 (telephone)
(301) 589-5175 (fax)
E-mail: info@musictherapy.org

Created in 1998 with the unification of the American Association for Music Therapy and the National Association for Music Therapy. Publishes Journal of Music Therapy and Music Therapy Perspectives. Offers the following membership categories: professional (those engaged in the professional use of music therapy, including music therapists, physicians, psychologists, administrators, educators, allied health professionals, and others), associate, student, retired professional, inactive music therapist, affiliate, and honorary life.

British Society for Music Therapy
25 Rosslyn Avenue
East Barnet
Herts England EN4 8DH

Publishes British Journal of Music Therapy.

APPENDIX

SUMMARY OF ACTION
METHODS PRESENTED

The information in this appendix was compiled from the chapters and has been supplemented by additional information from the chapter authors. The columns (with explanation where needed) are as follows:

1. Name of action method
2. Name of therapy using this action method
3. Chapter
4. Main purpose
5. Therapy modality in which action method is useful (presented in order of most to least useful):
   - I = Individual
   - G = Group
   - C = Couple
   - F = Family

Note: These action methods should not be viewed as technologies to be replicated. Successful use of action methods requires mature clinical judgment and sensitivity regarding particular clients and circumstances.

6. Training needed (uses an 8-point rating scale to represent the minimum level of preparation needed by a hypothetically average therapist, without prior specialty training in the method, to use it ethically and effectively):

    1 = Reading the chapter (or other source) description of the action method only

    2 = Seeing the action method demonstrated by a knowledgeable therapist

    3 = Having experienced the action method as a client or in a training simulation

    4 = Having previously used the action method once under the supervision of a knowledgeable therapist

    5 = Completing a 1/2- to 2-day specialized workshop in the action method

    6 = Completing a 4- to 8-week specialized course in the action method

    7 = Completing a 1-year specialized training program in the action method

    8 = Completing a specialized training program in the action method lasting more than 1 year

(Note that a number of authors point out that fuller use of their action methods requires more extensive training.)

7. Populations the action method is best used with
8. Prerequisite conditions for successful use of the action method
9. Contraindications and cautions

Name of action method	Name of therapy	Chapter	Main purpose	Modality	Training needed	Populations action method best used with	Prerequisite conditions for successful use of action method	Contraindications and cautions
Experimenting with locating feelings in the body and working with what emerges	Gestalt therapy	1	Foster emergence of authentic being through contact	I, G, C, F	8	Particularly effective with highly intellectualized persons with limited access to feelings	Client's body sense must be activated and therapist must be able to perceive depth and reality of clients' and own experiences.	Method is perceived as interruption of therapist–client contact.
Empty-chair work	Gestalt therapy	1	Create and externalize experience of person or object	I, G, C, F,	8	Works best with imaginative, expressive clients	Client should be willing to attempt it without pressure.	Extreme self-consciousness or too little sense of self
Simple use of self-esteem tool kit	Satir system	2	Move about terrain of self-esteem	I, G, C, F	5	Any individual, couple, family, or group sufficiently present for contact and new input regarding themselves, others, and their immediate context	Solid therapeutic alliance between client and therapist	(1) Client is unable to understand intended benefits of activity. (2) Some part of client system is unable to focus on process.
Complex use of self-esteem tool kit	Satir system	2	Move about terrain of self-esteem	G, C, F	7	Those who appreciate importance of family of origin as central to coping strategies and who are willing to enter domain of woundedness in group context	Therapeutic alliance with client, high level of safety and support between and among group members, sufficient time for immersive experience and full debriefing for role-players and observers	(1) Clients have no support to sustain changes. (2) Clients have not progressed in recovery from addictions or sexual abuse.
Out-of-session enactment of ritual	Therapeutic rituals	3	Help transition out of therapy as clients tap into own resources	I, G, C, F	5	Any	Therapist's own comfort and energy level	Symbols are not meaningful or metaphorical.

Appendix continues

Name of action method	Name of therapy	Chapter	Main purpose	Modality	Training needed	Populations action method best used with	Prerequisite conditions for successful use of action method	Contraindications and cautions
Action metaphor	Boundary sculptures	4	Explore personal and interpersonal boundaries	I, G, C, F	2, 5	All	Some practice and ease of the therapist in moving or using props; offering disclaimers that this could be "off the wall" or offer new information	Prior heightened vulnerability of client, which can be lessened by substituting rope sculpture for positioning of persons
Action metaphor	Rope sculpting and diagramming	4	Explore and assess interpersonal boundaries and connections between persons	I, G, C, F	1	All	Some practice and ease of the therapist in moving or using props; offering disclaimers that this could be "off the wall" or offer new information	Prior heightened vulnerability of client, which can be lessened by substituting rope diagramming for rope sculpting
Self-sculptures	Drama therapy	5	(1) Facilitate self-examination (2) Help clients achieve clarity and mastery	I, G, C, F	6	Mid- to high-functioning clients capable of insight and tolerant of emotional connectedness to internal worlds	(1) Established level of trust between group members and toward the therapist (2) Receptivity to deeper level of work (3) Established ease with dramatic processes and role-playing	Do not progress to later stages if client seems overwhelmed by initial witnessing of his or her sculpture.
Line repetition	Drama therapy	5	Free expression and containment of emotion	I, G, C, F	3	Any	Relevant physical warm-up and establishment of playful, expressive environment	Careful oversight when dealing with emotionally volatile clients

Technique				Purpose	Population	Requirements	Cautions
Parts of self empty-chair technique	6	I, G, C, F	5	Concretize and clarify internalized conflicts	Any person beyond the preteen years, but better for those somewhat cognitively intact (i.e., not significantly demented, delirious, or acutely psychotic)	(1) Assessment of clients' ability and readiness to explore problem systematically (2) Rationale, orientation, and warm-up (3) Formal operational reasoning (late preteen years on, or about minimum of 14-year-old level of intelligence)	Cognitive disarray, as awareness of who is in which role is needed
Intrapsychic action sociometry; presenting the inner world	6	I, G, C, F	6	(1) Externalize feelings to circumvent denial or minimization (2) Increase group cohesiveness (3) Warm up other group members to resonating issue in own lives	Any person beyond the preteen years, but better for those somewhat cognitively intact (i.e., not significantly demented, delirious, or acutely psychotic)	(1) Assessment of clients' ability and readiness to explore problem systematically (2) Rationale, orientation, and warm-up (3) Formal operational reasoning (late preteen years on, or about minimum of 14-year-old level of intelligence) (Empty-chair work is somewhat easier to use and keep track of who's who than multiple parts of self.)	Cognitive disarray, as awareness of who is in which role is needed
Single doubling	7	G	3	Reinforce behaviors selectively to strengthen therapeutic group processes	Clients with mental retardation, chronic psychiatric disabilities, or dual diagnosis of both	Therapist's familiarity with population and experience in conducting group psychotherapy	(1) Do not stand behind paranoid clients. (2) Do not use with issues of death and grieving unless therapist has specific training in managing these issues in group settings.

Appendix continues

Name of action method	Name of therapy	Chapter	Main purpose	Modality	Training needed	Populations action method best used with	Prerequisite conditions for successful use of action method	Contraindications and cautions
Multiple doubling	Interactive-behavioral therapy	7	(1) Enhance group feelings of support (2) Evoke belongingness and acceptance	G	3	Clients with mental retardation, chronic psychiatric disabilities, or dual diagnosis of both	Therapist's familiarity with population and experience in conducting group psychotherapy	(1) Do not stand behind paranoid clients. (2) Do not use with issues of death and grieving unless therapist has specific training in managing these issues in group settings.
Presents	Rehearsals for growth	8	Promote feelings of generosity between partners	C, G, F	4	Any dyad, including children over 4, in which participants are cognitively oriented to following instructions	Prior indication of attentiveness to other's words and actions, flexibility in interacting and accepting other's directions and suggestions, and validation of other's reality	(1) Psychotic functioning (2) Open hostility between partners
Puppets	Rehearsals for growth	8	Facilitate exploration, spontaneity, and cooperation in relationships	Dydadic client partners, C, G, F	5	Any dyad, including children over 5, in which nonerogenous touching between partners is not problematic	Prior indication of attentiveness to other's words and actions, flexibility in interacting and accepting other's directions and suggestions, and validation of other's reality	Active symptoms of psychosis or paranoid ideation; recent physical abuse between partners
Basic staccato breathing	Core Energetics	9	(1) Open up muscular blocks to enhance overall flow of energy (2) Help restore or maintain balance between active and receptive energies	I, G	5	Adolescents and adults of any age, including individuals with physical disabilities or illness or mood disorders (i.e., dysthymic disorder, depression, or anxiety)	Client's readiness for body psychotherapy and capacity for body-focused awareness	(1) Clients with lower back injuries should proceed cautiously (without arching the back). (2) Avoid with clients with medium to strong schizophrenic or schizotypical behavioral patterns or bipolar episodes.

Technique	Model		Purpose	Format		Indications	Requirements	Contraindications
Advanced staccato breathing	Core Energetics	9	(1) Change behaviors (2) Deepen emotional experiences (3) Add new coping mechanisms	I, G	6	Clients who have progressed past introductory stages and individuals with major energetic blocks and other energetic problems	Client's readiness for body psychotherapy and capacity for body-focused awareness	(1) Clients with lower-back injuries should proceed cautiously (without arching the back). (2) Avoid with clients with medium to strong schizophrenic or schizotypical behavioral patterns or bipolar episodes.
Body scanning	Phoenix Rising Yoga Therapy	10	Introduce new clients to body awareness techniques	I	5	All except those listed in "Contraindications"	Ability to stand and to focus on a guided body experience.	Severe distress when closing eyes and focusing on inner experience
Assisted posture with dialogue	Phoenix Rising Yoga Therapy	10	Introduce new clients to body awareness techniques	I, C, F	6	All except those listed in "Contraindications"	Ability to stand and to focus on a guided body experience.	Severe distress when closing eyes and focusing on inner experience
Family drawing	Family art therapy	11	Provide family with opportunity to visually represent dynamics or patterns in which it functions	C, F	6	Any conjoint therapy	Family members' willingness to explore meaning and embrace interpretative complexity	None when well handled by trained art psychotherapist
Communication collage	Family art therapy	11	Uncover problem areas (e.g., conflicts, defensive mechanisms, style of functioning)	G, C, F	6	Any conjoint therapy	System's willingness to share and communicate with other systems	None when well handled by trained art psychotherapist
Interactive family and group art project	Family art therapy	11	Include group dynamics as a strategy to support family treatment goals	G, C, F	6	Any therapy involving multiple systems (i.e., family, couples, or group therapy)	System's willingness to share and communicate with other systems	None

Appendix continues

Name of action method	Name of therapy	Chapter	Main purpose	Modality	Training needed	Populations action method best used with	Prerequisite conditions for successful use of action method	Contraindications and cautions
Spontaneous movement	Dance/movement therapy	12	(1) Retrieve disavowed self-identification pertaining to earlier ruptured significant relationships (2) Transform and reintegrate ruptured relationships in more benign form	I, G	8	(1) All ages, levels of emotional development, and degree of emotional disturbance (2) Adjunctively in the treatment of physical illness involving a strong bodily felt component (i.e., traumatic perceptual shifts in body image)	Client's willingness to move in self-directed, spontaneous way in presence of therapist	Some clients may find movement modality intolerable or extremely anxiety provoking.
Dream enactment through movement	Dance/movement therapy	12	Reclaim and integrate disavowed qualities in self	I, G	8	Mentally disturbed children, adolescents, and adults, with technical modifications that take into consideration age and emotional developmental level, capacity for insight, and tolerance for regression and reintegration	Emotionally supportive self-therapeutic environment	(1) Clients who need to continually shore up defenses to function in integrated fashion (2) Clients who are mentally retarded or brain-damaged (3) Clients who cannot avail themselves of long-term treatment

Method		Goals			Client population	Requirements/indications	Contraindications
Supportive music psychotherapeutic method	13	(1) Relieve depression and dementia (2) Improve memory and quality of life (3) Improve group cohesiveness	I, G, C, F	8	All, including psychiatric, neurological, rehabilitation, and geriatric clients; victims of sexual, physical, or emotional abuse; clients with eating disorders, substance abuse, or mental retardation; clients with mild to severe dementia and depression; clients who are isolated or physically impaired; clients with inter- and intrapersonal communication problems (adults and children)	Sufficient client focus to follow instructions and not be disruptive to group process	Clients who are psychotic or hallucinating
Insight music psychotherapeutic method	13	(1) Relieve emotions attached to trauma (2) Rebuild self-esteem (3) Reestablish feeling of being in control	I, G, C, F	8	All, including clients who have experienced physical, emotional, or sexual abuse	(1) Trusting therapist–client relationship (2) Client's readiness to face and relive trauma in safe environment	Clients not ready to face and relive trauma

AUTHOR INDEX

SUBJECT INDEX

Children (*continued*)
 dance/movement therapy and, 257
 developmentally disabled, 257
 drama therapy and, 116
 psychodrama and, 139
 self-esteem tool kit and, 37–40
 use of symbols, 55–56, 68
Chronic pain management, 209
Client–therapist relationship
 client disinterest, 72–73
 Gestalt, 5, 22, 23–24
 Satir system, 49–50
Cognitive networking, 148–149
Collage making, 230–233, 295
Commission on Psychiatric Therapies, 247
Communication collage, 230–233, 295
Communication stance, 32, 33
Community-based work, 6
Confluence, 4
Congruence, 31
Conjoint Family Therapy (Satir), 30
Consciousness, 184
Coping, 31
Core Energetics, 183–202
 action methods, 185–186
 empirical support, 200
 overview, 183–185
 versus predecessors, 186–188
 repeated and successive uses, 199–200
 resistance to, 198–199
 staccato breathing, 188–198, 294, 295
 stages, 186
 therapist characteristics and training, 201
Couples therapy, 173–175
Cybernetics, 228
Cycle of experience model, 6

Dance/movement therapy (DMT), 245–260
 action methods, 296
 empirical support, 256–258
 overview, 245–248
 practices, 248
 psychoanalytically informed application, 249–255
 resistance to, 255
 therapist characteristics and training, 258–259
Defensiveness, 43

Developmentally disabled, 139, 145–162, 257
Developmental transformations, 101, 102
Diagnostic and Statistical Manual of Mental Disorders, 21
Dialogue, 14, 16–19, 295
Disclosure, 132, 137
Divorce, 74
Doubling, 126, 132–133, 138, 149–150, 293, 294
Drama therapy
 action methods, 292
 for children, 116
 efficacy and research, 117–118
 integration with real life, 99–107, 116–117
 key approaches, 101–103
 line repetition, 103–107
 versus psychodrama, 100, 128–129
 resistance to, 115–116
 self-sculptures, 107–115
 therapist training, 118–119
Dream enactment, 296
Dreamwork, 274

Empowerment, 18
Empty chair work, 6, 13–20, 126, 131n, 134, 291
Enactment, 79, 125–126, 127, 149
Energy, 184–186
Existentialism, 228
Expressive arts therapy, 23
 analytical music, 263–283
 art making, 225–241
 dance/movement, 245–260
Extemporaneous improvisation, 168
Externalization, 47, 79–96

Family drawing, 228–230, 295
Family floor plan, 63–64
Family mapping, 33, 47
Family reconstruction, 32
Family Ritual Interview, 73–74
Family sculpting, 32, 83–84, 133
Family systems, 228
Family therapy, 30, 208, 225–241
Family Therapy With the Experts (McLendon), 34
Family traditions, 60–61

guiding principles, 169
methods, 166–168
research and empirical support, 177–178
resistance to, 175–177
therapist characteristics and training, 178–179
Relationship therapy, 165–179
Replay, 126
Resistance
to action methods, 137–138
art therapy, 236–239
Core Energetics, 198–199
dance/movement therapy, 255–256
drama therapy, 115–116
Gestalt therapy, 20
IBT, 158–159
music therapy, 279–280
psychodrama, 137–138
RfG games, 175–177
Satir system, 43, 46–47
yoga therapy, 216
Resonator function, 281
Retroflection, 4, 10, 14
Reubenfeld synergy method, 187
Risk taking, 167
Rites of passage, 58
Ritual therapy, 57–58, 65–66, 68–72
action methods, 291
client disinterest, 72–73
efficacy, 73–76
modification and design, 66–68
research, 73–74
Rituals
art materials and, 63
genogram, 65
pictures, 60–61
stories and, 64–65
symbols and, 61–62
as therapy resource, 56–57
triggering memories, 63–64
upcoming, 62–63
Role distance, 138
Role method, 101, 102–103
Role playing
action methods, 125–140
drama therapy, 100
group, 40–44
music therapy, 273
role-training and, 150
sculpting, 32–33
Role reversal, 100, 126, 135–136, 138

Role-training, 150
Roller, 186, 187
Rope sculptures, 91–94, 292
Ropes, 88–90

Safety, therapeutic, 176, 179
Satir Institute of the Southeast, 49
Satir system
case examples, 34–44
change process model, 44–48
goals, 31
history, 29–30
homework, 46
key methods, 32–34, 291
resistance to, 46–47
therapist training, 48–50
Scripted scenes, 100
Sculpting
as action process, 82, 83–84
boundary, 86–88
rope, 91–94, 292
Satir system, 32–33, 38, 41
Self-discovery, 84–85
Self-esteem, 16, 31
Self-esteem tool kit, 32, 33–34, 37–44, 291
Self-expression, 225
Self-massage, 186
Self Realization Fellowship, 206
Self-reflection, 130
Self-sculptures, 107–115, 292
Self-talk, 67
Self technique, 130–133
Self-trust, 85–86
Separation and/or divorce, 74
Sharing phase, 149
Significant others, 138
Single doubling, 150–154, 293
Social constructionism, 228
Sociodrama, 128, 148
Sociometry, 133
Soliloquy, 126
Somatic communication, 269, 273, 274–279
Somatic resonance, 9
Spirituality, 184, 187, 188
Splitting, 274, 278
Spontaneity, 167
Spontaneous movement, 296
Spontaneous regression, 268, 274, 276
Staccato breathing, 188–194, 294, 295

ABOUT THE EDITOR

Daniel J. Wiener, PhD, ABPP, Licensed Marriage and Family Therapist, Certified Group Psychotherapist, is a licensed psychologist in marital, family, and relationship therapy. He is associate professor at Central Connecticut State University, where he trains marriage and family therapists and maintains private practices both in Manhattan and Connecticut. He has extensive experience as a clinical trainer and supervisor, organizational consultant, and workshop presenter to both lay and professional audiences.

In addition to numerous articles and book chapters, he is the author of *Rehearsals for Growth: Theater Improvisation for Psychotherapists* (W. W. Norton, 1994). His hobbies include performing team improvisational comedy (Theater Sports), tennis, chess, travel, and madrigal singing.